ADVANCES IN
VETERINARY SCIENCE AND
COMPARATIVE MEDICINE

VOLUME 14

CONTRIBUTORS TO THIS VOLUME

ROBERT S. BRODEY

CHARLES H. CUNNINGHAM

P. B. ENGLISH

RICHARD A. FREEDLAND

R. J. W. GARTNER

RICHARD A. GRIESEMER

N. ST. G. HYSLOP

ROBERT O. JACOBY

JOHN W. KRAMER

STANLEY E. LELAND, JR.

R. A. LENG

M. MANSJOER

SOERATNO PARTOATMODJO

A. A. SEAWRIGHT

JOSEPH W. SKAGGS

KURT DIETER STOTTMEIER

ADVANCES IN
VETERINARY SCIENCE AND
COMPARATIVE MEDICINE

Edited by

C. A. Brandly
College of Veterinary Medicine
University of Illinois
Urbana, Illinois
and
College of Veterinary Medicine
Kansas State University
Manhattan, Kansas

Charles E. Cornelius
College of Veterinary Medicine
Kansas State University
Manhattan, Kansas

Volume 14

1970
ACADEMIC PRESS
NEW YORK AND LONDON

ACADEMIC PRESS, INC.
111 Fifth Avenue, New York, New York 10003

United Kingdom Edition published by
ACADEMIC PRESS, INC. (LONDON) LTD.
Berkeley Square House, London W1X 6BA

LIBRARY OF CONGRESS CATALOG CARD NUMBER: 53-7098

PRINTED IN THE UNITED STATES OF AMERICA

CONTENTS

Hypervitaminosis A of the Cat

A. A. SEAWRIGHT, P. B. ENGLISH, AND R. J. W. GARTNER

In Vitro Cultivation of Nematode Parasites Important to Veterinary Medicine

STANLEY E. LELAND, JR.

Use of Serum Enzymes as Aids to Diagnosis

RICHARD A. FREEDLAND AND JOHN W. KRAMER

Avian Infectious Bronchitis

CHARLES H. CUNNINGHAM

Immunologic Injury to Dogs

ROBERT O. JACOBY AND RICHARD A. GRIESEMER

Glucose Synthesis in Ruminants

R. A. LENG

The Epizootiology and Epidemiology of Foot and Mouth Disease

N. ST. G. HYSLOP

Canine and Feline Neoplasia

Robert S. Brodey

Veterinary Medicine in Indonesia

Joseph W. Skaggs, M. Mansjoer, and Soeratno Partoatmodjo

A Review of Recent Developments in Veterinary Science in the Federal Republic of Germany

Kurt Dieter Stottmeier

CONTRIBUTORS

Numbers in parentheses indicate the pages on which the authors' contributions begin.

ROBERT S. BRODEY, Department of Surgery and the Tumor Clinic, University of Pennsylvania School of Veterinary Medicine, Philadelphia, Pennsylvania (309)

CHARLES H. CUNNINGHAM, Department of Microbiology and Public Health, College of Veterinary Medicine, Michigan State University, East Lansing, Michigan (105)

P. B. ENGLISH, Veterinary School, University of Queensland, St. Lucia, Brisbane, Australia (1)

RICHARD A. FREEDLAND, Department of Physiological Sciences, School of Veterinary Medicine, University of California, Davis, California (61)

R. J. W. GARTNER, Animal Research Institute, Department of Primary Industries, Yeerongpilly, Brisbane, Australia (1)

RICHARD A. GRIESEMER, Department of Veterinary Pathology, The Ohio State University, Columbus, Ohio (149)

N. ST. G. HYSLOP, Animal Pathology Division, Health of Animals Branch, Canada Department of Agriculture, Animal Diseases Research Institute, Hull, Quebec, Canada (261)

ROBERT O. JACOBY, Department of Veterinary Pathology, The Ohio State University, Columbus, Ohio (149)

JOHN W. KRAMER, Department of Physiological Sciences, School of Veterinary Medicine, University of California, Davis, California (61)

STANLEY E. LELAND, JR., Department of Infectious Diseases, College of Veterinary Medicine, Kansas State University, Manhattan, Kansas (29)

R. A. LENG, Department of Biochemistry and Nutrition, School of Rural Science, University of New England, Armidale, N.S.W., Australia (209)

M. MANSJOER, Zoonoses Laboratory, Padjadjaran State University, Bandung, Indonesia (355)

SOERATNO PARTOATMODJO, College of Veterinary Science, Institute of Agricultural Sciences, Bogor, Indonesia (355)

A. A. SEAWRIGHT, Veterinary School, University of Queensland, St. Lucia, Brisbane, Australia (1)

JOSEPH W. SKAGGS, Kentucky State Department of Health, Frankfort, Kentucky (355)

KURT DIETER STOTTMEIER, National Communicable Disease Center, Atlanta, Georgia (365)

PREFACE

Review and evaluation of newer means for confronting the myriad disease-inducing factors and entities that beset the members of the animal kingdom comprise the content of this volume. This effort identifies substantial yields of progress from protracted, sophisticated research effort on primarily nonhuman animal disease that have transcending potential and direct value to the human as well as other species. Disease factors involving man or which may emerge as health problems to him are also dealt with. Thus, both the necessity and merit of the comparative medical approach to more abounding health for all species are reemphasized.

The subjects of the volume, which are presented in the various chapters by authorities, range from malnutritional, infectious, parasitic, and neoplastic to immunoaberrational disease. More sophisticated and precise methods and techniques, e.g., definition of specific enzyme profiles for exquisitely accurate diagnoses of specific disease states, and the multicompartmental analyses of incidence data, without which solution of a variety of disease enigmas would have been impossible, are also recognized and evaluated.

The pathways and implications of the basic phenomena of glucose synthesis in ruminant animals are related to both biologic demands of "physiologic" health and bioeconomics. Justified anticipation that all stages of nematodal animal parasites may be cultivated *in vitro* portends important progress, also.

Reemphasis of the impact of multiple environmental factors, e.g., diet source, age, and muscular activity on hypervitaminosis A in cats enlightens for us the interaction of many variables on disease outcome. Equally, the imperative need for elucidating the ecology of both host and parasite by further intensive research is restressed if such volatile contagions as foot and mouth disease and avian infectious bronchitis are to be denied their enormous toll on total health and well being. The sequence of dire economic concern and heroic eradication measures when foot and mouth epidemics strike and of early subsequent public and often official agency indifferences and apathy toward probable recurrence of this intolerable plague exemplify man's historic, never-justifiable, lack of reality.

The dramatic forward surge in understanding of the central role of immune mechanisms in hypersensitivity, autosensitivity, and transplantation, especially that to which extensive experimentation with dogs has contributed, has been ably evaluated by the authors.

Finally, the scope of this series of *Advances* has been enlarged by inclusion of concluding short chapters that report progress, both general and scientific, in veterinary medical endeavor in various selected countries. For this innovation, due appreciation is expressed to a member of the Advisory Board, Dr. James H. Steele.

In presenting this volume, the editors humbly solicit its critically constructive evaluation by the expanding readership. The editors reiterate their deep gratitude for the serious, competent, and dedicated effort of the contributors and for the high ability and cooperation of the staff of Academic Press, Inc.

CONTENTS OF PREVIOUS VOLUMES

Hypervitaminosis A of the Cat

A. A. SEAWRIGHT, P. B. ENGLISH, AND R. J. W. GARTNER*

*Veterinary School, University of Queensland; Animal Research Institute,
Department of Primary Industries, Queensland, Australia*

I. Introduction

Adult cats with a bone disease characterized by extensive, confluent exostoses of the cervicothoracic vertebrae are frequently encountered in urban areas of Australia. A similar bone disease was reported in 7 cats in Uruguay (Christi, 1957). Seawright and English (1964) named this condition "deforming cervical spondylosis."

The ingestion of large quantities of vitamin A in polar bear liver (Rodahl and Moore, 1943; Rodahl, 1949) and bovine liver (Herbst *et al.*, 1944; Pavcek *et al.*, 1945) had been shown to cause bone lesions in young rats. Most of the liver fed to cats in Australia is derived from sheep and cattle grazing pasture throughout the year, and it has higher concentrations of vitamin A (Gartner and Anson, 1966; Gartner *et al.*, 1968) than are reported in other countries. The livers from 2 affected cats contained extremely high concentrations of vitamin A, 28,125 and 24,688 micrograms per gram (μg./g.), respectively, compared with 83 μg./g. in an unaffected cat of the same age (Seawright *et al.*, 1965).

As a predominantly liver diet appeared to be common to all affected

* Drs. Seawright and English are Reader in Pathology and Professor of Veterinary Clinical Studies, respectively, at the Veterinary School, St. Lucia, Brisbane, Australia, and Mr. R. J. W. Gartner is Senior Chemist in the Animal Research Institute, Department of Primary Industries, Yeerongpilly, Brisbane, Australia.

cats, experiments were undertaken by feeding both raw liver and vitamin A (Seawright et al., 1965, 1967). The successful experimental production of the natural disease (English and Seawright, 1964; Seawright and English, 1964; English, 1969) confirmed that it was due to hypervitaminosis A. There are recent reports of the disease in Britain (Fry, 1968; Lucke et al., 1968; Baker and Hughes, 1968); it is also believed to occur in the United States of America (Riser, 1966) and in New Zealand (Dodd, 1966; Cordes, 1967).

Contributions on hypervitaminosis A in the cat, other than by the present authors, have added little new information except in relation to the world distribution of the disease. Accordingly, in order to avoid the repetition of certain references, observations unsubstantiated by references may be taken as having originated from previous papers by English and Seawright (1964), Seawright and English (1964), Seawright et al. (1965, 1967), and English (1969), or from previously unpublished observations of these workers.

II. Clinical and Pathologic Features

1. General Systemic Toxicity of Excess Dietary Vitamin A

In experiments to study deforming cervical spondylosis of the cat, 31 weanling kittens of both sexes, from 9 litters, were used. Also, observations of clinical and pathologic features have been made in an additional 30 naturally affected animals since papers describing these facets of the disease were written.

The age of affected cats presented for treatment has ranged from about 2 to 9 years (Christi, 1957; English and Seawright, 1964). The time of onset of clinical signs is influenced by the age at which excessive vitamin A feeding begins, the actual level of the vitamin A in the diet, and the duration of time over which it is fed. The disease can be produced in younger cats if vitamin A supplementation or liver feeding begins at the time of weaning. For example, when the amount of liver in the diet of newly weaned kittens was sufficient to ensure a vitamin A intake of 17 to 35 μg./g. body weight, daily, all animals had developed deforming cervical spondylosis within 10 months. The disease had not developed in this time in kittens receiving synthetic vitamin A daily, by gavage, at the rate of 15 μg./g. body weight, but had developed in animals receiving it at twice this rate. The toxic amounts for cats were thus similar to those required to produce hypervitaminosis A in rats (Rodahl and Moore, 1943; Herbst et al., 1944; Rodahl, 1950) mice, rabbits, guinea pigs and cockerels (Rodahl, 1950), calves (Grey et al., 1965), and pigs (Wolke et al., 1968).

Vitamin A supplied as liver was more potent for the cats than the same quantity of the synthetic preparation as, in the former case, there was a higher incidence of bone lesions, a greater proportion of the dose stored, and higher plasma concentrations produced (Seawright et al., 1967).

The clinical features following both liver feeding and dosing with excess synthetic vitamin varied in time of onset and severity.

Dickinson and Scott (1959) considered 0.6 μg./g. body weight an adequate daily quantity of vitamin A for cats. Our results showed that within 4 to 6 weeks marked signs of toxicity had developed in kittens with an average daily intake of vitamin A of 35 μg./g. body weight (diet of liver) and 150 μg./g. body weight (synthetic vitamin A as gavage). It took 15 weeks when the dose rate of synthetic vitamin A was 30 μg./g. Affected animals had malaise characterized by loss of appetite, lethargy, torpor, marked irritability, as well as exophthalmos, and scurfiness and dullness of the coat.

All cats consistently fed liver for a year or more showed the typical depression and irritability of chronic vitamin A toxicosis. At 41 weeks cats receiving 17 μg./g. body weight had developed only deforming cervical spondylosis; but irritability and depression were present in most of the naturally affected animals with advanced skeletal lesions.

Similar clinical manifestations of chronic hypervitaminosis A have been reported in rats (Rodahl, 1949, 1950) and in children (Caffey, 1951). Increase in cerebrospinal fluid pressure was found to occur in man (Marie and See, 1954), and clinical signs such as headache, nausea, and hydrocephalus were attributed to the pressure. It is probable that increased cerebrospinal fluid pressure occurs in the cat in hypervitaminosis A, and that it contributes largely to the signs of depression and irritability seen in such cases.

When vitamin A was removed from the diet or when liver was replaced by an alternative protein concentrate low in vitamin A, the signs of systemic toxicity in cats disappeared within a few weeks. Likewise, rapid improvement was observed in chronic hypervitaminosis A in man after cessation of dosing with excess of vitamin A (Caffey, 1951; Gerber et al., 1954).

2. Skeletal Lesions

a. Cervicothoracic Spine

The earliest indication of skeletal injury in kittens fed liver was increased sensitivity to palpation of the region of the base of the skull or the adjacent proximal part of the neck. Sensitivity was present for 2 to

3 weeks before any loss of flexibility due to exostoses of the cervical spine could be detected and, in some animals, as early as 15 weeks after the start of daily liver feeding. Radiographic studies of affected kittens at this stage indicated that new bone formation first occurred in the region of the diarthrodial joints between the second and third cervical vertebrae. Exostosis formation involving the atlas and occipital bone is also commonly observed in natural cases of the disease, but radiographic detection of this lesion in the early stages is difficult. These early osseous proliferations are followed within weeks by similar lesions on the dorsolateral margin of the more caudal cervical vertebrae and cranial thoracic vertebrae. They tend to coalesce to produce large confluent exostoses which are tumor-like in appearance (Fig. 1), as they encroach on and replace contiguous soft tissues (Seawright and English, 1964; Baker and Hughes, 1968). As the more anteriorly placed vertebrae fuse and the anterior spine becomes rigid, active new bone proliferation extends posteriorly where flexibility and movement are still possible. Extension of the process from the skull to the sacrum is seen in some severely affected animals. Similar, although less common, confluent exostosis formation may also occur on the ventral margin of the cervicothoracic spine rather than on the dorsolateral margins.

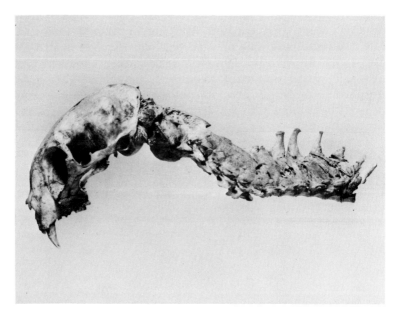

Fig. 1. Extensive exostosis formation on the cervicothoracic spine of a 4-year-old cat due to hypervitaminosis A.

b. *Extraspinal Sites*

Apart from the bone lesions on the cervicothoracic spine, which are almost universal in chronic hypervitaminosis A in the cat, exostoses are next most common in the forelimbs and the thoracic cage. Lesions in the forelimb originate in the fibro-osseous insertions of ligaments and tendons at the ends of the bones and in the vicinity of joints, thus restricting movement. Finally, they may grow together from either side, coalesce, and produce complete extraarticular ankylosis. The elbow joint is most frequently affected, and in many animals both elbow joints are completely fused in the flexed position.

Periarticular exostoses are next most common around the shoulder joints, while involvement of the carpal or more distal limb joints is rare. In individuals in which the cervicothoracic lesions are extensive, it is not unusual for the articulations of the ribs to be affected by osseous hyperplasia and for most, if not all, of the thoracic cage to be rigid (English and Seawright, 1964; Baker and Hughes, 1968). Hyperostoses cause a uniform enlargement of one or more ribs in some animals. Also, hyperostoses containing some cartilage are commonly seen as enveloping collar-like formations on rib cartilages. The process spreads to involve the sternum, which becomes misshapen as the sternal cartilages are overgrown by new bone depositions on adjacent rib cartilages and sternebrae. This causes the sternum to lose elasticity and become subject to depressed fractures.

Lesions of the hind limb and pelvic girdle are seen in some advanced cases of the disease. Sacroiliac ankylosis is the most common lesion, but exostoses around the hip joint, on the tuberosities and epicondyles of the femur, and on the tibia sometimes occur. Joints distal to the stifle joint are rarely affected.

c. *Histopathologic Changes*

Histopathologic changes affecting the cervical vertebrae and other bones were described by Seawright and English (1964), Seawright *et al.* (1967), and Baker and Hughes (1968). There is subperiosteal proliferation of new woven bone around the apophyseal joints of affected vertebrae which, with new proliferations of cartilage from the margin of the articular hyaline cartilage, over-grow the joint and replace the synovial membrane. There is associated resorptive erosion of contiguous cortical and cancellous bone, with disappearance of myeloid marrow and its replacement with fibrous marrow. At the reactive edge of the exostosis, the osteogenic field can be seen spreading into adjacent inter- and intramuscular connective tissues, resulting in replacement of the muscle by new woven bone. In older lesions the bridged vertebrae are largely re-modeled in the affected area, with replacement of osseous trabeculae by bone marrow often containing residual fragments of hyaline articular cartilage of an overgrown joint. The exterior surface appears smooth with normal fibrous periosteum.

d. Clinical Signs Associated with Skeletal Lesions

The earliest clinical signs of deforming cervical spondylosis are the consequence of development of exostoses on the cervical spine. These

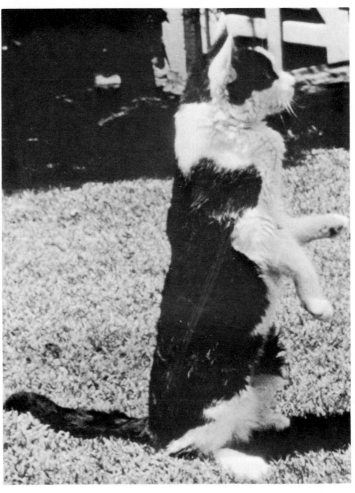

Fig. 2. The kangaroo-like posture adopted by a cat with advanced hyper-vitaminosis A.

include stiffness and rigidity of the head and neck (Christi, 1957; English and Seawright, 1964; Lucke *et al.*, 1968; Baker and Hughes, 1968) and an unkempt and matted coat (English and Seawright, 1964; Baker and Hughes, 1968).

Where the new bone formations have encroached on the intervertebral foramina affecting spinal nerves and ganglia, forelimb lameness, ataxia or paralysis, and hyperesthesia or anesthesia of the skin of the neck, base of the skull, and forelimb may be seen. In the very young animal, paralysis of individual muscles may result in unbalanced growth of the limb causing deformities of developing bones, such as the scapula, and joints. Trauma may precipitate marked and permanent lameness of an affected cat which otherwise had shown no obvious signs of the disease.

Affected cats frequently adopt a kangaroo-like sitting posture (Fig. 2). Extension of the cervical osseous lesions posteriorly results in an increase in the inclination of the whole thoracolumbar curvature (Tucker, 1964), which shifts the center of gravity of the body ventrally and posteriorly. The cat walks with its hind limbs flexed to maintain the new inclination of the thoracolumbar curvature. Cats with ankylosis of several cervical vertebrae must turn their entire body to change their field of vision. Movement of the eyeballs appears to be greatly reduced, in such cases, giving the animal a fixed stare.

In the advanced condition, many animals are emaciated (English and Seawright, 1964; Baker and Hughes, 1968). As the disease progresses, muscles of the trunk and limbs undergo disuse atrophy. This is possibly the main basis of the debility so frequently seen in cats that have been affected for prolonged periods.

e. Alterations of Cervical Lesions with Time

When liver was replaced with meat in the diet of young cats with cervical spinal exostoses, which had been fed on liver for a year, further encroachment of contiguous soft tissues ceased. In radiographs (Fig. 3), the edges of these lesions at this stage were irregular, indistinct, and poorly mineralized. After a further year on a diet free of liver, the new bone of the exostoses became denser and its edges smooth. After a further two years, during which time milk was absent from the diet, the bones generally became more porous, and the dense new bone formation became markedly reduced. However, the macerated spine at this stage revealed extensive remodeling similar to that in Fig. 1, and the vertebrae from the second to the seventh were completely fused, thus indicating that correction of the diet after the disease becomes established results in cessation of the progress of the lesions, but little significant reversal. The general clinical condition of the animals was nevertheless greatly im-

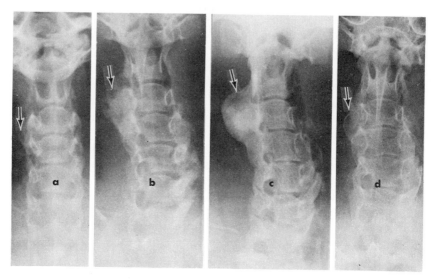

Fɪɢ. 3. Dorsoventral radiographs of an exostosis (arrow) on the cervical spine of an experimentally affected cat at 6 months (a), 12 months (b), 2 years (c), and at 4 years (d).

proved, as has been observed in similar animals by Lucke *et al.* (1968) and English (1969).

f. Special Bone Lesions due to High Excess Dosing with Vitamin A

When weanling kittens given 33 μg./g. of vitamin A daily for 4 weeks were allowed to grow for 13 more weeks on a diet free of vitamin A, a typically abnormal hind limb gait developed. Necropsy showed abnormality of development and permanent shortening of the femur with rotation of the distal epiphysis, and shortening of the tibia with dorsal prolongation of the tibial tubercle. This prevented normal extension of the stifle joints and, in walking, the hocks were displaced laterally, thus accounting for the characteristic gait observed. This degree of vitamin A supplementation for so short a period did not cause exostosis formation at any site on the skeleton, and the syndrome and gait were clearly quite different from those described for older, naturally affected cats with deforming cervical spondylosis. Other findings by Clark and Seawright (1968) included irregular shortening of the metatarsal bones which gave rise to digits of irregular length. Sometimes the malformation was symmetrical, affecting only the third digits (Fig. 4). Shortening of long bones was due to resorption and eventual disappearance of one or both carti-

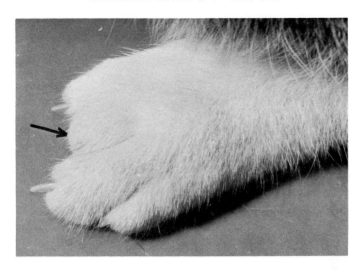

Fig. 4. Shortening of the third digit (arrow) of a hind foot of a kitten due to failure of growth of the third metatarsal in hypervitaminosis A.

laginous epiphyseal plates, preventing elongation of the bone with growth of the animal. Appositional bone growth occurred, but the metatarsals of hypervitaminotic A cats were thinner than comparable bones of control cats.

These findings suggested some suppression of osteoblastic activity as has been demonstrated in various bones in hypervitaminosis A in the young rat (Irving, 1949), calf (Grey et al., 1965), chicken (Baker et al., 1967), and pig (Wolke et al., 1968). Exophthalmos due to hypervitaminosis A in young rats was explained by Irving (1949) as being due to suppression of osteoblastic activity in intramembranous bones of the skull, in which remodeling and growth of the bones of the orbit failed to keep pace with the growth of the eyeball. This probably occurs also in the cat. However, the suppression of osteoblasts by the rat without affecting osteoclasts caused porosity and extreme fragility of the long bones followed by spontaneous fractures (Collazo and Rodriguez, 1933; Davies and Moore, 1934; Strauss, 1934; Wolbach and Bessey, 1942; Moore and Wang, 1943; 1945; Rodahl, 1950). This degree of suppression of osteoblasts in the cat does not appear to occur, and it might be related to the relatively slower growth rate of the kitten compared with the young rat. The main effect of hypervitaminosis A on the growing skeleton of the cat was on chondrocytes causing degeneration of the cells and lysis of matrix, as has been demonstrated both *in vivo* in rabbits (Thomas et al., 1960) and *in vitro* in cultured mouse bones (Fell and Thomas, 1960).

g. Mechanisms of Vitamin A Action on the Skeleton

Excess dietary vitamin A is thus associated with two distinctly different skeletal disorders in the growing cat.

Generally, the commonest cause of exostosis formation is trauma to the periosteum. Exostoses of toxic origin superficially similar to those present on the bones of these cats have been observed in the young of many species affected with osteolathyrism (Selye, 1957). Here the basic defect of collagen synthesis is such that musculotendinous insertions in the periosteum break down during normal muscular activity. Also in chronic hypervitaminosis A of the cat, it has been suggested that (Seawright et al., 1967) there was an increased sensitivity of the periosteum of trauma, and, further, that cervicothoracic location of the lesions was due to excessive muscular activity of this region in the act of coat cleaning. It has been established that excess vitamin A causes escape of lysosomal proteolytic enzymes capable of dissolving bone and cartilage matrix (Fell and Dingle, 1963). It has been suggested also that, because of its surface active properties, vitamin A increases the lability of the lipoprotein cytomembranes (Bangham et al., 1964), thus rendering them unstable and more prone to mechanical injury (Dingle and Lucy, 1962). If the osteogenic cells of periosteum of the cats were so affected, slight trauma due to normal muscular activity might then damage the tissues, thus provoking periosteal inflammation and exostoses as in osteolathyrism.

Cortical hyperostosis of long bones has not been observed in the limbs of cats as it has in children with hypervitaminosis A (Toomey and Morrissette, 1947; Caffey, 1951), although such lesions are occasionally found affecting the ribs, rib cartilages, and sternum of cats. Somewhat similar lesions of toxic origin occur in osteofluorosis of other species (Hodge and Smith, 1965). In the latter disease, degenerative changes in osteoblasts forming new cortical bone are responsible for the production of osteones of reduced capacity to bear mechanical stress, and extensive compensatory subperiosteal new bone is laid down accordingly. Although marked suppression of osteoblastic activity with osteoporosis has been recorded in hypervitaminosis A in some species, it does not seem to be so prominent in the cat. Nevertheless, it is logical to assume that to some extent, it also occurs in the latter species, and that the pathogenesis of exostoses and hyperostoses in hypervitaminosis A may well be similar to that of osteofluorosis. Supporting this view further is the fact that considerable exposure to toxic quantities of both these substances must occur before subperiosteal proliferation of new bone develops and that the exostoses or hyperostoses are located mainly on parts of the skeleton experiencing the most stress. Current studies by the authors of the turnover of cervical vertebral bone in hypervitaminosis A in the cat may clarify the pathogenesis of this lesion.

3. Oral Lesions

a. Gingival Tissues

When liver is the main component of the diet of cats from the time of weaning, the gums near the base of the teeth become swollen and hyperemic within 15 weeks. If liver feeding is sustained, the gums particularly about the molar teeth hypertrophy and large pink florid proliferations develop after 6 to 12 months (Fig. 5). These hypertrophic lesions of the gums tend to subside, and the gums become atrophied after about 15 months of liver feeding.

Supplementation of the diet of cats with excess vitamin A produced similar but not so severe gingival lesions as those observed in cats fed liver for the same period. It has been shown that irrespective of the route of administration to the rat, be it oral, subcutaneous, or percutaneous, the lesions of hypervitaminosis A were similar (Rodahl, 1950). Nevertheless, severe inflammatory changes occurred on the oral and labial

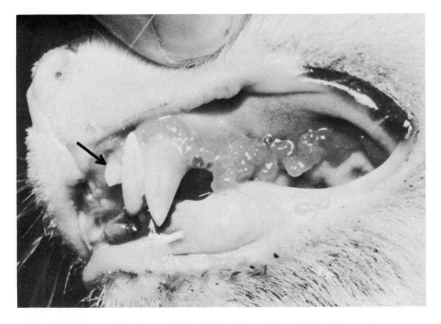

Fig. 5. The mouth of a cat after 45 weeks on liver diet; all except one upper incisor tooth (arrow) were lost, and the gums were florid and hypertrophic.

mucous membranes of rats given vitamin A concentrate by mouth (Rodah! and Moore, 1943). Some ovine liver fed to cats contains as much as 1200 μg./g., and it is possible that the direct effect of the vitamin in the food aggravated the gingival lesions of the animals fed liver.

b. Teeth

It has been observed in experimental cats that, soon after emergence of the permanent incisor teeth in the inflamed gums, the teeth disappeared one at a time so that by the age of 12 months animals were edentulous. Permanent molar teeth were dull yellow. Tartar was deposited on the crowns and carious change was evident, mainly at the neck near the bifurcation of the roots within 6 months of eruption. In some animals, caries became so widespread that the crowns of all molar teeth finally eroded away leaving only broken-off, necrotic root fragments in the jaws. Most cats that had been fed liver consistently for a year had only canine teeth remaining at 18 to 24 months of age.

c. Jaws

Some molar teeth developed pulpitis and apical root abscesses, and this was followed by chronic low grade osteomyelitis of the jaw, most commonly observed in mandibles on which a thick zone of radiating trabeculae of subperiostical new woven bone developed outside the old cortical cement line.

Despite the widespread and severe inflammation of the gums and degenerative changes of the molars, periodontal disease with alveolar pyorrhea in this part of the jaw was unusual.

Irving (1949) studied the alveolar bone associated with the incisor teeth of the hypervitaminotic A rats and recorded its abnormal narrowness and fragile appearance compared with jaws from control rats. It is possible then that similar defective development of bones composing the alveoli of the incisors occurred in the cats. Thus, a combination of the two factors, namely, extension of gingival inflammation so as to involve the periodontal membranes, and inadequate anchorage of the teeth in the maxillae and mandibles, probably led to early loosening and subsequent loss of the incisors in some cats with hypervitaminosis A.

4. Skin Lesions

Except for the unkempt condition of the coat due to inability or reluctance to clean it as a consequence of pain, or of restriction of movement of the head and neck, lesions of the skin did not occur consistently in cats with vitamin A toxicity. Inability of some animals to reach a certain part of the coat resulted in the appearance of wigs of hair.

The fur of the back and hindquarters of whole colored gray and black cats often had a reddish tinge after about 25 weeks of vitamin A supplementation or liver feeding, whereas a transient alopecia of the head, neck, and shoulders similar to that described in rats (Weslaw et al., 1938; Rodahl, 1950) occurred in 2 cats after a year on a diet of liver. In other cats, a proliferative dermatitis characterized by irregular, friable wart-like lesions were present after about a year, and these resolved within 3 weeks after substitution of the liver for meat. Skin lesions were described in experimental hypervitaminosis A in other animals (Domagk and Dobeneck, 1933; Moll et al., 1933; Weslaw et al., 1938; Rodahl and Moore, 1943; Studer and Frey, 1949; Rodahl, 1950; Niemann and Klein Obbink, 1954; Swerczek and Nielsen, 1967).

5. Changes in Parenchymatous Organs

a. Liver

The gross pathologic feature common to all cats with hypervitaminosis A was a fatty liver. The liver is the main storage organ of the vitamin. Pale green, fading autofluorescence (Querner, 1935; Popper and Greenberg, 1941) due to vitamin A was observed microscopically in frozen sections in the sites which stained for neutral fat (Seawright et al., 1967). These included Kupffer cells and periportal macrophages as well as the cytoplasm of periportal hepatocytes. The lipid-laden Kupffer cells and macrophages, both in the sinusoids and portal tracts, coalesced to form large multinucleated cells containing a pink foamy cytoplasm after prolonged high intake of vitamin A.

b. Kidney

The kidney tissue of cats fed vitamin A was more fatty than that of control cats, the lipid being contained mainly in the cytoplasm of the tubular epithelial cells. The degree of fatty infiltration increased until the cell walls of the tubular cells broke down, and the fat globules merged to form fatty cysts in long-standing cases. This was accompanied by interstitial fibrosis and mononuclear inflammatory infiltration. In contrast to the liver tissue, all areas of fat staining in the kidney did not show strong autofluorescence (Moore et al., 1963; Seawright et al., 1967), although a faint diffuse fluorescence of vitamin A could usually be demonstrated over the whole cortex.

c. Adrenal

Fatty changes were seen mostly in cortical cells immediately adjacent to the medulla, and small quantities of vitamin A were also present in this area.

d. Lung

The lung of cats with hypervitaminosis A had no gross pathologic changes. Microscopically, lipid and vitamin A were found in alveolar lining cells and in interstitial macrophages in the early stages. With time, the lipid-engorged cells aggregated and coalesced to form large foamy masses in some cats. These appeared as plaques under the visceral pleura, as nodules in the parenchyma when adjoining alveolar lumens filled up and coalesced, and as collars in peribronchial and perivascular connective tissues. In some older cats, masses consisting of these large foamy cells resembling cellular exudate were present in bronchial lumens.

e. Spleen

In long-standing cases of hypervitaminosis A, the spleen was usually paler than normal and slightly enlarged. There was lipid infiltration of the pulp and focal autofluorescence due to the vitamin around small blood vessels.

f. Lymph Nodes

The mesenteric and hepatic lymph nodes were usually enlarged due to infiltration of the cortex and medulla with greasy, yellowish caseous-like material when the liver was grossly affected with fatty infiltration. Microscopically, this tissue consisted of masses of large lipid-laden macrophages similar to those in the liver and lungs. Lymphoid follicles atrophied and almost disappeared.

Similar changes in parenchymatous organs of rats with hypervitaminosis A have been described (Domagk and Dobeneck, 1933; Collazo and Rodriguez, 1933; Drigalski and Laubmann, 1933; Uotilla and Simola, 1938; Noetzel, 1939; Rodahl, 1950), although the location of lipid in the rat kidney was in the capillary endothelial cells (Domagk and Dobeneck, 1933) rather than in the tubular epithelial cells as in the cat. The extensive infiltration of the reticulohistiocytic system with lipid in hypervitaminosis A has also been stressed by others (Niemann and Klein Obbink, 1954; Moore, 1957).

III. Some Aspects of Vitamin A Metabolism in Hypervitaminosis A

1. VITAMIN A VALUES IN BODY TISSUES AND FLUIDS

a. Liver

Values for vitamin A in both experimentally induced and natural cases of deforming cervical spondylosis of adult cats are shown in Table

TABLE I

TISSUE CONCENTRATIONS OF VITAMIN A IN EXPERIMENTALLY INDUCED AND IN
NATURAL CASES OF DEFORMING CERVICAL SPONDYLOSIS OF THE CAT

Cat	Liver vitamin A		Kidney vitamin A		Plasma vitamin A (μg./100 ml.)
	(μg./g.)	(Total mg.)	(μg./g.)	(Total mg.)	
Constant feeding of liver					
Naturally affected[a]	28,125	1,969	—	—	657
Naturally affected	17,730	1,808	264	6.6	675
Naturally affected	20,069	2,890	466	16.8	504
Naturally affected	22,135	2,523	1,337	29.4	227
Experimental cat 1	28,669	1,949	89	1.4	635
Experimental cat 7[a]	24,688	1,703	—	—	1,718
Experimental cat 8	22,441	1,997	496	11.4	947
No liver for past 3 years					
Experimental cat 2	2,695	552	36	1.2	260
Experimental cat 3	4,970	770	9	0.3	72
Experimental cat 5	2,424	484	44	1.6	1,810

[a] Seawright et al. (1965).

I. Liver was fed to produce lesions in the experimental animals, and it was the main component of the diet in the natural cases. It is evident that the liver vitamin A concentrations were comparable in both the natural and experimental cases, and that these were greater than the highest levels reported in mammals by Rodahl (1949).

In a survey to determine the incidence of hypervitaminosis A in Brisbane, Australia (Seawright et al., 1968), cats were placed in one of two groups according to vitamin A concentrations in their livers. One group (25 cats) had a geometric mean quantity of 11,000 μg./g. and the other group (75 cats) a geometric mean value of 200 μg./g. Nine of the cats of the first group had slight periosteal proliferations highly suggestive of early lesions of deforming cervical spondylosis, and the vitamin values of this group were comparable with those observed in natural and experimental cases. No lesions were present in the lower vitamin A reserve group, the liver values of which were similar to those reported by Moore et al. (1963) in cats fed on diets adequate in vitamin A for periods of up to 9 years.

By removing liver from the diet, a marked reduction of body reserves occurred after about 3 years (Table I). Only after such a period were the concentrations of vitamin A in the liver of our cats of the order reported for normal cats by Lowe et al. (1957) and Moore et al. (1963). The exceptionally high hepatic reserves which characterize the onset of cervical and other bone lesions thus may be subsequently depleted to normal levels after permanent lesions of the skeleton have been established.

b. Kidneys

Large amount of vitamin A are stored in the kidney of the adult cat (Table I). Lowe *et al.* (1957) found a mean concentration of 33 µg./g. in 9 cats. Moore *et al.* (1963) reported values of 3 to 177 µg./g. in 82 cats, with a mean of 50 µg./g.; Ferrando *et al.* (1966) reported values of 0 to 1266 µg./g. in 20 cats, with a mean of 188 µg./g. Seawright *et al.* (1968) found a geometric mean level of 21 µg./g., with a 66% range of 6 to 77.5 µg./g. in 100 cats. Heywood (1967) observed that the storage of vitamin A in the kidney was not characteristic of all felidae, and apart from the domestic cat, appreciable concentrations (about 20 µg./g.) were found in only the jungle cat and the caracal lynx.

c. Plasma

The plasma content of affected cats was very high, that of cat 7 (Table I) being comparable with the highest levels reported in hypervitaminosis A of human beings (Gerber *et al.*, 1954; Moore, 1957). These concentrations declined in 2 of the 3 cats taken off liver. However, cat 5 had the highest value recorded in these studies, but the reason for it is unknown.

Although liver feeding is clearly implicated in the etiology of hypervitaminosis A, there was no information initially about the quantity of the vitamin needed in the diet to cause such high reserves. Subsequently, we showed that, after 24 weeks of feeding liver containing an average vitamin A content of 453 µg./g., the mean liver, kidney, and plasma values of cats were 13,409 µg./g., 856 µg./g. and 926 µg./100 ml., respectively. When cats had eaten liver containing 286 µg./g. of vitamin A for 41 weeks, the mean liver, kidney, and plasma contents were 26,123 µg./g., 187 µg./g., and 766 µg./100 ml., respectively. Cats fed meat, for the same period as the latter animals, had mean values of the vitamin in the liver, kidney, and plasma of 714 µg./g., 87 µg./g., and 188 µg./100 ml., respectively.

Neither in all our analytical data, taken as a whole, nor in those of Moore *et al.* (1963) and Ferrando *et al.* (1966) was there any relationship between renal and hepatic reserves of vitamin A in the cat. It was suggested by Moore *et al.* (1963), however, that kidney vitamin A concentration reflects the turnover rate of the vitamin in the body. Possibly, the more severe effects of intoxication in cats given very high doses of vitamin A (Seawright *et al.*, 1967) were associated with high turnover rates of the vitamin.

d. Urine

Heywood (1967) found no vitamin A in the urine of some felidae, but normal dogs excrete substantial quantities (30 to 150 μg./ml.) in urine (Catel, 1938; Lawrie et al., 1941; Moore et al., 1963). The vitamin A concentration of the urine of both normal and affected cats is given in Table II, together with a value quoted by Moore et al. (1963). It is ap-

TABLE II

The Concentration of Vitamin A in the Urine of Cats Relative to the Concentration in Other Tissues

Urine (μg./100 ml.)	Liver (μg./g.)	Kidney (μg./g.)	Plasma (μg./100 ml.)	Remarks
Nil	388	58	—	Normal cat
37	31	77	—	From Moore et al. (1963)[a]
131	5429	212	198	Normal cat
190	11563	43	200	Experimentally induced hypervitaminosis A
588	19983	12	1223	Experimentally induced hypervitaminosis A

[a] Moore et al. (1963) found no vitamin A in the urine of 3 other cats.

parent that the value for urine is unrelated to the amount in the kidney, as the highest concentration found in the former was associated with the lowest value in the kidney. There are insufficient data to relate urine values to those of plasma, but in man (Sharman et al., 1966) relationships would vary markedly with variation in times of blood sampling after a liver meal.

2. Fertility of Affected Animals

When entire male and female cats with chronic hypervitaminosis A and with developed cervical spondylosis were kept together, pregnancy did not occur; however, the female became pregnant subsequently when mated with a normal male.

a. Males

The testes of the affected males were soft and flabby, although secondary male characteristics had developed normally. Single testes taken from males at the time of parturition of their female littermates revealed degenerative changes in the tubules, with failure of spermatogenesis. Testicular degeneration was apparent after 12 to 15 months on a diet of liver. When one of the male cats subsequently received a diet free of vitamin A for 6 months, testicular function returned to normal as judged by successful matings and by histologic evidence of normal spermatogenesis in the remaining testis. Similar testicular degeneration was reported in young rats by Maddock *et al.* (1953); it was not prevented by vitamin E and did not resolve when the rats were returned to a diet low in vitamin A. Differences between the cats and the rats are probably a matter of degree, the lesions being more severe in the latter.

b. Females

In the preliminary studies on fertility, 3 female siblings (cats 1, 3, and 4 in Table III) that had been fed liver for 12 to 15 months after weaning were successfully mated to a normal cat and produced 13 full-term kittens. The kittens of one cat, however, had to be delivered by hysterotomy. All but one kitten were delivered alive, although only 3 were reared to weaning age. No anatomic abnormalities of the kind attributed to excessive quantities of vitamin A at a critical period of gestation and described by Cohlan (1953), Giroud and Martinet (1955), Kalter and Warkany (1961), Marin-Padilla and Ferm (1965), and Wiersig and Swenson (1967) for rats, mice, golden hamsters, and dogs, were found in the kittens. Further evidence against congenital abnormalities being associated with hypervitaminosis A in cats is suggested by the fact that, although the latter condition is common in Brisbane (Seawright *et al.*, 1968), there was no associated high incidence of congenital abnormality.

3. Vitamin A Values for Kittens of Affected Mothers

Values for liver and kidney vitamin A in kittens born to the intoxicated cats, together with data on the mothers and values from deficient cats and their kittens are shown in Table III. Values in day-old kittens from cats with hypervitaminosis A were relatively high compared with those from deficient cats, with values of 6 and 1 μg./g. of liver and kidney in a full term fetus (Moore *et al.*, 1963) and with the value of 1 μg./g. in livers of newborn kittens (Van Eckelen and Wolff, cited by Moore, 1957). This indicates a substantial placental transfer of the vitamin when the concentration in the blood of the mother (e.g., cat 1) is high. Furthermore, the accumulation of high reserves of vitamin A in livers of 2- to 4-week-old kittens from cat 1 indicated that large amounts of the vitamin were secreted in the milk fat, as in the case of the rat (Rodahl, 1950). Excessive intake of vitamin A in the milk may also have contributed to the high mortality rate in the kittens of the affected mothers.

It is reasonable to assume that the values of vitamin A in cat 3, 12 to 15 months after receiving a daily diet of liver, were comparable with those of its littermates. These values were 28,699 μg./g., 89 μg./g., and 635

μg./100 ml. for the liver, kidneys, and plasma, respectively, of cat 1 and 24,688 μg./g. and 1,718 μg./100 ml. for the liver and plasma, respectively, of the first experimental cat (7) analyzed from this group (Table I). Values in cat 3, approximately 2½ years after being changed from liver to meat diet show substantial reduction of body reserves of vitamin A over this period. After her first litter, cat 3 was mated to the same male cat and produced 2 more litters, 45 and 63 weeks after the first one. The vitamin A reserves of these kittens were substantially lower than those of kittens of comparable age from cat 1. This difference was attributed to the vitamin A reserves of the respective mothers.

From limited data available (Table III) on hepatic concentrations in kittens of affected cats on liver diet, and assuming that the increase in hepatic concentrations with age is linear up to weaning, it can be estimated that these kittens would have had values of 2500 to 3500 μg./g. when 6 to 8 weeks old. The three kittens from these cats which reached weaning age had no signs of deforming cervical spondylosis or other skeletal lesions.

The kidney vitamin A values of our kittens were generally lower than those of domestic cats. However, the only value available to compare them with on an equivalent age basis was that of <1 μg./g. found by Moore *et al.* (1963) in a full-term fetus. These workers also found a higher concentration of vitamin A in kidneys than in liver in 31 of 82 cats, and Seawright *et al.* (1968) reported a similar finding in 11 of 100 cats.

Cats 10 and 12 were reared in the same environment as cats 1, 3, and 4, but they received meat rather than liver. They, too, were mated after 12 to 15 months, and only cat 10 became pregnant, but the kittens died soon after birth. As shown in Table III these kittens had no initial reserves of vitamin A, and the reserves in the cats were low. Nevertheless, the plasma levels of the cats were relatively high compared with that in cat 3 (Table I) with the values of 19 ± 12 to 68 ± 17 μg./100 ml. in cats receiving 145–195 μg. vitamin A/100 g. feed (Gershoff *et al.*, 1957), with the content of 75 μg./100 ml. for a normal cat (Seawright *et al.*, 1965) and with values of 187 to 189 μg./100 ml. in 3 vitamin A adequate experimental cats fed meat and milk (Seawright *et al.*, 1967).

The macerated skeletons of cats 10 (Fig. 6) and 12 had enlarged bones with coarse structure caused by formation of cancellous rather than compact bone, which is characteristic of vitamin A deficiency in the dog (Mellanby, 1944; Wolbach, 1947). This aberration was not observed by Gershoff *et al.* (1957), who did not study the bones in his vitamin A deficient cats. Another lesion suggestive of vitamin A deficiency was found in the lungs, namely focal squamous metaplasia of the terminal

TABLE III

TISSUE VITAMIN A VALUES OF EXPERIMENTAL CATS AND OF THEIR KITTENS

Animals	Age of kittens (days)	Liver vitamin A (µg./g.)	(Total µg.)	Kidneys vitamin A (µg./g.)	(Total µg.)	Plasma vitamin A (µg./100 ml.)	Remarks
Cat 4	—	—	—	—	—	—	Clinical hypervitaminosis A on diet of liver
Fetus	full term	141	520	nil	nil	—	
Kitten	1	68	145	9	12	—	
Kitten	1	23	81	2	3	—	
Cat 1	—	28,699	1,949,492	89	1,380	635	Clinical hypervitaminosis A on diet of liver
Kitten	15	1,007	11,125	35	84	—	Cat killed 10 weeks after producing this litter and tissues analyzed
Kitten	15	1,163	11,225	31	97	—	
Kitten	24	1,553	23,500	80	387	—	
Kitten	26	1,454	19,000	133	715	—	
Cat 3	—	—	—	—	—	—	Clinical hypervitaminosis A on diet of liver
Kitten	1	162	1,025	3	5	—	
Kitten	2	209	1,363	7	10	—	
Kitten	2	192	1,427	1	2	—	

Cat 3	—	—	—	—	—	No liver or vitamin A for 41 weeks
Kitten 1	143	636	1	2	—	Second litter born 45 weeks after first litter
Kitten 8	138	856	2	4	—	
Kitten 8	122	990	3	5	—	
Kitten 15	89	1,280	9	29	—	
Kitten 21	181	2,179	8	31	—	
Kitten 22	186	2,440	17	65	—	
Cat 3	4,970	770,350	9	315	72	No liver or vitamin A for 59 weeks
Kitten 1	82	452	2	2	—	Third litter born 18 weeks after second litter
Kitten 9	108	992	3	7	—	Cat 3 killed 83 weeks after producing this litter and tissues analyzed
Kitten 17	140	1,752	5	18	—	
Kitten 23	195	1,464	10	24	—	
Kitten 26	130	1,492	12	53	—	
Kitten 38	280	3,730	5	19	—	
Cat 10	1	120	21	500	167	Clinical hypovitaminosis A diet of meat and milk
Kitten 1	Nil	Nil	Nil	Nil	—	
Kitten 1	Nil	Nil	Nil	Nil	—	
Kitten 2	3	11	8	10	—	
Kitten 2	7	18	15	16	—	
Cat 12	3	319	5	103	247	Clinical hypovitaminosis A diet of meat and milk

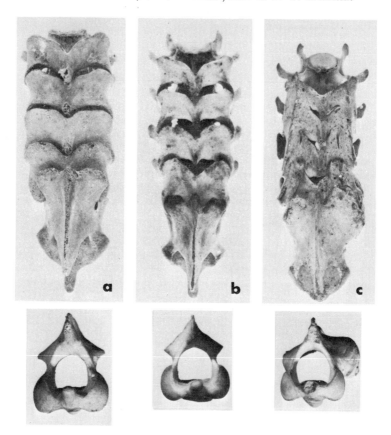

FIG. 6. Cervical vertebrae of an A hypovitaminotic cat (a), a normal cat (b), and an A hypervitaminotic cat (c); large coarsely modeled bones, normal bones, and confluent exostosis formation, which is indicative of the respective vitamin A status of each, are evident.

epithelium of some bronchioles and alveolae, as reported by Gershoff *et al.* (1957).

IV. Summary

Extensive exostoses of the cervical spine, causing crippling, is a fairly common condition of cats in Australia. The disease is caused by prolonged feeding of raw liver and has been shown to be due to hypervitaminosis A. It has also been reported in New Zealand, Great Britain, United States of America, and Uruguay.

Both experimentally induced and naturally occurring cases of the disease have a characteristic syndrome, with palpable rigidity of the cervical spine, hyperesthesia, lameness of one or both forelimbs, and abnormalities of gait. Clinical signs of hypervitaminosis A in affected animals improved markedly within a few weeks when liver or vitamin A was withdrawn from the diet.

Storage of large quantities of vitamin A in the body results in lipid infiltration of many organs such as the liver, kidneys, and lungs as well as the reticulohistiocytic system. Vitamin A is readily identified in these lipid deposits. The main toxic effect is on the skeleton, but lesions of teeth and skin may occur. Excess vitamin A chiefly affects cartilage cells and causes lysis of the matrix in the young animal. Osteoblasts also appear to be affected but to a lesser extent. The stress of persistent coat cleaning is believed to be the factor which causes exostoses to occur most commonly in the anterior region of the neck. With continued high intake of vitamin A, the lesions progress caudally and may cause ankylosis of the entire spinal column. The bone changes are permanent but affected bones become remodeled with time.

Australia has a large meat export industry. Liver is therefore plentiful and inexpensive and is often fed to cats. In addition, livers from grazing animals of Australia are reported to be generally higher in vitamin A than those of grazing animals of other countries.

Daily intake of vitamin A of 17 to 35 μg./g. body weight for 6 to 12 months is needed for the induction of bone lesions in the cat. Hepatic storage of the vitamin in affected cats varies from 2,500 to about 40,000 μg./g. Large quantities of the vitamin, up to 3000 μg./g., may occur in the kidney, and vitamin A may be found in the urine.

Intoxication with vitamin A causes testicular degeneration and temporary loss of fertility of males but not female cats. There is substantial transfer of vitamin A to offspring of affected cats in the milk but less via the placenta. Livers of kittens may contain as much as 3500 μg./g. of vitamin A at weaning, and this may predispose them to hypervitaminosis A if they are fed on liver or other diets high in vitamin A as adults.

References

Baker, J. R., and Hughes, I. B. (1968). A case of deforming cervical spondylosis in a cat associated with a diet rich in liver. *Veterinary Record* **83**, 44–45.

Baker, J. R., Howell, J. McC., and Thompson, J. N. (1967). Hypervitaminosis A in the chick. *British Journal of Experimental Pathology* **48**, 507–512.

Bangham, A. D., Dingle, J. T., and Lucy, J. A. (1964). Studies on the mode of action of excess of vitamin A. 9. Penetration of lipid monolayers by compounds of the vitamin A series. *Biochemical Journal* **90**, 133–140.

Caffey, J. (1951). Chronic poisoning due to excess vitamin A. *American Journal of Roentgenology, Radium Therapy* **65**, 12–26.

Catel, W. (1938). Klinische und tierexperimentelle Studien über die normale und pathologische Physiologie des A-Vitamins. *Monatsschrift für Kinderheilkunde* **73**, 316–344.

Christi, G. A. (1957). Osteo periostitis difusa anquilosante en el gato. *Anales de la Facultad de Veterinaria del Uruguay, Montevideo* **6**, 95–105.

Clark, L., and Seawright, A. A. (1968). Skeletal abnormalities in the hindlimbs of young cats as a result of hypervitaminosis A. *Nature* **217**, 1174–1176.

Cohlan, S. Q. (1953). Excessive intake of vitamin A as a cause of congenital anomalies in the rat. *Science* **117**, 535–536.

Collazo, J. A., and Rodriguez, J. S. (1933). Hypervitaminosis A. *Klinische Wochenschrift* **12**, 1732–1734.

Cordes, D. S. (1967). Personal communication. New Zealand Department of Agriculture, Ruakura, N. Z.

Davies, A. W., and Moore, T. (1934). The distribution of vitamin A in the organs of the normal and hypervitaminotic rat. *Biochemical Journal* **28**, 288–295.

Dickinson, C. D., and Scott, P. P. (1959). Nutrition of the cat. 1. A practical stock diet supporting growth and reproduction. *British Journal of Nutrition* **10**, 304–311.

Dingle, J. T., and Lucy, J. A. (1962). Studies ₋n the mode of action of excess of vitamin A. 5. The effect of vitamin A on the stability of the erythrocyte membrane. *Biochemical Journal* **84**, 611–621.

Dodd, D. C. (1966). Personal communication. School of Veterinary Medicine, University of Pennsylvania, Philadelphia, Pennsylvania.

Domagk, G., and Dobeneck, P. (1933). Über histologische Befunde bei der Überdosierung mit vitamin A-Konzentrat. *Archiv für pathologische Anatomie und Physiologie* **290**, 385–395.

Drigalski, W., and Laubmann, W. (1933). Über Schädigung durch vitamin A. *Klinische Wochenschrift* **12**, 1171–1174.

English, P. B. (1969). Clinical communication: A case of hyperostosis due to hypervitaminosis A. *Journal of Small Animal Practice* **10**, 207–212.

English, P. B., and Seawright, A. A. (1964). Deforming cervical spondylosis of the cat. *Australian Veterinary Journal* **40**, 376–381.

Fell, H. B., and Dingle, J. T. (1963). Studies on the mode of action of excess of vitamin A. 6. Lysosomal protease and the degradation of cartilage matrix. *Biochemical Journal* **87**, 403–408.

Fell, H. B., and Thomas, L. (1960). A comparison of the effects of papain and vitamin A on cartilage. II. Effects on organ cultures of embryonic skeletal tissue. *Journal of Experimental Medicine* **111**, 719–744.

Ferrando, R., Fourlon, C., Wolter, R., and Denois, M. (1966). Reserves hepatiques et renales de vitamin A du chat. *Recueil de Médicine vétérinaire* **142**, 1207–1210.

Fry, P. D. (1968). Cervical spondylosis in the cat. *Journal of Small Animal Practice* **9**, 59–61.

Gartner, R. J. W., and Anson, R. J. (1966). Vitamin A reserves of sheep maintained on mulga (*Acacia aneura*). *Australian Journal of Experimental Agriculture and Animal Husbandry* **6**, 321–325.

Gartner, R. J. W., Alexander, G. I., and Bewg, W. P. (1968). Seasonal fluctuations of hepatic vitamin A reserves in beef cattle grazing unimproved pastures. *Queensland Journal of Agriculture and Animal Sciences* **25**, 225–233.

Gerber, A., Raab, A. P., and Sobel, A. E. (1954). Vitamin A poisoning in adults with description of a case. *American Journal of Medicine* **16**, 729–745.

Gershoff, S. N., Andrews, S. B., Hegsted, D. M., and Lentini, E. A. (1957). Vitamin A deficiency in cats. *Laboratory Investigation* 6, 227–240.

Giroud, A., and Martinet, M. (1955). Hypervitaminosa A et anomalie chez le foetus des rat. *Internationale Zeitschrift für Vitaminforschung* 26, 10–18.

Grey, R. M., Nielsen, S. W., Rousseau, J. E., Calhoun, M. C., and Eaton, H. D. (1965). Pathology of skull, radius and rib in hypervitaminosis A of young calves. *Pathologia Veterinaria (Basel)* 2, 446–467.

Herbst, E. J., Pavcek, P. L., and Elvehjem, C. A. (1944). Telang livers and vitamin A toxicity. *Science* 100, 338–339.

Heywood, R. (1967). Vitamin A in the liver and kidney of some felidae. *British Veterinary Journal* 123, 390–395.

Hodge, H. C., and Smith, F. A. (1965). Biological properties of inorganic fluorides. *In* "Fluorine Chemistry" (J. H. Simons, ed.), Vol. 4. Academic Press, New York.

Irving, J. T. (1949). The effects of avitaminosis and hypervitaminosis A upon the incisor teeth and incisal alveolar bone of rats. *Journal of Physiology (London)* 108, 92–101.

Kalter, H. G., and Warkany, T. (1961). Experimental production of congenital malformations in strains of inbred mice by maternal treatment with hypervitaminosis A. *American Journal of Pathology* 39, 1–21.

Lawrie, N. R., Moore, T., and Rajagopal, K. R. (1941). Excretion of vitamin A in urine. *Biochemical Journal* 35, 825–836.

Lowe, J. S., Morton, R. A., and Vernon, J. (1957). Unsaponifiable constituents of kidneys in various species. *Biochemical Journal* 67, 228–234.

Lucke, V. M., Baskerville, A., Bardgett, P. L., Mann, P. G. H., and Thompson, S. Y. (1968). Deforming cervical spondylosis in the cat associated with hypervitaminosis A. *Veterinary Record* 82, 141–142.

Maddock, C. L., Cohen, J., and Wolbach, S. B. (1953). Effect of hypervitaminosis A on the testes of the rat. *Archives of Pathology* 56, 333–340.

Marie, J., and Sée, G. (1954). Acute hypervitaminosis A of the infant: Its clinical manifestations with benign acute hydrocephalus and pronounced bulge of the fontanel. *American Journal of Diseases of Children* 87, 731–736.

Marin-Padilla, M., and Ferm, V. H. (1965). Somite necrosis and developmental malformations induced by vitamin A in the golden hamster. *Journal of Embryology and Experimental Morphology* 13, 1–8.

Mellanby, E. (1944). Nutrition in relation to bone growth and the nervous system. *Proceedings of the Royal Society* B132, 28–46.

Moll, T., Domagk, G., and Laquer, F. (1933). Über das vitamin A-Konzentrat, Vôgan und seine Wertbestimmung. *Klinische Wochenschrift* 12, 465–467.

Moore, T. (1957). "Vitamin A." Elsevier, Amsterdam.

Moore, T., and Wang, Y. L. (1943). The toxicity of pure vitamin A. *Biochemical Journal* 37, viii–ix.

Moore, T., and Wang, Y. L. (1945). Hypervitaminosis A. *Biochemical Journal* 39, 222–228.

Moore, T., Sharman, I. M., and Scott, P. P. (1963). Vitamin A in the kidney of the cat. *Research in Veterinary Science* 4, 397–407.

Niemann, C., and Klein Obbink, H. J. (1954). The biochemistry and pathology of hypervitaminosis A. *Vitamins and Hormones* 12, 69–99.

Noetzel, H. (1939). Morphologische Untersuchungen bei vitamin A Überdosierung. *Zeitschrift für die gesamte experimentelle Medizin* 105, 83–88.

Pavcek, P. L., Herbst, E. J., and Elvehjem, C. A. (1945). The nutritional value of telang livers. *Journal of Nutrition* **30**, 1–9.

Popper, H., and Greenberg, P. (1941). Visualization of vitamin A in rat organs by fluorescence microscopy. *A. M. A. Archives of Pathology* **32**, 11–32.

Querner, F. R. (1935). Der microscopsche Nachweis von Vitamin A im animalen Gewebe. Zur Kenntnis der paraplasmatischeh Leberzellinschlüsse (III Mitteilung). *Klinische Wochenschrift* **14**, 1213–1217.

Riser, W. H. (1966). Personal communication. School of Veterinary Medicine, University of Pennsylvania, Philadelphia, Pennsylvania.

Rodahl, K. (1949). The toxic effect of polar bear liver. *Norsk. Polarinstitutt,* No. 92.

Rodahl, K. (1950). Hypervitaminosis A—a study of the effect of vitamin A in experimental animals. *Norsk. Polarinstitutt,* No. 95.

Rodahl, K., and Moore, T. (1943). The vitamin A content and toxicity of bear and seal liver. *Biochemical Journal* **37**, 166–168.

Seawright, A. A., and English, P. B. (1964). Deforming cervical spondylosis in the cat. *Journal of Pathology and Bacteriology* **88**, 503–509.

Seawright, A. A., English, P. B., and Gartner, R. J. W. (1965). Hypervitaminosis A and hyperostosis of the cat. *Nature* **206**, 1171–1172.

Seawright, A. A., English, P. B., and Gartner, R. J. W. (1967). Hypervitaminosis A and deforming cervical spondylosis of the cat. *Journal of Comparative Pathology* **77**, 29–39.

Seawright, A. A., Steele, D. P., and Clark, L. (1968). Hypervitaminosis A of cats in Brisbane. *Australian Veterinary Journal* **44**, 203–206.

Selye, H. (1957). Lathyrism. *Revue canadienee de biologie* **16**, 1–82.

Sharman, I. M., Moore, T., and Tietzner, Z. A. (1966). The absorption of vitamin A after a meal of liver. *Proceedings of the Nutrition Society (England and Scotland)* **25**, xxxii–xxxiii.

Strauss, K. S. (1934). Beobactungen bei Hypervitaminose A. *Beiträge zur pathologischen Anatomie und zur allgemeinen Pathologie* **94**, 345–352.

Studer, A., and Frey, J. R. (1949). Über Hautveränderungen der Ratte nach grossen oralen Dosen von Vitamin A. *Schweizerische medizinische Wochenschrift* **79**, 382–384.

Swerczek, T. W., and Nielsen, S. W. (1967). Skin lesions produced by hypervitaminosis A in calves. *Laboratory Investigation* **16**, 639–640.

Thomas, L., McClusky, R. T., Potter, J. L., and Weissmann, G. (1960). Comparison of the effects of papain and vitamin A on cartilage. I. Effects in rabbits. *Journal of Experimental Medicine* **111**, 705–718.

Toomey, J. A., and Morrissette, R. A. (1947). Hypervitaminosis A. *American Journal of Diseases of Children* **13**, 437–480.

Tucker, R. (1964). Contributions to the biomechanics of the vertebral column I. Biomechanical characteristics of the thoraco-lumbar curvature. *Acta Theriologica* **8**, 45–72.

Uotilla, U., and Simola, P. E. (1938). Über die Bezieungen zwischen den Vitaminen und dem Reticuloendothelialen System. *Archiv für pathologische Anatomie und Physiologie* **301**, 523–534.

Weslaw, W., Wronski, B., Wroblewski, A., and Wroblewski, B. (1938). Symptomatologie und Verlauf der A-hypervitaminose bei Ratten infolge enterler, subcutaner und percutaner Darrichung von Vitamin A-Konzentraten. *Klinische Wochenschrift* **17**, 777–781.

Wiersig, D. O., and Swenson, M. J. (1967). Teratogenicity of Vitamin A in the canine. *Federation Proceedings* **26**, 486.

Wolbach, S. B. (1947). Vitamin A deficiency and excess in relation to skeletal growth. *Journal of Bone and Joint Surgery* **29**, 171–192.

Wolbach, S. B., and Bessey, O. A. (1942). Vitamin A deficiency and excess in relation to skeletal growth. *Physiological Reviews* **22**, 233–289.

Wolke, R. E., Nielsen, S. W., and Rousseau, J. E. (1968). Bone lesions of hypervitaminosis A in the pig. *American Journal of Veterinary Research* **29**, 1009–1024.

In Vitro Cultivation of Nematode Parasites Important to Veterinary Medicine *

STANLEY E. LELAND, JR.†

Department of Infectious Diseases, Kansas State University, Manhattan, Kansas

* Contribution V No. 126, Department of Infectious Diseases, Kansas Agricultural Experiment Station, Manhattan. Supported in part by NSF Research Grant GB 7532 and contributing to Regional Project W-102-Biological Methods of Control for Internal Parasites.

† The author is Professor of Parasitology, and Acting Head of the Department of Infectious Diseases, College of Veterinary Medicine, Kansas State University, Manhattan, Kansas.

I. Introduction

1. IMPORTANCE AND PURPOSE

The *in vitro* cultivation of parasitic nematodes and ultimately the development of media of known constitution will undoubtedly open important new experimental approaches in the field of helminthic diseases.

Unlike the bacteriologist, who can in many cases cultivate his organisms in suitable media, or even the virologist who can resort to the chicken embryo or tissue culture technique, the parasitologist must conduct his investigations in the presence of the complicating influence of the host. No Trichostrongyle parasite of a vertebrate host has been cultivated throughout its life cycle, including multiplication (see Appendix). Although contributions concerning the cultivation of free-living, self-fertilizing, hermaphroditic soil nematodes (Dougherty, 1959) and the parasitic nematodes of arthropods (Stoll, 1959) are both numerous and important, this discussion will consider only the nematode parasites of vertebrates.

One of the cardinal requirements for an organized study of a disease-producing organism is the maintenance or availability of the organisms in the laboratory and preferably with an *in vitro* method of cultivation. This requirement has not been fully satisfied in the case of the parasitic nematodes of domestic animals. For the maintenance of pure cultures of the species which parasitize domestic animals, the situation resolves itself, almost entirely, to one of raising susceptible hosts from birth in a worm-free environment and infecting these hosts with pure cultures of the worm to be studied. For parasites of the large domestic animals, this procedure is expensive and time consuming.

The development of media of known composition would also provide means for making accurate and precise measurements of the exchange of substances, between the parasite and the medium, and provide a better method for reproducing the exact conditions of a given experiment. It would be possible to determine exactly what substances are required by the parasite as essential nutrients. It would make possible precise metabolic studies of the parasite and thus provide a rational approach to the development of anthelmintics. In addition, the scientist equipped with knowledge of the essential metabolism and *in vitro* growth requirements would be able to incorporate radioactive material in the synthetic media with the ultimate goal of tagging the parasite. This would conceivably make possible the tracing of the parasite's migration through the host and thus contribute information concerning the life cycle and disease-producing properties of the parasite.

The *in vitro* cultivation of the parasitic stage of nematodes will be valuable in the study of their morphogenesis, as constant observation is possible.

Studies on the parasites of certain wildlife and marine species will be facilitated by *in vitro* cultivation systems, since many of these hosts are generally unavailable, difficult to raise in captivity, or make extensive and essentially unknown global migrations.

These systems will assist in evaluating the influence of certain host habits on parasitism such as hibernation.

Since the immune response to helminthic infection is thought by many to be a response by the host to the excretory or secretory products, or both, of the living worm, *in vitro* cultivation of the parasite would facilitate production and collection of these materials for antigenic and immunologic studies. Furthermore, the isolation of these products will make possible evaluation of their disease-producing potential. Inasmuch as parasitic nematodes cause tissue changes which range from necrosis to proliferation (Foster, 1942; Leland *et al.*, 1961), some of which are not due to mechanical damage (biting, chewing, etc.), the role of these products is of basic interest to the pathologist.

It is reasonable to assume that advances in the immunology of diseases caused by nematodes will be equally as exciting as those which followed the development of culture techniques for viral, bacterial, and protozoan parasites.

The ultimate completion of the entire *in vitro* life cycle of parasites of vertebrates, including multiplication, would seem to be largely a function of the amount of effort that is directed toward elucidation of the remaining problems. The outlook could be rated as optimistic since, within the last 12 years, an increasing number of Trichostrongyle parasites have been cultivated to the egg-laying (infertile) stage (Weinstein and Jones, 1956; Leland, 1961, 1965a,b, 1967a,b, 1968, 1969) (Figs. 1–6).

Recent reviews by Silverman (1965) and Taylor and Baker (1968) included annotated bibliographies which adequately compiled the fund of information relating to *in vitro* cultivation of parasitic helminths. Readers desiring historic and detailed reference citations are directed to these reviews.

The purpose of this treatise is to present the author's concept of developments in the field of *in vitro* cultivation of nematode parasites and to review the progress in cultivation research carried out by the author and his associates. No attempt has been made to accumulate an exhaustive bibliography and only citations relative to the discussion are included.

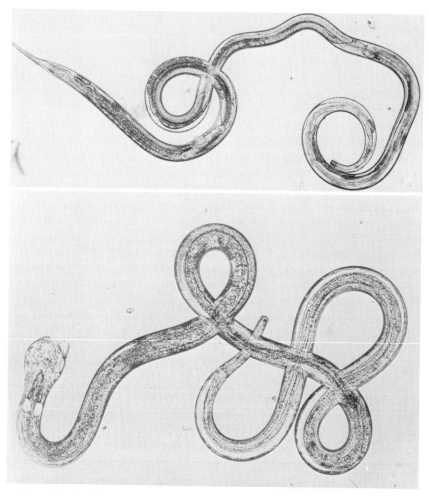

Fig. 1 (*top*). *Cooperia punctata,* sexually mature adult female produced *in vitro* showing eggs in all stages of development. $\times$ 65.

Fig. 2 (*bottom*). *Cooperia punctata,* sexually mature adult male produced *in vitro.* $\times$ 90.

2. Suggestions on Terminology

It is to be expected that, as a new field of investigation emerges, specialized terminology becomes necessary. Terms from other disciplines are often brought into usage; and, in the course of events, their original meaning becomes altered or expanded and can no longer be regarded as equivalent.

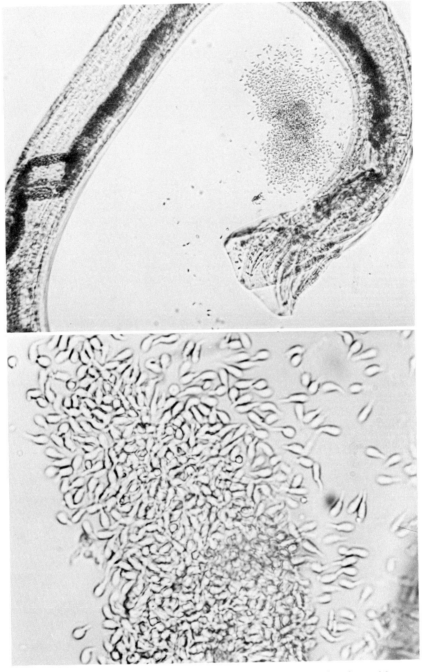

FIG. 3 (*top*). *Hyostrongylus rubidus,* adult male produced *in vitro* with sperm mechanically ejaculated. × 133.

FIG. 4 (*bottom*). Higher magnification of sperm in Fig. 3. × 680.

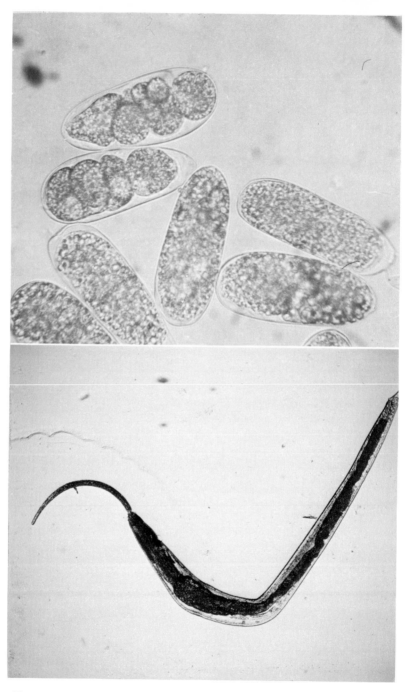

Fig. 5 (*top*). *Hyostrongylus rubidus*, eggs produced by female worms grown *in vitro* showing two eggs undergoing cleavage. × 431.

Fig. 6 (*bottom*). Fourth-stage *Oesophagostomum* sp. ingesting *Cooperia* sp. in culture. × 94.

The term "axenic" (from Greek, without foreign life) was originally introduced by Baker and Ferguson (1942) to characterize maintenance of platyfish free from any other demonstrable organisms. An axenic organism was defined as "a species free from any life apart from that produced by its own protoplasm." The term axenic, as used in reference to nematode cultivation, has lost some of its original specificity. It has been applied to nematode cultures whose microbial populations are kept under static control by antibiotics. In addition, the question of whether or not the cells of the nematode itself are free of virus or rickettsia appears to have been largely ignored in cultures designated as axenic. Because the correct use of the term depends on the inability to demonstrate the presence of other organisms, the degree of sophistication used in their detection is essentially the determining factor.

It would, therefore, appear that the use of the term axenic in relation to metazoan cultivation should be discouraged. This view is shared, at least in part, by Stoll (1959) and Silverman (1965).

The term *"in vitro"* appears more appropriate in reference to cultures of parasitic nematodes, particularly in the context of an artificial environment rather than the direct translation "in glass." The extent to which other forms of life have been excluded from cultures should be indicated with each situation. The state of the science has now reached a point where development of parasitic nematodes in culture is often compared with that in the host so both the terms *"in vitro"* and *"in vivo"* are particularly useful.

Dougherty (1953, 1959) introduced terminology that essentially classified culture medium according to the degree of its chemical definition. We have found no particular advantage in the use of this terminology and have considered a medium, either chemically defined in which case the chemical structure is known for *all* constituents, or complex, where the chemical structure of one or more of the constituents is unknown. Furthermore, we recognize no validity in attempts to merge the two definitions. Reference to a "supplemented chemically defined medium" where the supplementation consists of a substance chemically (structurally) undefined should be avoided. This designation of medium has resulted in confusion and misquotation.

II. Media

1. REQUIREMENTS

Advances in the field of tissue culture have contributed greatly to the development and success of *in vitro* cultivation of parasitic nematodes. However, for tissue culturing the *in vitro* requirements of only the particular type of cell must be known for successful cultivation, whereas, in the *in vitro* cultivation of parasitic nematodes, the requirements of many types of cells, organs, and even systems must be considered. A further complication is that the requirements at one stage of the parasite are not necessarily identical or even similar to those of another stage. Appropriate steps must be taken to provide the optimal population density and sex ratio in the culture system. With most gastrointestinal nematode parasites, one should recall that from relatively primitive infective larvae, with no genital system and little excretory system, there evolves an adult worm in three weeks or less possessing a complicated reproductive system capable of producing large numbers of eggs. Thus, the parasite, though like the cell in that it is incapable of unaided independent survival, is considerably more complex as are its *in vitro* growth requirements.

It is therefore not surprising that in the current state of the science, the parasitologist does not enjoy the advantages of a chemically defined medium for *in vitro* cultivation of nematode parasites of vertebrates. There is reason to be optimistic, however, if one recalls that the first successful cell or tissue cultures were realized with complex media and only after considerable time and effort did chemically defined media evolve. In many respects, the present state of *in vitro* nematode cultivation is comparable to that of tissue culture achievements of 15 or 20 years ago. As with early cell culture, media successful in parasitic nematode culturing have included such complex components as tissue extracts, proteins, and serum.

Based on titrations with *Cooperia punctata* as a monoinoculant or mixtures of gastrointestinal nematodes, a medium designated Ae (Leland, 1963a) has evolved which, with slight modification for the particular species concerned, can support growth of eight species to the adult stage, seven of these to egg-laying period plus eight others to fourth stage (Tables I to IV).

Medium Ae consists of chicken embryo extract, serum, sodium caseinate plus cystine, vitamins, a liver extract, and antibiotics in a balanced salt solution. In the following discussion, each of these components are considered in terms of their influence on culturing.

2. Chicken Embryo Extract

Originally in tissue culturing and currently in nematode culturing, chicken embryo extract (CEE) was a common denominator for growth and metamorphosis. One might well surmise that the highly nutritious nature of embryonic tissue plus low content of inhibitory substances ac-

TABLE I

THE EXTENT OF *in Vitro* DEVELOPMENT IN Ae MEDIUM OR MODIFIED Ae MEDIUM BY BOVINE PARASITES

Parasites from bovine	Nonparasitic stages					Parasitic stages					Produced *in vitro*	
	Egg	Stage 1	Molt	Stage 2	Molt	Inf.[a] Stage 3	Molt	Stage 4	Molt	Stage 5	Eggs	Sperm
Cooperia punctata	+	+	+	+	+	+	+	+	+	+	+	+
Cooperia pectinata	+	+	+	+	+	+	+	+/[b]	+	+	+	+
Ostertagia ostertagi						+	+	+/[b]	+	+	+	
Cooperia oncophora	+	+	+	+	+	+	+	+				
Haemonchus placei						+	+	+				
Oesophagostomum radiatum	+	+	+	+	+	+						
Trichostrongylus axei	+	+	+	+	+	+						

[a] Inf. = Infective stage.

[b] / = Cultivation to this point from fertile eggs.

TABLE II

THE EXTENT OF *in Vitro* DEVELOPMENT IN Ae MEDIUM OR MODIFIED Ae MEDIUM BY PORCINE PARASITES

Parasites from swine	Nonparasitic stages					Parasitic stages					Produced *in vitro*	
	Egg	Stage 1	Molt	Stage 2	Molt	Inf.[a] Stage 3	Molt	Stage 4	Molt	Stage 5	Eggs	Sperm
Hyostrongylus rubidus						+	+	+	+	+	+	+
Oesophagostomum quadrispinulatum						+	+	+	+	+		+
Ascaris lumbricoides var suum	+	+	+	+	+	+						

[a] Inf. = Infective stage.

TABLE III

THE EXTENT OF *in Vitro* DEVELOPMENT IN Ae MEDIUM OR MODIFIED Ae MEDIUM BY OVINE PARASITES

Parasites from ovine	Nonparasitic stages					Inf.[a]		Parasitic stages				Produced in vitro	
	Egg	Stage 1	Molt	Stage 2	Molt	Stage 3	Molt	Stage 4	Molt	Stage 5	Molt	Eggs	Sperm
Ostertagia circumcincta						+	+	+	+	+	+	+	
Ostertagia trifurcata						+	+	+	+	+	+	+	
Oesophagostomum sp.		+	+	+	+	+	+	+					
Nematodirus sp.	+			+	+	+	+	+					
Haemonchus contortus	+					+	+						

(*Oesophagostomum* sp. and *Nematodirus* sp. nonparasitic stages — in Earle's Solution)

[a] Inf. = Infective stage.

TABLE IV

THE EXTENT OF *in Vitro* DEVELOPMENT IN Ae MEDIUM OR MODIFIED Ae MEDIUM BY EQUINE, CANINE, AND FELINE PARASITES

Parasites	Nonparasitic stages						Inf.[a]	Parasitic stages			
	Egg	Stage 1	Molt	Stage 2	Molt	Stage 3	Molt	Stage 4	Molt	Stage 5	
From equine:											
Cyclicostephanus sp.						+	+	+			
From canine:											
Ancylostoma caninum						+	+	+[b]			
From feline:											
Ancylostoma tubaeforma[c]	+	+	+	+	+	+	+	+	+	+	

[a] Inf. = Infective stage.
[b] Three specimens to fourth stage.
[c] Slonka and Leland (1969).

count for the growth-promoting properties of CEE. Weinstein and Jones (1956) apparently first recognized the potential value of CEE for culturing nematodes and successfully utilized it to cultivate the rat parasite *Nippostrongylus brasiliensis* (=*N. muris*). However, Silverman (1959) and Leland (1963a) were unsuccessful in utilizing the medium of Weinstein and Jones (1956) for cultivating certain gastrointestinal nematodes of ruminants although Leland (1963a) repeated the cultivation of *N. brasiliensis*. Silverman (1959) was of the opinion that the preparation of the liver extract was responsible for unsuccessful application of the Weinstein and Jones medium. However, after using the same commercial preparations of liver extract of Weinstein and Jones (1959), Leland (1963a) concluded that the kind of CEE preparation was the critical factor in cultivating the gastrointestinal nematodes of ruminants. Weinstein and Jones (1957) obtained best results with *N. brasiliensis* by omitting liver concentrate and increasing their CEE.

Leland (1963a) observed that with the media of Weinstein and Jones (1956, 1957) the CEE tended to precipitate and there was a lack of clarity after the long periods of cultivation necessary with the domestic animal parasites. Diamond and Douvres (1962) also observed this lack of clarity. Leland (1963a) reported a method of preparation, handling, and incorporation of CEE in Ae medium that considerably reduced precipitation. The omission of CEE from Ae medium resulted in complete loss of growth-promoting activity, and any experimental variation in Ae medium causing precipitation likewise resulted in partial to complete loss of activity. Also passage of Ae medium through a Millipore GS filter (pore size $0.22 \mu \pm 0.002 \mu$) resulted in 91% reduction in the number of adult worms that developed, and no eggs were produced (Leland, 1964). This finding indicates that the CEE in Ae medium ideally must exist in a state where the particulate material does not precipitate but that its components do not pass through a filter of 0.22μ pore size. In addition, CEE can vary in composition, depending upon breed and nutrition of the hen which produced the egg, age of the embryos extracted, diluent used for extracting, ratio of diluent to embryo volume, degree of centrifugation, concentration when frozen, and possibly other undetermined factors. The preparation of CEE may be likened to a fingerprint in that probably no two products are exactly alike. Therefore, until a more uniform substitute for CEE becomes available, it is important that, for preparing CEE from recorded formulas or for defining a modified preparation, precise and detailed descriptions be given.

Embryo extract has been prepared from species other than the chicken (Leland, 1959; Diamond and Douvres, 1962), but with no particular advantage demonstrated thus far. The time and cost necessary to produce embryos of large domestic mammals has discouraged investigators from using them.

3. SERUM

As was the case with early attempts at tissue culture, serum was found to be a beneficial or required component of media for cultivating the parasitic stages of many nematode species (Weller, 1943; Weinstein and Jones, 1956, 1959; Silverman, 1959; Leland, 1961, 1963a,b, 1965a,b,c, 1967a; Douvres, 1962a,b, 1966). Douvres (1962b) considered bovine serum a required component of medium used to culture *Oesophagostomum radiatum* to the fourth molt. More generally, inclusion of serum in media has had an enhancing effect, e.g., there were more and larger adult *C. punctata* that laid eggs (Leland, 1963a). However, medium Ae, which was suitable for both development of *C. punctata* from third- stage larvae to adults that laid infertile eggs, and for hatching fertile eggs from host feces, was inadequate or inhibitory for development of the first and second nonparasitic larval stages. The inhibitory nature of Ae medium involved its serum component, because omission, or heat inactivation of the serum, allowed development of these nonparasitic stages. The critical influence of serum on the nonparasitic stages is not surprising when one considers that these stages do not naturally come in contact with serum.

Weinstein and Jones (1959) obtained increased yields of adult *N. brasiliensis* when a basal medium of CEE was supplemented with human rather than rat serum. Leland (1963a,b, 1965a,b,c, 1967a) observed superior development in medium containing host-homologous serum rather than host-heterologous serum.

As precipitation reactions can occur, both *in vivo* and *in vitro,* between living larvae and serum from infected hosts (Sarles, 1938; Otto, 1939), the serum incorporated in media is generally obtained from young helminth-free animals. Because a continuing supply of young helminth-free animals is needed to produce monospecific infections of nematodes being studied, the same animals can serve as serum donors before infection. Douvres (1960), however, was unable to demonstrate precipitates on larvae of *Oesophagostomum radiatum* grown in medium containing sera from immune hosts, but he observed retardation in larval growth.

4. SODIUM CASEINATE PLUS CYSTINE

Weinstein and Jones (1956) found that sexually mature adult *N. brasiliensis* developed only in medium composed of CEE, rat serum, sodium caseinate plus cystine, and liver extract. Weinstein and Jones (1959) reported that adult *N. brasiliensis* could be produced without the liver extract and sodium caseinate plus cystine. Although Weinstein and Jones (1956, 1959) did not comment on the possible function of sodium caseinate plus cystine in their original medium, Leland (1963a) observed a solubilizing effect on his Ae medium in that the omission of sodium caseinate resulted in considerable precipitation during incubation. One might postulate that sodium caseinate serves as a source of amino acids for nematodes in culture, and its selection was influenced by the fact that the composition has been carefully studied and was known to be similar to several other proteins (Block and Bolling, 1945). However, it now seems probable that there are serious shortcomings in the amino acid balance of casein for metazoa of rapid metabolism, e.g., the cystine and cysteine content of casein is usually low as compared to most other animal proteins (Block and Bolling, 1945; Haurowitz, 1950). This presumably accounts for the supplementation with cystine. Cystine and cysteine are freely interconverted in most biologic systems and appear to form an oxidation–reduction (redox) system. Berntzen and Mueller (1964) used cysteine and glutathione (reduced), in a related manner, in an effort to control the redox of medium used to cultivate tapeworms. However, the significance of cystine on the redox potential of media in nematode culturing has not been determined.

5. VITAMINS

Nematode cultivators have logically assumed that the parasite must have vitamin requirements. Undoubtedly, these are supplied to some extent by the complex extracts that are included in most media. The general approach to provide the vitamin requirement has been to supplement media with blocks of eight or more vitamins with the objective of improved development. In the selection, balance, and concentration of vitamins employed for nematode cultivation there is again seen the influence of cell culture experience.

Weinstein and Jones (1959) observed that a vitamin mixture had a growth-promoting effect for the parasitic stages of *N. brasiliensis*. The vitamin mixture in micrograms per milliliter of final medium consisted of thiamine hydrochloride, 2.5; pyridine hydrochloride, 2.5; calcium pantothenate, 2.5; nicotinic acid, 2.5; *p*-aminobenzoic acid, 2.5; folic acid, 1.25; riboflavin, 0.75; and choline chloride, 10.

Douvres (1962a) using the same vitamin mixture enhanced the rate of development of *O. radiatum* through all stages to fourth molt but produced no increase in yields of late fourth-stage and fourth-molt larvae in his medium.

In Ae medium, the vitamin mixture consists of biotin, choline, folic acid, nicotinamide, pantothenic acid, pyridoxal, and thiamine all at 5.0

μg./ml. and riboflavin at 0.5 μg./ml. of final medium. This vitamin content is qualitatively and proportionately identical, but it is five times the concentration of the vitamins in Eagle's basal medium for tissue culture. In titrations with *C. punctata*, the inclusion of this mixture and concentration of vitamins in Ae medium resulted in improved development, greater size, and egg production (Leland, 1963a).

In medium used to culture *Trichinella spiralis* from its stage in muscle to sexually differentiated adults producing juveniles *in vitro*, Berntzen (1965) utilized a vitamin mixture composed of thiamine hydrochloride, riboflavin, calcium pantothenate, pyridoxine, *p*-aminobenzoic acid, niacin, folic acid, *i*-inositol, all at 2.5 mg./154 ml. medium (16.2 μg./ml. final medium), biotin 1.25 mg./154 ml. medium (8.1 μg./ml. final medium), choline chloride 25.0 mg./154 ml. medium (162.3 μg./ml. final medium), and B_{12} 60 units/154 ml. medium (0.39 units/ml. final medium). For purposes of comparison, the vitamin concentrations used by Berntzen were converted to micrograms per milliliter of final medium, and they appear above within the parentheses. The vitamin concentrations used by Berntzen are the highest successfully used to cultivate nematodes to the adult stage. Berntzen did not, however, indicate whether the final concentration of vitamins was arrived at by titration or whether the concentration was selected to insure a surplus. Weinstein and Jones (1959) and Leland (1959) have found that vitamins beyond a certain concentration did not improve the growth-promoting effect.

6. Liver Extract

In addition to CEE, various preparations of liver extract (LE) have been used with varying degrees of success in cell and nematode culturing. Where successfully employed in nematode culturing, various preparations of LE usually have had an enhancing effect on a basic medium (Stoll, 1940; Weinstein and Jones, 1956; Silverman, 1959; Douvres, 1962a; Leland, 1963a; Eckert, 1967). However, a toxic influence has been detected in certain methods of preparation or with concentrations exceeding an apparent optimal level (Lapage, 1935; Stoll, 1940; Weinstein, 1953; Silverman, 1959; Leland, 1959).

Investigators have generally titrated LE to an optimal concentration in order that the growth-promoting properties would outweigh any toxic effects.

In developing Ae medium, a number of fresh and commercial liver preparations were tested. A commercially available liver concentrate (Sigma No. 202-20) was most consistent in its enhancing ability. According to the manufacturer, the concentrate is produced by making a hot aqueous extract of hog liver and removing the major contaminants other than nucleotides and degradation products by chromatography. Approximate partial assays by the manufacturer are: "CoA, 1–3%; TPN, 5–10%; DPN, 10–20%; plus guanosine, uridine, cystidine, phosphates and other coenzymes."

Eckert (1967), in a modification of medium Ae, utilized a desiccated beef liver extract (Oxoid) in place of the Sigma preparation and also obtained development of *C. punctata* third-stage larvae to the egg-laying or sperm-containing adult.

7. ANTIBIOTICS

In selecting the particular stage of the parasite to be inoculated in a culture system, the problem of separating the nematode from the multitude of microorganisms consistently present in the natural habitat must be given appropriate consideration. In many cases, the stages desired for inoculation in culture are associated with stomach or intestinal contents, or feces. Since the culture medium is highly nutritious, even small numbers of uninhibited microorganisms soon overgrow the culture system to the detriment of the nematodes.

In preparing the nematodes for inoculation, three operations are necessary for removal or suppression of the associated microorganisms and the culturist usually employs all three. The procedures consist of (1) mechanical removal of microorganisms by repeated centrifuging, settling, or utilizing the Baermann process with sterile solutions; (2) exposure to appropriate concentrations of antiseptic solutions not injurious to the nematode, e.g., $HgCl_2$, sodium hypochlorite, merthiolate, or formalin; and (3) incubation in antibiotics prior to inoculation or incorporation of antibiotics in the culture medium or preferably both. It is, of course, necessary to determine beforehand the appropriate time of exposure and concentration of the antiseptics and antibiotics used in a particular system, as these agents can produce adverse effects on nematodes *in vitro* even at low concentrations.

Cultivation from the adult stage of the nematode is particularly difficult because it is necessary to kill or suppress the microorganisms within the complex alimentary canal of the nematode.

The egg stage is generally more amenable to the use of antiseptics and antibiotics for removing associated microorganisms, but it is more difficult to separate and recover the eggs from the feces.

The ideal stage of the gastrointestinal nematode for introduction *in vitro* is the infective third stage, as the larvae are easily recovered from fecal cultures by the Baermann procedure and, due to their relatively simple morphologic composition, more effective use of antiseptics and antibiotics is possible. Once the life cycle, including multiplication, is accomplished *in vitro*, the problem of excluding microbial associates will not be as great and subculturing from any stage will be possible. For the present, however, it is necessary to incorporate antibiotics in medium used for nematode culturing to prevent the destructive overgrowth of undesirable microorganisms. A mixture of antibotics which is active against gram-positive and gram-negative bacteria, yeasts, and fungi is usually employed.

Penicillin, dihydrostreptomycin, and mycostatin are routinely incorporated in Ae medium. When the proper preinoculation procedures are employed, this antibiotic mixture is only rarely inadequate. Consistent contamination usually can be traced to inoculum originating from a particular batch of feces or animal where the contaminant is not sensitive to these antibiotics. It is then necessary to determine, by appropriate antibiotic sensitivity tests, which antibiotic must be added without detrimental effect on the nematodes (Leland, 1969).

8. BALANCED SALT SOLUTIONS

A number of balanced salt solutions (BSS) used for tissue culture have been employed in nematode culturing. All are elaborations of the formulation of Ringer (1895). In nematode culturing a BSS helps perform certain basic functions, such as (1) maintenance of pH of medium within defined limits by providing buffer systems, (2) the bicarbonate–carbon dioxide buffer system of many BSS is also thought to provide the stimulus causing larval exsheathment of some nematode species (Section III,8,*b*), (3) BSS helps maintain osmotic pressure within defined limits, and (4) BSS provides a source of inorganic ions for normal cell metabolism.

In developing Ae medium (Leland, 1959), Earle's BSS was found better than Tyrode's or Hank's BSS as a diluent for the medium components. The superiority of Earle's BSS was evident both in more advanced development of *C. punctata* and in improved medium stability, particularly of its pH. The greater buffer capacity and increased concentration of CO_2 and carbonic acid of Earl's BSS are at least partially responsible for such effects on medium and organism. Furthermore, Earle's BSS is designed for use with a 5% CO_2 gas phase, whereas Tyrode's and Hank's BSS are designed for an air gas phase.

It is generally conceded that NaCl solutions alone are unfavorable to animal tissues and much inferior to balanced salt solutions. The toxic effect of NaCl was observed for the nematode *Haemonchus contortus* (Stoll, 1940). The evidence therefore favors the use of BSS in the medium as well as for preinoculation processing of larvae. In this respect, we have also refrained from using 0.85% NaCl in the Baermann procedure and have used tap water instead.

9. INDICATORS

When color changes create a problem with the basic purpose of an experiment, e.g., as with vital staining procedures or spectrophotometric analysis, use of indicators in a culture system may be contraindicated. Otherwise an acid–base indicator can serve as a valuable monitor of culture conditions. The change in color of phenol red in Ae medium readily indicates the overgrowth of acid-producing contaminants or excessive loss of CO_2 from a faulty culture vessel. In longevity trials where Ae medium is not replaced, the slow accumulation of acid by-products is signaled by the indicator. In tests with *C. punctata*, the inclusion or exclusion of phenol red in Ae medium had no detectable influence on the development of the nematode.

The inclusion of phenol red in BSS, used for suspending, diluting, or extracting various experimental ingredients, is also helpful in predicting the influence of additives on the basal medium. If, for example, the pH of an ingredient to be added differs markedly from the basal medium, adjustment prior to its addition may be desirable to avoid depletion of buffer capacity.

III. Physicochemical Conditions

1. GENERAL REQUIREMENTS FOR CULTIVATION

It is necessary for successful *in vitro* nematode cultivation to provide an environment that is suitable for both the organism and the essential nutrients provided in the medium. A nematode may be capable of surviving at a particular pH, temperature, or redox potential yet the essential nutrients may be in an unavailable or rapidly denaturing form.

In its habitat in the alimentary canal, the parasite is subjected to regular physiologic changes relative both to the feeding habits of the host and the specific location in the gut. In the latter case, certain species apparently depend on these differing conditions in that development to a certain stage occurs at an anterior station of the gut, whereas continued development depends on relocation at a posterior site. The nematode can take up residence at a location along the gut where physicochemical conditions are suitable and essential, yet rapidly degrading nutrients are continually supplied. To provide these conditions *in vitro*, researchers have periodically or continually replaced the medium, made periodic alterations in its composition, and/or adjusted the physicochemical environment of the culture to correspond with conditions normally encountered in the life cycle in the host. Some of the pertinent physicochemical conditions and their relation to *in vitro* culturing are reviewed in the following sections.

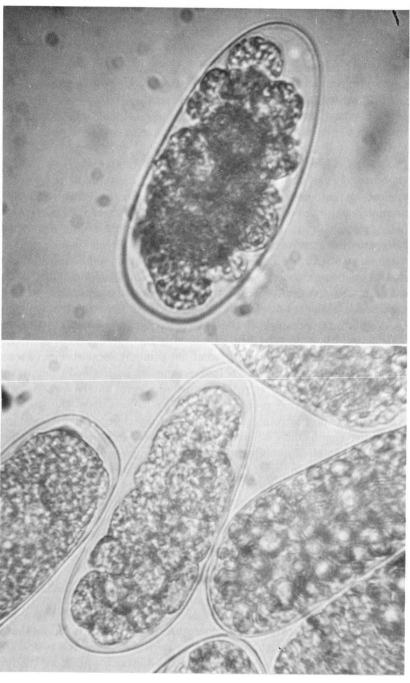

Fig. 7 (*top*). *Cooperia punctata*, egg in 32-cell stage of cleavage produced by female worm grown *in vitro*. × 862.

Fig. 8. (*bottom*). *Hyostrongylus rubidus*, egg in 32-cell stage of cleavage produced by female worm grown *in vitro*. × 862.

cysted larvae to adults which produced progeny *in vitro* (Berntzen, 1965).

With a free-living nematode, Fatt (1967) found that following heat shock in distilled water extra vitamins and salts were needed in culture medium for the organism to reproduce.

A further point concerns optimal temperature for *in vitro* development. The assumption that the internal temperature of the nematode is the same as the body temperature of the host needs verification.

5. HYDROGEN-ION CONCENTRATION

From her review of the literature, Hyman (1951) concluded that parasitic nematodes possessed a wide tolerance to alterations of hydrogen-ion concentration, although some correspondence with that of their natural habitat was evident. Adult Trichostrongyles of sheep endure a pH range of about 4 to 9. *Haemonchus contortus* tolerated a pH range of 3.2 to 9.0 but did not survive better in strongly acid media although its natural environment is highly acid (Davey, 1938). Silverman (1963) also concluded that *in vivo* conditions were not necessarily a guide to *in vitro* requirements of parasites. He observed that *H. contortus* underwent optimal development *in vitro* at pH 6.4 to 6.5, whereas *in vivo* it developed in the gastric mucosa at pH 1.0 to 1.2.

The possibility, as mentioned in Section III,1, that certain essential nutrients or biologic triggering mechanisms are more sensitive in their pH requirements than are the nematodes cannot be ignored. These factors would account for the long survival periods but lack of development of nematodes in certain media. Carrying the point further, the likelihood cannot be dismissed that an alternating pH may be essential to meet all the requirements for development of the nematode.

6. OSMOTIC RELATIONS IN CULTURING

Hyman (1951) considered parasitic nematodes capable of varying the osmotic concentration of their internal fluids in response to that of the external medium but exercising some control over the passage of substances through the body wall. Von Brand (1966) considered nematodes generally more resistant to variations in environmental osmotic concentration than cestodes or acanthocephalads. These observations, however, pertain to ability to survive and do not necessarily relate to requirements for growth and development *in vitro*. As pointed out by Silverman (1963), the maintenance of tonicity by nematodes is an energy process, and differences between the osmotic pressure of the medium and the isosmotic point of a parasite may result in dissipation of reserves that might otherwise be used for growth and development.

Although inorganic ions make a major contribution to osmotic pressure, the other components and conditions of the culture medium are not without some influence. For example, protein molecules in the medium contribute in terms of their number, not size. Furthermore, the osmotic pressure of the culture medium is affected by pH change because the number of anionic and cationic groups in the protein molecule depends on pH. Thus, dialyzable anions and cations are required to balance the charge on the proteins, and an unequal distribution of these ions inside and outside the nematode could conceivably prevail (Donnan effect). The osmotic relationship that exists between the external culture medium and the internal fluids of the nematode are obviously complex, and only conjectural information is available for experimental design.

Considering only the contributions to osmotic pressure made by salts, investigators have approached the problem empirically in the following ways: In designing media both the total concentration and relative proportions of the various salts employed have been based on the composition of vertebrate body fluids (equivalent to 0.85 to 0.90% NaCl). Some workers considered that such a concentration was hypertonic to nematode body fluids and that the ion proportions were probably not suitable for nematode tissues (Rogers, 1945; Hobson, 1948). In this respect, the pseudocoel fluid of ascarids served as a basis (0.38% NaCl plus small amounts of other salts). However, with a salt medium designed to imitate pseudocoel fluid, Baldwin and Moyle (1947) found that nematodes survived no longer than in certain other salt solutions.

In light of the vast array of nutrients that are generally added to a basic salt medium, some thought should be given to the effect of the resulting osmotic conditions on the nematode. It is advisable to test a prospective medium empirically over a wide range of osmotic conditions for each species.

Finally, the optimal osmotic conditions for *in vitro* growth and development may prove to be a compromise between the optimal conditions for nematode survival and integrity of the nutrients.

7. OXIDATION–REDUCTION POTENTIAL

In seeking additional clues to successful growth and development of nematodes *in vitro*, cultivationists have considered the oxidation–reduction (redox) potential of the medium as a possible parameter. Berntzen (1966) found that optimal *in vitro* growth of *T. spiralis* occurred in his medium M126 at a redox potential of +100 to +50 millivolts. The redox potential is a quantitative expression of the tendency of reduced substances to become oxidized and is a measure of intensity and not of the amount of oxidation or reduction of which the system is capable. As used with measurements on complex culture media, the redox potential gives an overall estimate of the numerous oxidation–reduction systems. However, the state of oxidation of all substances is not measurable by methods employing a meter and noble-metal electrode (Hopkins, 1967). Meter measurements provide information concerning certain systems including three which are important to culturing, namely, the glutathione, cysteine, and ascorbic acid systems.

In looking to the redox potential of a particular *in vivo* environment as a guide or starting point, the culturist is again faced with questions similar to those encountered with pH, namely, is the *in vivo* potential necessarily the ideal one for the *in vitro* environment? What are the luminal versus paraluminal potentials?

Hopkins (1967) recommended wary evaluation of redox data concerning media but acknowledged usefulness of measurements of a medium both initially and following the cultivation period. He reasoned that the redox range within which good cultures were obtained could thus be determined empirically.

8. GASEOUS PHASE OF THE CULTURE ENVIRONMENT

A culture system in which a nematode is to be introduced generally consists of three phases: the liquid phase, composed of soluble components (Section II); the solid phase, consisting of particulate matter (Section II,1), cells, or supporting matrix (Section III,3); and the gaseous phase.

a. Oxygen

All parasitic nematodes studied thus far respire aerobically when oxygen is present regardless of whether they lead a predominantly aerobic or anaerobic life *in vivo*. They would, therefore, seem to be facultative aerobes. The oxygen consumption varies with species, stage, age, degree of motility, size (larger parasites have lower metabolic rates than small ones), temperature, hydrogen ion concentration of the medium, and oxygen tension of the environment. Eggs of nematodes of the digestive tract generally do not develop far within the host because of a lack of oxygen and unfavorable temperature.

Oxygen tension also varies at the different *in vivo* locations. Parasites of the respiratory tract and those with access to the blood of the host have available a rich supply of oxygen. The bile ducts and intestinal lumen of the large vertebrates are poor in oxygen content or completely oxygen-free. However, there is significant diffusion of oxygen from the mucosa to the lumen. The oxygen is used rapidly by the microflora of the intestine, resulting in a gradient from the mucosa to the center of the lumen. The existence of such a gradient plus the ability to tolerate absence of oxygen for varying periods of time gives the parasite considerable latitude in satisfying its oxygen requirements. The provision for such a gradient in an *in vitro* system could produce interesting results.

Some nematodes of the alimentary tract possess a hemoglobin with a high affinity for oxygen. Hemoglobin of *Nematodirus*, for example, has a greater affinity than human myoglobin for oxygen (Lee, 1965). Hemoglobin in the body wall of some nematodes not only may serve to store oxygen during periods of anoxia, but also may function in the transfer of oxygen from the environment to their cuticle and, thence, to the body fluid. This situation would account for the manner in which nematodes gather and distribute oxygen in the absence of specialized organs such as gills and circulatory systems.

In culturing *T. spiralis*, Berntzen (1965) obtained the maximal results with a gas phase of 85% N–5% CO_2–10% O_2, whereas multiple molting occurred in over 50% of the adults with 95% air–5% CO_2 with the same medium. The adults were unable to free themselves from their sheaths and no embryos were produced by sheathed females.

The evidence for making oxygen available to nematodes during *in vitro* cultivation is therefore rather convincing.

b. Carbon Dioxide

The extrapolation of information from metabolic experiments suggests that inclusion of CO_2 in the gas phase is desirable also. Carbon dioxide fixation is known to be an important feature of the metabolism of intestinal nematodes such as *Heterakis gallinarum* (Fairbairn, 1954), *Ascaris lumbricoides* (Saz and Vidrine, 1959), and *Trichuris vulpis* (Bueding *et al.*, 1960). Deprivation of CO_2 may retard glycolysis and inhibit glycogenesis. Fairbairn *et al.* (1961) reported that fermentation and glycogen synthesis were effectively inhibited when phosphate was substituted for bicarbonate as buffer, suggesting that CO_2 may be an essential nutrient for the tapeworm, *Hymenolepis diminuta*.

Silverman *et al.* (1966) observed an enhancing effect of CO_2 which was apparently independent of pH change. The number of third-stage larvae converted to fourth stage (*Dictyocaulus viviparus* and *H. contortus*) was also greater when free CO_2 was added as compared to nongassed cultures, even when calculations suggested that the H^+ and HCO_3^- ions were the same in the two test cultures. Maples (1969) found the concentration of CO_2 required for the optimal development of *H. contortus* larvae was dependent on the pH of the medium. At a low pH the optimal pCO_2 was low, and larvae were less sensitive to a range of CO_2 concentrations than at a pH near neutrality. Sommerville (1966) found the greatest number of fourth-stage *H. contortus* in solutions under a 40% CO_2 gas phase after incubation for 72 hours.

Leland (1961, 1963a) recognized the value of CO_2 in his earliest formulation of Ae medium. The medium was gassed with sterile CO_2 until the pH was 7.2 to 7.3 at 38.5°C. and atmospheric exposure was kept at a minimum. During the culturing period, a CO_2 equilibrium between the liquid and gas phases was presumed to develop within the sealed culture tube. By this empirical method, the conversion of *H. contortus* larvae from third to fourth stage in two cultures of 2825 and 3075 worms was 100% in medium Ap (Ap = Ae medium with swine serum substituted for calf serum). Fourth-stage larvae were first observed on day 11 of cultivation. Nearly all the larvae were dead when the cultures were terminated after 39 days (Leland, 1964).

As previously mentioned (Section II,8) CO_2 is a constituent of the CO_2/HCO_3^- buffer system and may provide the stimulus for larval exsheathment of some nematode species (Sommerville, 1964; Silverman and Podger, 1964).

There would seem to be little doubt that the inclusion of CO_2 in culture systems is desirable, although, as in the case of tapeworm cultivation (Hopkins, 1967), its optimal amounts for culturing nematodes are not precisely known.

IV. Some Intrinsic Characteristics of the Nematode in Culture

When a parasitic organism is cultured *in vitro*, it may reveal characteristics that differ in kind or degree from those *in vivo*. Nematodes cultured *in vitro* required a longer period of development than they did *in vivo*, and adults were smaller in size than those obtained *in vivo* (Weinstein and Jones, 1956; Leland, 1961, 1963a, 1967a,b, 1968, 1969).

The morphogenesis may be altered in culture. Douvres and Alicata (1962) observed that the development of the germinal primordium lagged behind somatic differentiation in cultured *C. punctata*.

The inoculation of Trichostrongyle nematodes in culture does not result in the simultaneous development of all individuals to the next stage. If *C. punctata* third-stage larvae are inoculated in Ae medium, egg-laying adults are observed as early as 21 days. However, active third- and fourth-stage larvae are also present. This is also the case with cultures of several months' duration. One might speculate that the presence of a certain number of adults in the culture may inhibit further development of third- and fourth-stage larvae. This phenomenon apparently has its parallel in cell culture and *in vivo*. Osgood (1957) postulated that cells have an inhibitory effect on one another in culture. When mature cells are present they inhibit multiplication of immature cells, but if the mature cells are removed, multiplication occurs. Michel (1963) observed that if adult Ostertagia were present in the abomasal

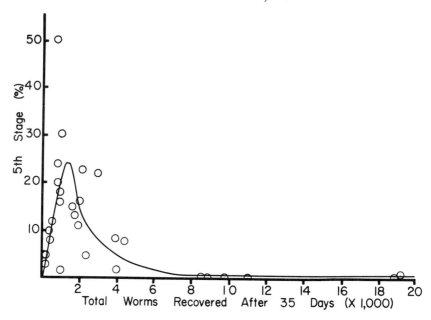

Fig. 9. Within a given set of culture conditions, i.e., amount of medium, size of culture vessel, and so forth, there exists an optimal population at which fifth-stage *C. punctata* are most efficiently produced. This phenomenon has its counterpart *in vivo* in the so-called "crowding effect."

lumen, the fourth-stage larvae buried in the mucosa did not migrate to the lumen and develop to adults until the existing adults were removed.

There appears to be limited but detectable cannibalistic and predatory activity (Fig. 6) by some nematode species in culture (Leland, 1963a).

It is not known whether all the above characteristics are limited to *in vitro* culture. The culturing process may facilitate detection or may actually intensify an *in vivo* characteristic. The so-called "crowding effect" seen *in vivo*, where overpopulation of worms within an organ retards nematode development or acts antihelmintically, can be demonstrated *in vitro* (Fig. 9).

V. Summary and Conclusions

Progress in cultivating some nematodes of domestic animals has shown that it is possible to produce realistic numbers of the parasitic stages *in vitro*. Successful cultivation can now be measured in terms of growth and development rather than simple survival. Media are complex and require preparation procedures which are similar in sophistication to the procedures used in tissue culture. The components of Ae medium are discussed in terms of selection and ability to support nematode growth and development *in vitro*. The essential physicochemical conditions and their relation to *in vitro* culturing are reviewed. The conditions necessary for successful cultivation appear to consist of an environment suitable both for the organism and for the essential nutrients in the medium.

Although the practical production of these organisms through several generations *in vitro* has not been achieved, the question now appears not to be whether, but how soon this will also be accomplished. The progress in cultivation has been essentially the result of empirical experimentation. Logically, the direction of research should now shift to qualitative and quantitative determinations of essential nutrients and optimal physicochemical conditions.

A practical cultivation procedure will not, in itself, solve all problems associated with a disease condition, but, when judiciously used in conjunction with other established procedures, it should provide the parasitologist a valuable new approach to the host–parasite relationship. It will be necessary for the parasitologist to proceed cautiously with any extrapolations of observations obtained *in vitro* to situations *in vivo*. The need for caution in relating *in vitro* and *in vivo* organismic behavior is evident from the experience of bacteriologists and virologists who have considerable experience in cultivating their parasites *in vitro*. In considering the disease condition or host–parasite relationship, it will be necessary to use *in vitro* procedures in conjunction with *in vivo* methods.

The results obtained from *in vitro* cultivation will provide answers to many, but not all, long-standing questions; and, perhaps of equal value, a basis has been provided for formulating new and more searching questions. In any event, the efforts sown in developing cultivation procedures should reap a harvest of valuable information which will have an influence on many facets of parasitology.

Appendix

Recently, Zimmerman and Leland (1969) announced the *in vitro* cultivation of *C. punctata* from third-stage larvae to adults which produced eggs that hatched and developed to second-stage larvae. Thus the production of fertile eggs, hatching, and multiplication have all been accomplished *in vitro* for this species.

REFERENCES

Baker, J. A., and Ferguson, M. S. (1942). *Growth of platyfish (Platypoecilus maculatus)* free from bacteria and other microorganisms. *Proceedings of the Society for Experimental Biology and Medicine* **51**, 116–119.

Baldwin, E., and Moyle, V. (1947). An isolated nerve-muscle preparation from Ascaris. *Journal of Experimental Biology* **23**, 277–299.

Berntzen, A. K. (1965). Comparative growth and development of *Trichinella spiralis* in vitro and in vivo, with a redescription of the life cycle. *Experimental Parasitology* **16**, 74–106.

Berntzen, A. K. (1966). A controlled culture environment for axenic growth of parasites. *Annals of the New York Academy of Sciences* **139**, 176–189.

Berntzen, A. K., and Mueller, J. F. (1964). *In vitro* cultivation of *Spirometra mansonoides* (Cestoda) from procercoid to the early adult. *Journal of Parasitology* **50**, 705–711.

Block, R. J., and Bolling, D. (1945). "The Amino Acid Composition of Proteins and Foods. Analytical Methods and Results." Thomas, Springfield, Illinois.

Bueding, E., Kmetec, E., Swartzwelder, C., Abadie, S., and Saz, H. J. (1960). Biochemical effects of dithiazanine in the canine whipworm, *Trichuris vulpis*. *Biochemical Pharmacology* **5**, 311–322.

Davey, D. G. (1938). Studies on the physiology of the nematodes of the alimentary canal of sheep. *Parasitology* **30**, 278–295.

Diamond, L. S., and Douvres, F. W. (1962). Bacteria-free cultivation of some parasitic stages of the swine nematodes *Hyostrongylus rubidus* and *Oesophagostomum quadrispinulatum* (*O. longicaudum*). *Journal of Parasitology* **48**, 39–42.

Dougherty, E. C. (1953). Problems of nomenclature for the growth of organisms of one species with and without associated organisms of other species. *Parasitology* **42**, 259–261.

Dougherty, E. C. (1959). Introduction to axenic culture of invertebrate metazoa: A goal. *Annals of the New York Academy of Sciences* **77**, 27–54.

Douvres, F. W. (1960). Influence of intestinal extracts and sera from cattle infected with *Oesophagostomum radiatum* on the *in vitro* cultivation of this nematode: Preliminary report. *Journal of Parasitology* **46**, Suppl., 25–26.

Douvres, F. W. (1962a). The *in vitro* cultivation of *Oesophagostomum radiatum*, the nodular worm of cattle. I. Development in vitamin-supplemented and non-supplemented media. *Journal of Parasitology* **48**, 314–320.

Douvres, F. W. (1962b). The use of infective larvae and *in vitro*-grown parasitic larvae of *Cooperia punctata* to detect antibodies in serum of a calf infected with this nematode. *Journal of Parasitology* **48**, Suppl., 15.

Douvres, F. W. (1966). *In vitro* growth of *Oesophagostomum dentatum* (Nematoda Strongyloidea) from third-stage larvae to adults with observations on inhibited larvae development. *Journal of Parasitology* **52**, 1033–1034.

Douvres, F. W., and Alicata, J. E. (1962). Development *in vitro* of the parasitic stages of *Cooperia punctata*, an intestinal nematode of cattle. *Journal of Parasitology* **48**, Suppl., 35.

Douvres, F. W., Tromba, F. G., and Doran, D. J. (1966). The influence of NCTC 109, serum, and swine kidney cell cultures on the morphogenesis of *Stephanurus dentatus* to fourth stage, *in vitro*. *Journal of Parasitology* **52**, 875–889.

Eckert, J. (1967). *In vitro*—Entwicklung invasionsfahiger nematoden—Larven zu parasitischen Stadien. *Zeitschrift fur Parasitenkunde* **29**, 242–274.

Fairbairn, D. (1954). The metabolism of *Heterakis gallinae*. II. Carbon dioxide fixation. *Experimental Parasitology* **3**, 52–63.

Fairbairn, D., Wertheim, G., Harpur, R. P., and Schiller, E. L. (1961). Biochemistry of normal and irradiated strains of *Hymenolepis diminuta*. *Experimental Parasitology* **11**, 248–263.

Fatt, H. V. (1967). Nutritional requirements for reproduction of a temperature sensitive nematode, reared in axenic culture. *Proceedings of the Society for Experimental Biology and Medicine* **124**, 897–903.

Foster, A. O. (1942). Internal parasites of horses and mules. *In* "Keeping Livestock Healthy," 1942 Yearbook of Agriculture (A. Stefferud, ed.), pp. 459–475. United States Department of Agriculture, Washington, D.C.

Haurowitz, F. (1950). "Chemistry and Biology of Proteins," p. 32. Academic Press, New York.

Hobson, A. D. (1948). The physiology and cultivation in artificial media of nematodes parasitic in the alimentary tract of animals. *Parasitology* **38**, 183–227.

Hopkins, C. A. (1967). The *in vitro* cultivation of cestodes with particular reference to *Hymenolepis nana*. *In* "Problems of In Vitro Culture" (A. E. Taylor, ed.), Vol. 5, pp. 27–47. Blackwell, Oxford.

Hyman, L. H. (1951). *In* "The Invertebrates: Acanthocephala, Aschelminthes, and Entoprocta. The pseudocoelomate Bilateria," Vol. III, pp. 389–439. McGraw-Hill, New York.

Lapage, G. (1935). The behaviour of sterilized exsheathed infective trichostrongylid larvae in sterile media resembling their environment in ovine hosts. *Journal of Helminthology* **13**, 115–128.

Lee, D. L. (1965). "The Physiology of Nematodes," pp. 56–59. Freeman, San Francisco, California.

Leland, S. E., Jr. (1959). Unpublished data.

Leland, S. E., Jr. (1961). The *in vitro* cultivation of the parasitic stages of *Cooperia punctata, Cooperia oncophora, Ostertagia ostertagi, Ostertagia circumcincta*: A preliminary report. *Journal of Parasitology* **47**, Suppl., 21.

Leland, S. E., Jr. (1962). The *in vitro* cultivation of *Cooperia punctata* from egg to egg. *Journal of Parasitology* **48**, Suppl., 35.

Leland, S. E., Jr. (1963a). Studies on the *in vitro* growth of parasitic nematodes. I. Complete or partial parasitic development of some gastro-intestinal nematodes of sheep and cattle. *Journal of Parasitology* **49**, 600–611.

Leland, S. E., Jr. (1963b). *In vitro* cultivation of fourth and fifth stages of the swine nodular worm *Oesophagostomum quadrispinulatum*. *Journal of Parasitology* **49**, Suppl., 58–59.

Leland, S. E., Jr. (1964). Unpublished data.

Leland, S. E., Jr. (1965a). *Cooperia pectinata. In vitro* cultivation of the parasitic stages including egg production: A preliminary report. *Journal of Parasitology* **51**, Suppl., 46.

Leland, S. E., Jr. (1965b). *Hyostrongylus rubidus. In vitro* cultivation of the parasitic stages including the production and development of eggs through five cleavages: A preliminary report. *Journal of Parasitology* **51**, Suppl., 47.

Leland, S. E., Jr. (1965c). *Oesophagostomum quadrispinulatum. In vitro* cultivation of parasitic adults including the formation of spermatogonia and oogonia. *Journal of Parasitology* **51**, Suppl., 47.

Leland, S. E., Jr. (1967a). Cultivation of *Cooperia pectinata in vitro* including egg production. *Journal of Parasitology* **53**, 630–633.

Leland, S. E., Jr. (1967b). The *in vitro* cultivation of *Cooperia punctata* from egg to egg. *Journal of Parasitology* **53**, 1057–1060.

Leland, S. E., Jr. (1968). *In vitro* egg production of *Cooperia oncophora*. *Journal of Parasitology* **54**, 136.

Leland, S. E., Jr. (1969). Cultivation of the parasitic stages of *Hyostrongylus rubidus in vitro,* including the production of sperm and development of eggs through five cleavages. *Transactions of the American Microscopical Society* **88**, 246–252.

Leland, S. E., Jr., Drudge, J. H., Wyant, Z. N., and Elam, G. W. (1961). VII. Some quantitative and pathologic aspects of natural and experimental infections of the horse. *American Journal of Veterinary Research* **22**, 128–138.

Maples, C. J. (1969). The development of *Haemonchus contortus in vitro.* I. The effect of pH and pCO₂ on the rate of development to the fourth-stage larva. *Parasitology* **59**, 215–231.

Michel, J. F. (1963). The phenomena of host resistance and the course of infection of *Ostertagia ostertagi* in calves. *Parasitology* **53**, 63–84.

Osgood, E. E. (1957). Observations on human leukemic cells in culture. *In* "The Leukemias: Etiology, Pathophysiology, and Treatment" (J. W. Rebuck, F. H. Bethell, and R. W. Monto, eds.), p. 277. Academic Press, New York.

Otto, G. F. (1939). The reaction between hookworm *Ancylostoma canium,* larvae and immune serum. *Journal of Parasitology* **25**, Suppl., 29.

Ringer, S. (1895). Further observations regarding the antagonism between calcium salts and sodium potassium and ammonia salts. *Journal of Physiology (London)* **18**, 425.

Rogers, W. (1945). Studies on the nature and properties of the perienteric fluid of ascaris. *Parasitology* **36**, 211–218.

Sarles, M. P. (1938). The *in vitro* action of immune rat serum on the nematode *Nippostrongylus muris* in the rat. *Journal of Infectious Diseases* **65**, 183–195.

Saz, H. J., and Vidrine, A. (1959). The mechanism of formation of succinate and propionate by *Ascaris lumbricoides* muscle. *Journal of Biological Chemistry* **234**, 2001–2005.

Silverman, P. H. (1959). *In vitro* cultivation of the histotrophic stages of *Haemonchus contortus* and Ostertagia *spp. Nature* **183**, 197.

Silverman, P. H. (1963). *In vitro* cultivation and serological techniques in parasitology. *In* "Techniques in Parasitology" (A. E. Taylor, ed.), Vol. 1, pp. 45–67. Blackwell, Oxford.

Silverman, P. H. (1965). *In vitro* cultivation procedures for parasitic helminths. *In* "Advances in Parasitology" (B. Dawes, ed.), Vol. 3, pp. 159–222. Academic Press, New York.

Silverman, P. H., Alger, N. E., and Hansen, E. L. (1966). Axenic helminth cultures and their use for the production of antiparasitic vaccines. *Annals of the New York Academy of Sciences* **139**, 124–142.

Silverman, P. H., and Podger, K. R. (1964). *In vitro* exsheathment of some nematode infective larvae. *Experimental Parasitology* **15**, 314–324.

Slonka, G. F., and Leland, S. E., Jr. (1969). *In vitro* cultivation of *Ancylostoma tubaeforme* from egg to fourth stage and maintenance of adults. *Journal of Parasitology* **55**, Suppl., 65.

Sommerville, R. I. (1964). Effect of carbon dioxide on the development of third stage larvae of *Haemonchus contortus in vitro. Nature* **202**, 316–317.

Sommerville, R. I. (1966). The development of *Haemonchus contortus* to the fourth stage *in vitro. Journal of Parasitology* **52**, 127–136.

Stoll, N. R. (1940). *In vitro* conditions favoring ecdysis at the end of the first parasitic stage of *Haemonchus contortus* (Nematoda). *Growth* **4**, No. 4, 383–406.

Stoll, N. R. (1959). Conditions favoring the axenic culture of *Neoaplectana glaseri,* a nematode parasite of certain insect grubs. *Annals of the New York Academy of Sciences* **77**, 126–136.

Taylor, A. E. R., and Baker, J. R. (1968). "The Cultivation of Parasites *In Vitro*." Blackwell, Oxford.

von Brand, T. (1966). "Biochemistry of Parasites," p. 26. Academic Press, New York.

Weinstein, P. P. (1953). The cultivation of the free-living stages of hookworms in the absence of living bacteria. *American Journal of Hygiene* **58**, 352–376.

Weinstein, P. P., and Jones, M. F. (1956). The *in vitro* cultivation of *Nippostrongylus muris* to the adult stage. *Journal of Parasitology* **42**, 215–236.

Weinstein, P. P., and Jones, M. F. (1957). The development of a study on the axenic growth *in vitro* of *Nippostrongylus muris* to the adult stage. *American Journal of Tropical Medicine and Hygiene* **6**, 480–484.

Weinstein, P. P., and Jones, M. F. (1959). Development *in vitro* of some parasitic nematodes of vertebrates. *Annals of the New York Academy of Sciences* **77**, 137–162.

Weller, T. (1943). Development of the larvae of *Trichinella spiralis* in roller tube tissue cultures. *American Journal of Pathology* **19**, 503–515.

Yasuraoka, K., and Weinstein, P. P. (1969). Effects of temperature on the development of eggs of *Nematospiroides dubius* under axenic conditions relative to *in vitro* cultivation. *Journal of Parasitology* **55**, 44–50.

Zimmerman, G. L., and Leland, S. E., Jr. (1969). *In vitro* cultivation of *Cooperia punctata* from third-stage larvae to adults which produced eggs that hatched and developed to second-stage larvae. *Journal of Parasitology* **55**, Suppl., 65.

Use of Serum Enzymes as Aids to Diagnosis

RICHARD A. FREEDLAND* AND JOHN W. KRAMER†

*Department of Physiological Sciences, School of Veterinary Medicine,
University of California, Davis, California*

I. Introduction

Clinical enzymology has expanded considerably since serum alkaline phosphatase was first recognized as being of diagnostic significance in the 1920's. Now, many more serum enzymes are known to have a significant

* Professor of Physiological Chemistry.
† Postdoctoral Trainee in Clinical Pathology, Supported by USPHS Grant GM633.

relationship to specific disorders in both human and veterinary medicine. Although a number of the enzymes to be discussed here are not in common use now, it is our purposes to familiarize the reader with the broad potential of enzymes in clinical medicine and experimental biology. The techniques required for determining activities of certain enzymes are expensive and complicated and, thus, may be carried out only in laboratories associated with institutional clinics and research. However, as the demand for them has become greater, some techniques have been modified to lessen their expense and complexity and to give a reasonable estimate of enzymic activity for clinical purposes. There appears little doubt that this demand will continue, and as the clinical veterinarian and researcher become more familiar with the potential of serum enzyme profiles in monitoring degenerative process, they will put them to greater use.

It is apparent that with the large mass of pertinent information both from work in human medicine and veterinary medicine, particularly from domestic animals in their conventional environments, and from experimental animals, that a somewhat selective and critical evaluation of investigations as well as discussions related to methodology, causes of enzyme release, importance of the rate of removal of enzymes, and uses of enzymic measurements of cerebral spinal fluids as well as in blood, will be desirable and helpful. This will be the objective of our presentation.

The greatest value in using the enzymes as diagnostic aids is in the specificities of their activities and presence in various tissues. There is considerable information on these specificities in man, and a growing body of knowledge from many domestic animals. During necrosis or degeneration of any given organ, only those enzymes contained within the organ can be released. It has generally been shown that the enzymes with the highest activity in a given tissue appear to leak from them to the greatest extent, although this is not always the case. There are several complicating factors in enzyme leakage with which we will deal in the section on mechanism of release and on importance of subcellular localization.

In general, elucidation of enzyme tissue specificity and, recently, the growing knowledge and use of isoenzymes, has enabled the clinician to obtain various profiles of serum or plasma enzymes which may be indicative of certain diseases. The term "enzyme profile" refers to the activities, particularly the changes in activities, of several enzymes in serum or plasma. Information on these changes is particularly important in cases where the enzymes occur in more than one tissue or organ. An increase in a given 4 of a certain 7 enzymes, for example, may be fairly indicative of damage to only a single tissue which has relatively high content of these 4 enzymes and a lower quantity of the other 3 enzymes that can be detected and measured.

1. NOMENCLATURE

As in any field, enzymology has a vocabulary of its own. However, nomenclature can become confusing and varied. Confusion has occurred in the use of differing nomenclatures by clinically oriented enzymologists and strictly research-oriented enzymologists. We will use the terminology that is most often used in clinical work. However, we think it will be worthwhile for the reader to understand why and where some major difficulties may occur, particularly so that he can be prepared to read literature with nomenclature somewhat different from that to which he has become accustomed.

An International Commission on enzymic nomenclature was formed by the International Union of Biochemistry in an attempt to categorize, catalogue, and systematize the nomenclature of various enzymes. Enzymes have been named generally for the reactions that they catalyze. However, the International Union of Biochemistry felt that a more systematic method of categorizing the enzymes in general classes would be useful, e.g., lactic dehydrogenase (LDH) is the name commonly used clinically for the particular enzyme that catalyzes the dehydrogenation of lactic acid to form pyruvic acid. It catalyzes the reaction in a reversible fashion; thus, it can convert lactic acid to pyruvic acid as well as pyruvic acid to lactic acid. In each of these reactions, a coenzyme is required which accepts hydrogen, in the case of the conversion of lactate to pyruvate, and donates hydrogen, in the case of the conversion of pyruvate to lactate as depicted in the following equation:

$$\text{Lactic acid} + \text{NAD} \rightleftharpoons \text{pyruvic acid} + \text{NADH} + \text{H}^+$$

The International Union of Biochemistry has preferred to call all such reversible dehydrogenases "oxidoreductases," since they can oxidize or reduce their respective substrates. Therefore, the official name is L-lactate: NAD-oxidoreductase, thus indicating that the substrates are lactate and NAD in the direction of oxidation. In much of the literature, the designation NAD (nicotinamide adenine-dinucleotide) will be substituted by the older term DPN (diphosphopyridine nucleotide), a term which is still used by research workers and by clinical investigators.

Much of the International Commission's work to standardize nomenclature as well as methods of reporting activity has been extremely worthwhile. However, the Commission has completely ignored the approach to clinical enzymology in several instances. This problem will be apparent later in this review, in dealing with two enzymes that are widely used in diagnostic work, namely, glutamic-pyruvic transaminase (GPT) and glutamic-oxaloacetic transaminase (GOT). We feel GPT and GOT were adequately descriptive of these enzymes, since there is a transamination between glutamic acid and pyruvic acid to form alanine and α-keto-glutarate according to the following formula (a), and the same for GOT in formula (b):

$$\text{(a)} \quad \text{Glutamic acid} + \text{pyruvic acid} \xrightleftharpoons{\text{(GPT)}} \alpha\text{-ketoglutarate} + \text{alanine}$$

$$\text{(b)} \quad \text{Glutamic acid} + \text{oxaloacetic acid} \xrightleftharpoons{\text{(GOT)}} \alpha\text{-ketoglutarate} + \text{aspartate}$$

Two names used for GPT and GOT are incorrect even from a technical viewpoint: GPT and GOT have been called glutamic-alanine transaminase and glutamic-aspartic transaminase, in both cases by research biochemists rather than clinical enzymologists. Both terms appear to be incorrect and unacceptable, since glutamic acid and alanine will not transaminate as there is no acceptor. Neither alanine nor glutamic acid has a keto group to accept the amino group. In order to clear up such confusions as will arise from the use of the term glutamic-alanine transaminase, the International Commission felt that it would be desirable to call both of these enzymes, aminotransferases, as they are indeed. They catalyze transfer of the amino group from one carbon skeleton to the other. However, the Commission's choice was a rather unfortunate one for the clinical enzymologist, since the official names designated by the International Union of Biochemistry for these two enzymes are now alanine amino transferase and aspartic amino transferase, with the understanding that, in both cases, α-ketoglutarate is the acceptor of the amino group. This situation immediately leads to the problem of the abbreviations for these clinically important enzymes. The abbreviation for both is AAT instead of GOT and GPT. Hence, we feel that the clinical enzymologist should continue to use GPT and GOT, although they are unacceptable names according to the International Union of Biochemistry Nomenclature Committee. We will continue to use the terms GPT and GOT in our work in clinical enzymology, since we believe that they are here to stay. Those terms which we feel are most common in this field will be used in this review so as to acquaint the reader with the terms he is most likely to see rather than those that may be preferable to the research biochemist.

2. Methods of Reporting Results

Obviously, if investigators and clinicians are to communiate effectively, their various definitions for units as well as terms must be easily convertible by those in different laboratories. If every laboratory group were to make up its own definitions for units of activity no other laboratory could be sure that any given value were indicative of normal or elevated activity of enzymes. Hence, we feel that the International Union of Biochemistry Committee on Nomenclature has made a definite and substantial contribution to clinical enzymology. The recommendation is that a unit of activity be defined as that quantity of enzyme that will cause the conversion of a μmole (micromole) of substrate or the production of a μmole of product per minute. This unit is referred to as an International Unit (IU), and as international units per milliliter or international units per liter or per 100 milliliters. The use of this unit will allow the conversion of activity with any corresponding activity anywhere in the world, and thus considerably reduce the prevailing confusion in this field. For example, there are 7 different designations of units for acid or alkaline phosphatase. It would be much simpler if everyone were to accept the use of International Units, since it appears to be the inevitable result. Delay will magnify the effort required to translate unitages from the accumulated literature.

Zimmerman *et al.* (1965) have reported, in international units, values for 8 serum enzymes in 21 species (Table I). In this review we discuss changes in levels on the basis of relative rather than absolute values so that there is no need to convert the different units used in the original publications.

3. Determination of Enzymic Activity

In general, enzymic activity is measured by incubating the enzyme with its substrate in a buffer solution and measuring the amount of product formed. In many cases this necessitates the stopping of the reaction usually with either acid, base, or some organic reagent, and then colormetrically estimating the amount of product formed. In other cases, it is feasible to measure the activity of the enzyme continuously over a short period of time. This is particularly true when either the substrate or the product is a chromaphore (i.e., absorbs light). This light absorption can occur in the visible range, near ultraviolet, or the ultraviolet itself. However, most of the reactions that are of importance to clinical enzymology have chromaphores or products which can be reacted to form a chromaphore which absorb between 340 and 700 mμ. Therefore, it is advantageous to have a spectrophotometer that has the flexibility of reading at any wavelength between these limits, and it is particularly important to make sure the instrument can read absorbancies at 340 mμ. The reason for this will become apparent shortly.

4. Sensitivity

To illustrate the specificity and sensitivity of enzymic methods, an example of lactic dehydrogenase may be used. If there is released approxi-

TABLE I.[a] MEAN[b] LEVELS OF 8 SERUM ENZYMES IN 22 ANIMAL SPECIES

Species	No.[c] of animals	GOT Karmen method	GOT Reitman-Frankel method	GPT Karmen method	GPT Reitman-Frankel method	Lactate dehydrogenase (LD)	Aldolase (ALD)	Phosphohexoisomerase (PHI)	Malic dehydrogenase (MD)	Isocitric dehydrogenase (ICD)	Glutathione reductase (GR)
Man	100 (S)	9 ± 3	11 ± 4	7 ± 3	10 ± 4	58 ± 16	2.0 ± 0.9	63 ± 16	43 ± 16	5.2 ± 2.4	52.0 ± 12
Monkey	3 (S)	12	11	11	12	111	8.7	349	85	22.0	74.4
Range[b]		(10-13)	(2-20)	(4-18)	(8-15)	(107-115)	(5.5-13.0)	(218-480)	(41-128)	(8.5-35.0)	(62.4-86.8)
Dog	24 (S)	9 ± 2 (6)[c]	15 ± 3	11 ± 4 (6)[c]	10 ± 2	38 ± 8	15.3 ± 2.8	151 ± 72 (7)[c]	126 ± 66 (7)[c]	10.0 (3)[c]	8.2 ± 5 (5)[c]
Range[b]										(9.0-11.0)	
Ferret	9 (S)	46 ± 9	—	14 ± 3	—	109 ± 22	32.8 ± 11.8	486 ± 93	405 ± 129	33.5 ± 7.9	20.0 ± 7.4
Cat	10 (S)	13 ± 2	23 ± 1	12 ± 8	18 ± 6	95 ± 45	11.9 ± 4.0	498 ± 154	125 ± 55	9.7 ± 2.7	11.8 ± 5.7
Rat	18 (P)	52 ± 18	26 ± 6	7 ± 2	7 ± 2	105 ± 28	9.5 ± 2.1	126 ± 35	113 ± 35	13.0 ± 11.0	5.2 ± 5.0
Mouse	5 (P)	29 ± 5	23 ± 8	9 ± 3	2 ± 1	195 ± 22	18.2 ± 3.9	209 ± 88	320 ± 50	20.0 (3)[c]	19.6 ± 11.3
Range[b]										(10.0-35.0)	
Guinea pig	10 (P)	23 ± 8	24 ± 10	13 ± 2	10 ± 2	38 ± 6	9.3 ± 1.5	750 ± 37	416 ± 151	94.0 ± 54.0	7.7 ± 3.1
Hamster	40 (P)	39 ± 14 (5)[b]	49 ± 14	13 ± 5 (5)[b]	30 ± 8	78 ± 22	31.5 ± 8.2	981 ± 292	830 ± 157	41.0 ± 27.0	52.0 ± 38.0
Rabbit	21 (P)	16 ± 6	8 ± 6	14 ± 4	11 ± 2	116 ± 57	23.9 ± 8.7	361 ± 182	310 ± 153	91.0 ± 30.0	31.0 ± 18.0
Pig	24 (S)	30 (2)[c]	46 ± 18	24 (2)[c]	25 ± 7	199 ± 46	54.8 ± 20.2	738 ± 367	521 ± 162	17.2 ± 7.1	22.1 ± 5.5
Range[b]		(25, 35)		(13, 36)							
Cow	100 (S)	33 ± 8	55 ± 12	19 ± 3	15 ± 6	473 ± 97	28.2 ± 7.4	487 ± 130	524 ± 170	64.0 ± 17.0	79.0 ± 33.0
Sheep	45 (S)	35 ± 21 (5)[c]	62 ± 28	8 ± 3 (5)[c]	9 ± 2	302 ± 58	23.1 ± 15.8	358 ± 119	340 ± 146	13.0 ± 5.6	18.6 ± 3.5
Goat	4 (S)	21	19	5	5	176	8.0	389	194	25.0	10.7
Range[b]		(15-29)	(17-20)	(Single value)	(4-6)	(133-198)	(2.2-16.4)	(261-640)	(150-290)	(Single value)	(6.7-19.7)
Horse	17 (S)	62 ± 21	97 ± 21	5 ± 1	6 ± 4	148 ± 58	13.4 ± 5.3	213 ± 109	280 ± 101	30.6 ± 11.2	94.0 ± 35.5
Goose	10 (S)	13 ± 5	24 ± 12	5 ± 2	10 ± 5	118 ± 25	11.9 ± 6.6	188 ± 98	2863 ± 479	25.3 ± 17.4	NDA[d]
Duck	7 (S)	21 ± 16	35 ± 19	6 ± 2	16 ± 4	159 ± 74	16.7 ± 12.5	352 ± 106	283 ± 91	30.0 ± 14.0	NDA[d]
Chicken	11 (S)	48 ± 13	91 ± 30	8 (2)[c]	8 ± 2	133 ± 30	12.9 ± 3.7	1012 ± 161	240 ± 54	18.7 ± 7.7	NDA[d]
Pigeon	10 (S)	49 ± 18	69 ± 13	15 ± 12	5 ± 5	148 ± 18	9.6 ± 5.5	235 ± 100	3018 ± 1110	15.4 ± 5.7	NDA[d]
Snake	3 (P)	15	9	12	NDA[d]	57	7.7	141	144	NDA[d]	NDA[d]
Range[b]		(10-25)	(2-15)	(4-20)		(26-87)	(0.2-13.3)	(70-212)	(50-238)		
Alligator	6 (S)	56 ± 11	84 ± 35	6 ± 2	7 ± 3	45 ± 18	2.2 ± 2.4	228 ± 107	231 ± 77	6.1 ± 5.6	8.5 ± 4.4
Carp	5 (S)	52 ± 20	—	8 ± 4	8 ± 4	137 ± 44	78.9 ± 10.8	762 ± 307	1318 ± 241	24.4 ± 6.7	11.5 ± 1.1

[a] From Zimmerman et al. (1965).

[b] Mean values and standard deviation are given for levels derived from serum (S) or plasma (P) samples of 5 or more animals. Values derived from less than 5 animals are shown as the average, and the range is indicated in the line below the value. Values expressed in International Units per liter.

[c] For the values derived from fewer animals than the number indicated in the second column, the number on which the particular value was based is shown in parentheses after the mean value.

[d] No demonstrable activity.

mately 0.10 mg. of this enzyme per 100 ml. blood, it would be almost impossible to measure the quantity by any normal protein method. Because the normal background content of serum protein is approximately 5 g./100 ml. plasma, i.e., 5000 mg., a change of 0.10 mg. in 5000 mg. would be difficult to detect. However, since the protein for which we are looking has enzymic specificity, its measurement can be accomplished with little difficulty, e.g., if the usual 3 ml. cuvette is used for assay, and the change in absorbance at 340 mμ due to the utilization of DPNH is measured with 0.10 ml. of serum per 3 ml. cuvette, a change in OD of 0.083 per minute can be observed. The change in density is the same as a change of 0.83 in 10 minutes. Such a large change in absorbance would be easy to estimate with reasonable accuracy, whereas, as observed before, it would be most difficult to estimate the degree of increase for this particular protein in the presence of all other serum proteins. In fact, we can appreciate the sensitivity of the method by considering that, even if no protein were present in the serum, it would be rather difficult to measure 0.10 mg. protein per 100 ml. by most standard techniques for measuring concentrations. This situation illustrates the sensitivity of a given enzymic activity for estimation of its concentration in serum rather than requiring determination by chemical methods.

5. TEMPERATURE

Most measurements that consist of continual readings over short periods of time are usually conducted at 25°C., or in many cases at room temperature which is conventionally near 22°C. Measurements of many enzymic activities, where the reaction is stopped and the amount of product estimated, are conducted around 37°C., although both of these types of determinations can easily be made at 25°C. or room temperature. Of prime importance when reporting results is the indication of temperature at which the reaction was conducted since, in many of the enzymic reaction examinations for clinical medical purposes, there is about a twofold increase in activity with a temperature rise from 25° to 37°C.

6. SUBSTRATE

One of the difficulties in correlating results among laboratories, besides that of the various units of measurement, arises from the use of different substrates, e.g., an alkaline phosphatase determination can be conducted by measuring the hydrolysis of α-glycerol phosphate and then by estimating the quantity of inorganic phosphate released. Another method of estimation uses p-nitrophenol phosphate. The latter method has the advantage that, on the removal of the phosphate group, p-nitrophenol particularly at the basic pH values used in the alkaline phosphatase determination is a chromophore absorbing strongly at 400 to 410 mμ. The problem in these determinations arises from the fact that alkaline phosphatases do not split α-glycerol phosphate and p-nitrophenol phosphate at the same rate. Therefore, even when using international units, two laboratories measuring samples of exactly the same degree of activity would be reporting quite different results depending on the choice of substrate.

7. KINETICS

The kinetics of the reaction must approximate zero order to obtain accurate results. Zero-order kinetics in this context simply means that the amount of product formed or substrate utilized over the period examined is directly proportional to time and concentration of enzyme. Thus, when the amount of enzyme is doubled, tripled, or increased tenfold the same rise in activity should be observed. This is not quite as critical in some clinical work since a marked elevation, without having an absolute value, may tell one what he wants to know, i.e., the clinician's interest is often really not whether a given enzyme has increased 40-fold or 80-fold, because, in any event, the lesion is pinpointed and may be considered serious. However, in many cases, particularly with enzymes that have equilibriums of approximately one, such as the transaminases, it is imperative that the kinetics be checked to a reasonable degree. The fact that a reaction has an equilibrium of one means that there will be equal quantities of each of the products at equilibrium, e.g., if one puts into the glutamic-pyruvic transaminase (GPT) system, equal quantities of alanine and α-ketoglutarate, at equilibrium the pyruvate and alanine concentrations will be equal and the α-ketoglutarate and glutamic acid concentrations will be equal. Therefore, if the reaction were too rapid, the best one could hope to obtain would be an equilibrium. This equilibriation may occur within 3 minutes, although the reaction may proceed for 15 minutes. If this were to happen one would estimate the enzymic activity at only 20% of its actual potential. In cases where one is attempting to estimate the severity of damage by the estimated activity of enzyme in the serum, this underestimation can be a complicating factor. In most cases, it is suggested by those presenting methods which require end-point determinations that the enzyme should be diluted tenfold and examined a second time where the activity exceeds a certain value.

As stated previously, many enzymes can be measured directly and continuously by the formation or removal of a chromophore. Two compounds that are particularly advantageous for use in this respect are NAD and NADP. The reduced forms of these coenzymes (i.e., NADH and NADPH) absorb light very strongly at 340 mμ; thus, any enzymes whose reaction can be directly or indirectly linked to coenzymes can be easily estimated with a spectrophotometer that will measure absorbance at 340 mμ. Several reactions in which these coenzymes can be directly linked to the enzymes in question are as follows: (1) lactic dehydrogenase, (2) glutamic dehydrogenase, (3) isocitric dehydrogenase, and (4) sorbitol dehydrogenase.

Several other enzymes can be measured by linking the product of the first reaction to a second reaction which consumes or produces NADH or NADPH. These multistep reactions are referred to as linked determinations, and some examples follow:

1. GPT utilizes the following principle:

$$\text{Alanine} + \alpha\text{-ketoglutarate} \overset{\text{(GPT)}}{\rightleftharpoons} \text{pyruvate} + \text{glutamate}$$

$$\text{Pyruvate} + \text{NADH} + \text{H}^+ \overset{\substack{\text{excess}\\ \text{LDH}}}{\rightleftharpoons} \text{lactate} + \text{NAD}^+$$

2. GOT uses this principle:

$$\text{Aspartate} + \alpha\text{-ketoglutarate} \overset{\text{(GOT)}}{\rightleftharpoons} \text{oxaloacetate} + \text{glutamate}$$

$$\text{Oxaloacetate} + \text{NADH} + \text{H}^+ \overset{\substack{\text{excess}\\ \text{MDH}}}{\rightleftharpoons} \text{malate} + \text{NAD}^+$$

3. An example of an enzyme where two reactions as well as the enzyme being measured are linked together in order to allow the estimation of DPNH utilization is creatine phosphokinase, which is assayed in this way:

$$\text{Creatine} + \text{ATP} \overset{\text{(CPK)}}{\rightleftharpoons} \text{creatine phosphate} + \text{ADP}$$

$$\text{ADP} + \text{Phosphoenolpyruvate} \overset{\substack{\text{excess}\\ \text{(pyr-kinase)}}}{\rightleftharpoons} \text{ATP} + \text{pyruvate}$$

$$\text{Pyruvate} + \text{NADH} + \text{H}^+ \overset{\substack{\text{excess}\\ \text{(LDH)}}}{\rightleftharpoons} \text{lactate} + \text{NAD}^+$$

It is important in the case of reactions with linked enzymes, that there be an excessive concentration of the second or third enzyme as in the case of creatine phosphokinase, in order to obtain estimates of activity. The use of linked enzyme determinations has been discussed in detail by Bergmeyer (1963). There are many sources of full details of methods for estimating enzymic activity; some are those of Wilkinson (1962), Henley *et al.* (1966), and Bergmeyer (1963) as well as those described in the pamphlets available from Sigma Chemical Co., St. Louis, Missouri on the estimation of many clinically important enzymes.

8. Quality Control

Because of infrequent demands for enzymic assays, inexperience of the analysts, and perishability of reagents, it is necessary that some form of quality control be carried out each time an unknown serum sample is assayed. This can be done by conducting an assay of a known or standard serum sample in parallel with the unknown. Since the standard's enzyme value is known, failure to reproduce it would suggest some error in the technique or possibly in the standard. Standard serum samples for enzyme assay are commercially available; however, they too are perishable and the directions of the manufacturer must be followed. Most enzyme assay kits now manufactured for use in clinical medicine are to determine end-point values. For this reason, it is important to realize the limitation of their use when dealing with samples of high enzymic activity. If the enzymic activity is high the substrate may have been consumed to a point that the rate of the reaction is limited (or reached) before the allotted time period has elapsed. In such cases, the values obtained will be lower than the true serum values. It may also be that the optical density is too great for reading on the spectrophotometer. In the latter case, the final preparation cannot be diluted and read. If a numerical value is required in both instances, the assays should be repeated with a diluted serum sample. However, should all the knowledge the clinician requires be that the activity is elevated beyond a certain point, repetition would not be necessary since the value obtained would not be erroneous on the high side, and the value could be expressed as "greater than an absolute numerical value."

9. Practicability and Cost

There is no question that the use of serum enzymes as diagnostic aids has great value. However, a practical question for the veterinarian is that of either doing the tests in his own laboratory or incurring the high costs adjusted with service by commercial laboratories. The cost factor is much more limiting in veterinary medicine than in human medicine because if the costs run too high, the veterinarian is likely to be asked whether the animal would recover without treatment or to euthanize it. The veterinarian may reduce the cost factor by expanding his own clinical laboratory to include a spectrophotometer which measures wavelengths as low as 340 mμ and as high as the visible range of at least 660 mμ. With this instrument many routine clinical tests as well as enzymic assays can be conducted. Other aids which are increasing in use are commercially produced kits for estimation of enzymic activity. Several of these kit procedures require a number of simple steps, and the tests give reasonable estimates of activity. However, it is obvious that there will be even a greater variety of tests for estimation of enzymic activities in the relatively near future; and that these will be as simple as those being used for the estimation of urinary sugar values. A possibility here would be to have test kits for sera. Such systems could contain all the linking enzymes, cofactors, and dyes needed for a particular assay; the clinician would need only to add a certain volume of buffer and 0.1 ml. of serum, and to incubate the mixture for a certain length of time in order to ascertain the degree of dye reduction followed by comparison with a standard chart. This procedure would give reasonable estimations of enzymic activity and only in the case of extremely high activity would greater dilutions be needed. However, it is obvious that with samples of high activity a diagnosis would be definitely confirmed. Such kits would have to be made available at costs as low as $.50 to $1.00 a test, and little effort would have to be involved. There would also be the obvious advantage of being able to run such tests within a 10- or 15- minute period in a clinical laboratory compared that of 24 to 48 hours before the receiving results from commercial laboratories. Thus, earlier diagnosis and, of course, earlier treatment would be possible. Some of these rapid tests are already available and there will be more.

10. COLLECTION AND STORAGE

For most enzymic work for diagnostic purposes, either serum or plasma is acceptable. The choice will be dependent on the clinican's interest in obtaining information on other parameters. Obviously, when the blood is collected care should be taken to avoid hemolysis, which releases to the plasma or serum rather high concentrations of certain enzymes such as transaminases and particularly lactic dehydrogenase. Escape of several other enzymes with hemolysis of the erythrocytes may also lead to serious test errors. Arginase is an example. Normally, it is extremely low in the plasma or serum and its presence may be very useful for diagnosis, since the activity of this enzyme increases very rapidly in liver damage, and is cleared at a rapid rate. The large quantity of this enzyme in erythrocytes makes avoidance of hemolysis even more critical.

The anticoagulant used to collect plasma must not interfere with the enzymic determination. For example, oxalate has an inhibitory effect on lactic dehydrogenase activity and also inhibits that of amylase slightly. Citrate inhibits amylase but not lactic dehydrogenase. Possibly the best of the anticoagulants to use in enzymic determinations on plasma is heparin, which inhibits the activity of very few enzymes. If fluoride is included in the samples, which may be desirable for glucose determination, this ion may interfere with a number of glycolytic enzymic activities.

However, the enzymes inhibited by fluoride generally are not those that are of diagnostic importance. After collection of the serum or plasma, one should avoid vigorous shaking, exposure to elevated temperature, or repeated freezing and thawing, since all of these tend to denature proteins and decrease enzymic activities. To store a portion for enzymic determination over a period of time, it is best to freeze the serum or plasma once, and hold it in this state. However, some activity is lost during the storage period even after freezing, and, since the degree differs among enzymes and possibly species, one should determine the loss during storage. More information will be of great help to the veterinary clinician, especially that on storage stability of serum or plasma enzymes from different animal species. After freezing at −18 to −20°C., the activity loss is generally no greater than 20 to 30% over a 3-week period.

II. Origin and Removal of Serum Enzymes

1. Origin of Serum Enzymes

The activities of any serum enzyme is a function of the rate of release of the enzyme from any given tissue, and the rate of its removal from the circulation. Thus, when leakage of a given enzyme occurs at a rate greater than that of normal removal, its activity will show an increase. An attempt will be made to cover both of these aspects in some detail in the remainder of this section.

It is usually assumed that enzymic leakage occurs because of damage to the cells of particular organs. Even in good health, it is apparent that there is some release of enzymic activity to the serum, which indicates that, under almost all conditions, damage to the cell is followed by leakage of enzymes and necrobiosis. However, it appears that with necrobiosis degradation would result from intracellular lysosomal activity after death of the cells.

There is evidence, particularly in the case of the transaminases in serum, that the concentration of these enzymes from a given target tissue is related to the dose of toxins involved (Wroblewski and LaDue, 1955; Molander et al., 1955; Bruns and Neuhaus, 1955). There is a correlation between the concentration and pathogenicity of injected viruses and enzyme content of the serum (Friend et al., 1955). However, in most of these and in other cases that we will be discussing, the concept that the injured cells are simply bags of enzymes that are released to the serum on literal explosion of the cells is completely untenable. The basis of this rationale is the great difference between the pattern of enzymic activity of the serum after damage to a particular organ and the concentration of these same enzymes in the tissue. The rate of removal of the enzymes is not sufficient to account for this difference. Therefore, it appears that the damaged tissues of various organs may actually be leaking out or even that enzymes are actively pumped through a damaged membrane into the serum while, at the same time, the organs are synthesizing more enzymes. Hence, we should be able to detect considerable amounts of enzyme in the serum without there necessarily being similar decreases in the various tissues. It should be pointed out, however, that in some cases, there is concomitant loss of enzymic activity by the tissue, concurrent with observed increases by the serum. The release of enzymes from cells has been firmly established by observations which include those on isolated organs (Zierler, 1958a,b; Sibley, 1958). There has been good agreement, in many studies, between the properties of enzymes occurring in serum with those of the enzymes of certain damaged organs (Wieland *et al.*, 1959; Vessel and Bearn, 1961) and, as has been previously mentioned, a decrease of the enzymic activity in the damaged tissues has been observed in some of these cases (Dreyfus *et al.*, 1956; Wroblewski, 1958; Schmidt *et al.*, 1958; Strandjord *et al.*, 1959).

There was good correlations in several cases between the degree of necrosis and the release of enzymes to the serum (Merrill *et al.*, 1956; Zelman *et al.*, 1959). However, some cases have revealed lack of correlation between these two parameters (Sibley, 1958; Siekert and Fleisher, 1958). There is considerable evidence that even slight damage to the cell, which injury cannot be detected morphologically, can cause release of enzymes from it to the serum. This happens after hypoxia, the enzymic activity of the serum rising in a relatively short time (Schmidt *et al.*, 1958; Hess and Raftopulo, 1957). The use of perfused hypoxic rat liver has also demonstrated this phenomenon (Schmidt *et al.*, 1966; Schmidt and Schmidt, 1967). In fact, in the latter experiment with perfused rat liver, where severe degrees of hypoxia could be obtained without causing effects on the central nervous system as would occur *in vivo*, it was shown that the enzymes located in the cytoplasm leaked from the liver in inverse proportion to their molecular weight. This result might be expected if there were simple membrane instability due to the anoxia and passive diffusion. The smaller molecules diffuse more rapidly than the larger. This phenomenon appeared to characterize a range of enzymes varying in molecular weight from around 40,000 to 140,000. Leakage was further indicated to be of passive nature, since the quantity that leaked to the serum was not only dependent on molecular weight of the enzyme but also on concentration of the enzyme in the tissue. Therefore, these experiments revealed that a predictable percentage of the enzyme present in the tissue would leak to the serum during each time unit, depending on molecular weight. However, the enzymes of mitochondrial origin took considerably longer to leak out of the tissue; also, they did not follow the simple diffusion kinetics of the soluble enzymes. We feel that these experiments which made use of a simple disfunction of the plasma cell membrane, the latter probably due to lack of energy resulting from inadequate oxygen supply, were important in showing that the percentage leakage of enzyme under these conditions was inversely proportional to molecular weight.

It has been shown in many species of higher animals that similar enzymes in similar tissues have approximately the same molecular weights. For example, the molecular weights of the lactic dehydrogenases of almost all animals examined were about 140,000; this fits in well with the theories of evolution, since the likelihood that various proteins of species as closely related as is supposedly true for most higher animals should not be too diverse in size. If simple leakage of enzymes by diffusion, without any selectivity, were to occur during liver damage, it would be easy to predict the content of enzymes in the serum of almost any species. However, this is definitely not the case; in fact, the serum enzyme profile obtained varies with different types of liver disease or necrosis. Therefore, there is strong suggestion that, in various diseases, there are changes in membrane permeability or systems of enzyme synthesis that leak certain enzymes preferentially from the cell. An example of such disorder could be accounted for by the observation of Redman (1968). He observed that enzymes normally found in the soluble fraction within the cell are synthesized in polysomes not adjacent to the endoplastic reticulum. In the liver, the synthesis of proteins such as serum albumin, which are readily and rapidly transported to the blood stream, takes place on ribosomes, which are in firm contact with the endoplastic reticulum leading into the circulatory system. Therefore, in addition to resultant specific changes in membrane permeability, damage which would lead to a translocation of the synthesis of certain enzymes could account for a greater output of freshly synthesized enzymes to the circulation. To our knowledge, this possibility has not been examined; however, it could be explored by using pulse labeling techniques and examining the rate and degree of labeling of the serum enzymes that are present during various disorders.

The fact that normal breakdown does not cause elevated enzymic activity in the serum is consistent with the fact that there are usually no changes in enzymic activity in the serum during starvation (White, 1958) or in some neuromuscular atrophies (Pearson, 1957; Dreyfus et al., 1958). In contrast, severe damage to cell metabolism, as in congenital muscular dystrophy, causes readily observable changes in enzyme content of the serum (Dreyfus and Shapira, 1954). These few general considerations involve a few possible causes of enzyme breakage in the cell, including changes in metabolism as well as factors such as toxins, disease states, dystrophy, poisoning, virus infection, which can alter membrane permeability.

2. Removal of Enzymes from the Blood

After enzymes have been released to the serum, the rate of their removal from the blood stream appears to be a first-order reaction, particularly when concentrations are extremely elevated. It has been shown that the protein is actually taken out of the bloodstream, and not simply inactivated (Massarrat, 1965). This fact was established by injecting radioactive enzymes in an animal and examining the disappearance of both enzymic activity and radioactivity. Both disappeared from the serum simultaneously, and the disappearance rate approached that of first-order kinetics, i.e., a given percentage of the enzyme was removed from the serum during a unit of time. There is surprisingly little information on the rates of clearance of autonomous enzymes from the bloodstream of experimental and domestic animals as well as human beings. Much of the information has been obtained from or calculated by the rate of disappearance of activity after severe injury or single insult, such as carbon tetrachloride poisoning. However, the half-life of the enzyme in serum in many cases may have been greatly overestimated due to the fact that the half-life was estimated by measuring the rate of return to normal after the peak was reached. However, there is no assurance that leakage of enzyme from the tissue to the bloodstream is not continuous, although assuredly not at a maximal rate during that time. Such a situation would lead to overestimation of half-life, since the assumption is made that there is no further significant release of enzyme to the bloodstream.

Some examples of half-lives reported for certain enzymes in various species are listed in Table II. There are many possible ways for clearance of enzymes from the serum. Among them, obviously, are the bile and urine routes, although very low levels of activity have been observed for urine, even when enzymic activity of the serum is high, suggesting that this is not a primary means of removal. There is also evidence that removal via the bile is probably not a major mechanism for removal of activity (Cleeve, 1962). In the case of kidney and urine, digestive enzymes such as amylase and pepsinogen, the precursor of pepsin, are excreted in the urine in appreciable quantities, but only traces of other enzymes with diagnostic potential can be detected despite their high concentration in serum in the absence of kidney damage (Rosalki and Wilkinson, 1959). These authors showed that the total 24-hour disappearance of transaminase and lactic dehydrogenase from serum compared to the low values in the urine suggested that the kidneys play only a minor role in con-

TABLE II

ESTIMATED HALF-LIVES FOR CLEARANCE OF ENZYMES FROM SERUM OR PLASMA

Enzyme	Species	$T_{1/2}$	Reference
LDH	Rabbit	150 Min.	Amelung (1960)
GPT	Rabbit	308 Min.	Amelung (1960)
GOT	Dog	12 Hrs.	Fleisher and Wakim (1956)
GOT	Dog	263 Min.	Zinkle et al. (in preparation)
GPT	Dog	20 Hrs.	Reichard (1959)
GPT	Dog	149 Min.	Zinkle et al. (in preparation)
LDH	Dog	<6 Hr.	Strandjord et al. (1959)
LDH	Dog	105 Min.	Zinkle et al. (in preparation)
ICD	Dog	<60 Min.	Strandjord et al. (1959)
Sorbitol D	Dog	232 Min.	Zinkle et al. (in preparation)
CPK	Dog	210 Min.	Cardinet et al. (in preparation)
Arginase	Calf	80 Min.	Cornelius et al. (1963b)
CPK	Horse	108 Min.	Cardinet et al. (1967)

trolling the serum levels of enzymic activity in the absence of renal disease. It is possible that the organs of the reticuloendothelial system may be responsible for the removal of enzymes from the serum as well as removal of circulating red blood cells and foreign bodies from the blood.

It is apparent that identification of differences in removal rates of enzymes from the plasma or serum can be useful for diagnostic purposes. Slow rates of removal of an enzyme from the serum may be an indication not only of a prevailing disease condition, but also of a prior one, e.g., a considerable amount of a particular enzyme is released to the serum as a result of liver damage; removal of the enzyme is slow, and elevated activities can be observed by testing serum or plasma during the active phase of liver damage and also for several days to a week or more after the damage has subsided (Cornelius et al., 1962). Therefore, enzymic activity is a useful criterion of whether the animal has recently had significant liver damage. Obviously, many cases of such damage are normally repaired rapidly and completely. Here, of course, active therapy treatment should not be the same as if the disease was progressing. To evaluate the situation further, tests can be conducted for another liver-specific enzyme such as arginase which is removed rather rapidly from the serum; if arginase content is elevated, the liver damage may be continuing or has subsided very recently. Therefore, it may pay to again test for these two enzymes, recognizing that transaminase is removed slowly and arginase more rapidly over the following 3 days or so. In continuing necrosis of the liver, the activities of both enzymes will remain high during this period. However, in cases where the liver is undergoing repair, marked decreases in arginase activity should occur, although the functional decrease of the transaminases may be expected to be much less marked. An illustration of such decreases came from the work of Cornelius *et al.* (1962).

In order to examine the feasibility of an explosive disruption of the cell as an explanation of serum enzyme activity, we can use theoretical calculations, as well as measurement of activity in a given tissue, if we know the apparent half-life of an enzyme in the serum. The results will show how much tissue would have to disintegrate for complete release of the enzyme. Such data indicate that there is probably a selective diffusion of enzymes through the membrane. Let us, for example, take arginase activity, the half-life of which is relatively short in sheep. Using the formula $T_{1/2} = 0.693/K$ where K is the fractional removal per unit time, it can be observed that if enzyme levels are maintained constantly over a long period of time, 69.3 of every 100 units of activity are removed during every half-life of arginase. Therefore, in order to maintain the observed constant activity, 69.3 units of each 100 units of observed activity must be released from the tissue to the blood stream during each effective half-life. We can examine this phenomenon by using arginase and sheep as examples. Assuming that the liver and plasma each total about 3% of the sheep's body weight, the liver's maximal contribution to plasma arginase can be estimated. The calculation will show that complete disruption of the cell with concomitant release of cellular enzymes cannot account for the sustained levels of arginase observed in sheep plasma (Cornelius *et al.* 1962). For ease of calculations, the following assumptions are made:

1. Constant arginase activity is 200 units per milliliter of plasma.
2. Liver arginase activity is 6,600 units per gram of liver (Cornelius *et al.*, 1962).
3. $T_{1/2}$ of arginase of plasma is 80 minutes (estimated from values for the calf; Cornelius *et al.*, 1962).

Therefore:

(a) 200 units/ml. $\times$ 0.693/80 minutes = units removed/time
(b) 140 units/ml./80 minutes = 420 units/ml./4 hour or 2520 units/ ml./day are removed.
(c) In 3 days 7560 units/ml. are removed.
(d) Since milliliters of plasma = grams of liver (3% of body weight each) more arginase would be removed from the plasma than would be present in the liver.
(e) Therefore, complete disruption and release could not account for the phenomenon, since levels of over 200 units/ml. have been observed for periods of at least 3 days (Cornelius *et al.*, 1962).

III. Isoenzymes

It has become apparent recently that many enzymes, i.e., proteins which catalyze a specific reaction, are made up of more than one type of protein. These protein types, catalyzing similar reactions, have been called isozymes, and the approved term by the International Union of Biochemistry is now isoenzymes. The isoenzymes can be separated on both physical and chemical bases. This is done most commonly by means of electrophoresis, a method which involves the use of electrical charges across a buffered medium; the latter can vary from starch to acrylamide to simple paper, and separation of the isoenzymes by this procedure depends on the various charges which they carry since, in many cases, the isoenzymes have similar molecular weights. However, if the other physical properties such as solubility in various concentrations of ammonium sulfate or organic solvents vary, these solubility differences can provide a means of separation. If the molecular weights of the various isoenzymes species should vary, Sephadex can be used to separate them. For most cases in clinical medicine, the zymogram is of considerable value. Zymograms are usually obtained by electrophoretic separation followed by specific staining. Specific staining can result from direct production of a colored product, such as in identification of phosphatases or by linking the reaction to some dye acceptor as is the case with many dehydrogenases. Some of the early work on phosphatases and esterases was conducted by Hunter and Markert (1957). It was followed shortly by a series of studies by Augustinsson (1958, 1959a,b,c, 1961), who examined the esterase activity in various mammalian and nonmammalian species including man. He observed that one type of esterase designated as esterase-A was the predominant isoenzyme in mammalian plasma such as that of man, monkey, dog, and of ruminant species and that it was absent from lower species such as bird, reptile and amphibian. A second isoenzyme, known as esterase-β, was present in lower vertebrates but absent in higher mammalian species. Since that time, numerous isoenzymes of esterases have been identified in various tissues. Depending on electrophoretic mobility and substrate specificity, the number of detectable isoenzymes can reach complex proportions, as demonstrated by Hunter and Burstone (1960), who observed and characterized 30 different isoenzymes of esterases in mouse liver. Paul and Fortrill (1961) examined the phosphoesterase isoenzymes of 8 mammals and a bird.

The distribution of these isoenzymes in specific tissues may be helpful in establishing a diagnosis. We stated earlier that various serum enzymes can serve as diagnostic aids depending on their tissue specificity and that a marked increase in a particular enzyme from a given tissue or organ may very well indicate that the tissue has been damaged. Various species of isoenzymes also may be limited to one or two tissues. While the enzymic activity itself may be fairly ubiquitous, a single isoenzyme may be organ specific and, therefore, useful for diagnostic purposes as a tissue-specific enzyme. Of course, the examination of an isoenzyme or a zymogenic pattern is more difficult than demonstration of the activity of a given enzyme. The patterns of different isoenzymes of various species of animals have not clearly been established, whereas the general enzymic components of many individual tissues have been more clearly determined. Recognizing these limitations clearly, discussion of various isoenzymes and their possible use can continue.

Determination of phosphatase values (mainly alkaline phosphatase) has been of considerable benefit for diagnosis of human disease, and there is no reason why such determinations may not become more applicable to recognition of veterinary medical disorders. These enzymes appear as multiple isoenzymes in most animals. Acid phosphatases (the isoenzymes) of a number of animal tissues have been studied by Markert and Moller (1959), who showed them to be a family of enzymes which have characteristic yet overlapping specificities for certain substrates. Alkaline phosphatase which has been used intensively for aiding diagnosis, particularly of hepatitis, biliary obstruction and skeletal diseases, may find considerable use in veterinary medicine. Stevenson (1961) encountered wide variations between the isoenzymes of alkaline phosphatase in young and old dogs; Owen and Stevenson (1961) showed that the isoenzyme present particularly in dogs with osteogenic sarcoma migrated toward the cathode whereas isoenzymes of their normal bone migrated toward the anode.

A family of isoenzymes can readily be found in the dehydrogenases. Members are lactic dehydrogenase, malic dehydrogenase, isocitric dehydrogenase, and glutamic dehydrogenase. If lactate dehydrogenase is examined, it can be observed to be made up of 5 isoenzymes, the quantity of each depending on the source of tissue from which they are derived. Apella and Markert (1961) showed that 5 isoenzymes of lactic dehydrogenase are composed of two types of subunits, 4 subunits being capable of forming an active lactic dehydrogenase molecule. This phenomenon can be visualized by the following:

$$\begin{array}{ccccc} \text{HHHH} & \text{HHHM} & \text{HHMM} & \text{HMMM} & \text{MMMM} \\ H_4 & H_3M & H_2M_2 & HM_3 & M_4 \end{array}$$

It has been shown that if subunit H_4, which stands for the isoenzyme of greatest concentration observed in the heart, and pure M_4 enzyme, which stands for the isoenzyme most concentrated in the skeletal muscle, are mixed together and subjected to electrophoresis, M_4 and H_4 isoenzymes are obtained in the amounts added. However, if this mixture is frozen in the presence of a high ionic concentration of salt, the subunits will disassociate and reassociate in a random manner so that the predominant isoenzyme will be the H_2M_2 isoenzyme, with the expected amounts of H_3M, M_3H, H_4, and M_4 (Markert, 1963). In this random recombination, there is relatively little of the pure M_4 or H_4 with which we started. It appears that the relative quantities of the isoenzymes in any given tissue depend on the relative amounts of M and H subunits synthesized in each tissue. The advantage of these isoenzymes, at least in human medicine, is quite apparent, but it will have to be evaluated much further to ascertain whether the distribution is the same or similar in all the species of domestic animals. An example of their advantage follows: Let us assume that we have observed increased activity of GOT, isocitric dehydrogenase (ICD), lactic dehydrogenase, and creatine phosphokinase without concomitant increase in GPT or sorbitol dehydrogenase. We would then have reason to suspect some muscular damage. It would be most illuminating if we could narrow this suspicion to that of injury to cardiac muscle or skeletal muscle. Differentiation could be established by examining the isoenzymic pattern of lactate dehydrogenase. If the predominant isoenzyme in the serum were the M_4 isoenzyme, it would be an indication of skeletal muscle damage; if the predominant isoenzyme were H_4, it would indicate cardiac damage.

Electrophoresis is not the only means for characterization of the lactate dehydrogenase, which acts on α-hydroxybutyric acid. The latter is similar to lactic acid but has an extra methylene group. It has been shown that the relative activity of the M_4 and H_4 isoenzymes toward the second substrate α-hydroxybutyric acid for NADH formation or α-ketobutyrate for NADH oxidation, when compared to a ratio of NADH formation or oxidation using either lactic acid or pyruvic acid as substrate, varies considerably depending on the isoenzyme of lactic dehydrogenase (Rosalki, 1963). The relative activity toward α-hydroxybutyric acid as compared to lactic acid is much greater for the H_4 isoenzyme than for the M_4. Therefore, it may be practicable to examine the relative activity toward each of these substrates in order to ascertain whether the predominant isoenzyme released is M_4 or H_4. The results may be useful when we suspect muscular damage and, if it has occurred, when we attempt to ascertain whether it is of cardiac or skeletal origin, but are not equipped to examine the isoenzyme pattern by electrophoresis.

Malic dehydrogenase has at least two dominant enzyme forms. However, unlike lactic dehydrogenase, where both forms are cytoplasmic and the variation in enzymes is with particular tissues, Thorne (1960) as well as Grimm and Doherty (1961) have shown that the two isoenzymes of malic dehydrogenase are a cytoplasmic form and a mitochondrial form. Therefore, it would be expected, as has been shown with GOT (Schmidt and Schmidt, 1967), that the predominantly cytoplasmic isoenzyme would increase in the serum during early stages of the damage and would be followed by the appearance of mitochondrial isoenzymes after the destruction of this subcellular particle were more complete. In the case of both malic dehydrogenase and GOT, the relative proportions of cytoplasmic to mitochondrial isoenzymes may be an indication of the severity of the disease as well as the degree of increase in enzyme activity.

That the two isoenzymes of isocitric dehydrogenase are not truly isoenzymes in the same sense as are lactic dehydrogenase and malic dehydrogenase was pointed out in previous discussion. The substrates and cofactors of the latter enzymes are identical, but there is variation in their kinetic properties, i.e., the K_m values are different (K_m value being the amount of substrate required to obtain $\frac{1}{2}$ maximal velocity). The cofactor requirement of isocitric dehydrogenase varies for the two supposed isoenzymes. In one case, the coenzyme is NAD; in the second, the coenzyme is NADP. However, the fact that this enzyme occurs as an isoenzyme is not of great significance in clinical medicine, since in almost all cases it is the NADP-linked enzyme, which is normally cytoplasmic in origin, that is used for clinical purposes, not the NAD-linked enzyme.

Glutamic dehydrogenase occurs in at least two isoenzymic forms. This enzyme may be of considerable use in clinical tests. It has the advantage of being low in the serum normally and of being a mitochondrial enzyme, the presence of which would be strongly indicative of cellular damage causing disruption and leakage of mitochondrial protein to the serum. Both of the two isoenzymes are located in the mitochondria, but one is readily released from the mitochondria on disruption and is water soluble. This water extractable form is probably the major isoenzyme released to the serum after disruption of mitochondria. The second isoenzyme of glutamic dehydrogenase requires detergent action to release it from the surface of the mitochondria under experimental conditions (Hirschberg and Osnos, 1962). It would be expected that this enzyme would not be released readily until the mitochondrial fragments were digested intercellularly. At this point, it is questionable whether the enzymic activity would be able to avoid proteolytic destruction. In the case of glutamic dehydrogenase, an increase in activity has been observed ranging from 3-fold to 20-plus-fold depending on the species (Freedland et al., 1966) by conducting the assay in the presence of ADP, which appears to keep the enzyme in a more active form. This, of course, has the advantage of a three-fold or more increase in sensitivity of the estimation of this enzymic activity, and is particularly important since its normal activity is low and its increase during tissue damage, although manyfold greater, is great in absolute or total activity.

Glutamic oxaloacetic transaminase, an important enzyme from the clinical standpoint, occurs in the form of isoenzymes. These isoenzymes are of both cytoplasmic and mitochondrial origin (Boyd, 1962b). There are also isoenzymes of the cytoplasmic form of GOT which depend on tissue specificity, as in the case of lactic dehydrogenase as well as isoenzymes of GOT, which occur within a single tissue, due to subcellular localization such as in cytoplasm and mitochondria. This situation is similar to that with malic dehydrogenase.

IV. Clinical Aspects

1. MYOPATHIES

The use of serum creatine phosphokinase (CPK) has specificity in the clinical diagnosis of acute myocardial infarctions and skeletal muscle myopathies of human beings, horses, and dogs and should be valuable for diagnosis of forms of myopathies in other mammals, this enzyme being relatively specific to striated muscle (Cook, 1967; Cardinet et al., 1967; Eshchar and Zimmerman, 1967; Gerber, 1964a,b). In the case of cattle in prolonged recumbency, serum CPK and GOT values may be of value in establishing a prognosis (Bjorsell et al., 1969). As muscular degeneration and necrosis develop, enzymes are released to the general circulation in sufficient quantity to be detected and a prognosis may be attained by serial interval determinations of both serum CPK and GOT. Serum CPK values generally return to normal in 2 to 3 days following insult, those of GOT, in 4 to 5 days. If the serum levels are not reduced, the condition may be regarded as progressive.

Myocardial infarction in man produces a serum enzyme profile of relatively specific type. Similar lesions in other animals also produce specific profiles, but they have been primarily reported only for experimental cases. Though similar profiles develop in experimentally produced myocardial infarctions of dogs, seldom is myocardial infarction recognized as a clinical entity. In dogs with experimentally produced acute myocardial infarctions, the serum enzyme content of GOT and GPT may be increased more than ten- and fourfold, respectively. Serum lactate dehydrogenase is also increased, but, because of wide normal fluctuations, significance can be attached only to very high levels of this enzyme. It may be suggested that the increase in serum GPT is of hepatic origin, as the result of cardiac insufficiency and hepatic congestion, but the rise occurs within 24 hours of the infarction, and there is close correlation between the total increase in serum activity and the loss of cardiac GPT from the infarcted area (Crawly and Sevenson, 1963; Nydick et al., 1957; Ruegsegger et al., 1959; Siegel and Bing, 1956). Gerber (1964b) reported that in horses with degenerative changes of cardiac muscle, increases occurred in serum GPT, GOT, and CPK.

Cardinet et al. (in preparation) have compiled normal serum CPK values for dogs and reported significant age and sex variations. Dogs of less than 8 months had two to three times higher serum CPK levels than older dogs, and males had 50% greater serum CPK activity than females. Holliday (1969) has observed significant increases in serum CPK and GOT levels in some cases of atrophic myositis and toxoplasmic myositis. However, he pointed out that treatment of atrophic myositis with corticosteroids results in the serum CPK returning to normal. This finding is of particular importance when dealing with referral cases that have incomplete histories, and it is of assistance in establishing a prognosis after treatment has been initiated.

The need for differential diagnosis is of particular concern in two myopathies of the horse. Myoglobinemia and the "tying up" syndrome of horses produce significant increases in serum GOT, LDH, and CPK content. These disease conditions appear to be similar in many ways although different in severity. In the "tying up" syndrome, increases in serum enzymes occurs prior to the onset of clinical signs. The serum enzymes mentioned increase in both conditions to many times their normal level. If the injury does not persist, the serum CPK value returns to normal in 2 to 3 days, those of GOT and LDH in 6 to 7 days, depending on the height of the initial rise (Cardinet et al., 1963; Cornelius et al., 1963a; Crawly and Sevenson, 1963; Gerber, 1964c). Attempts to differentiate the two diseases from liver necrosis on the basis of serum LDH isoenzyme patterns has not met with success (Gerber, 1966; Carper and Hanson, 1967). Exercise also produces a one- to fourfold increase in these serum enzymes, and its effect must be considered in differential diagnosis (Cardinet et al., 1963; Cornelius et al., 1963a). In horses with clinical signs of tetanus, significant increases in serum GOT, LDH, and CPK were reported by both Gerber (1964b) and Wurzner (1964).

Myopathies of nutritional origin are associated with abnormal serum enzyme patterns. One of the earliest reported was White Muscle Disease of sheep and cattle (Blincoe and Dye, 1958). Prior to the onset of clinical signs, 22-fold increases in serum GOT and LDH activity have occurred. These increases persisted along with the clinical signs and returned to normal following treatment and regression of the myopathies (Blincoe and Marble, 1960; Kuttler and Marble, 1958; Lagace et al., 1964; Swingle and Young, 1959). Pigs with nutritional muscular and hepatic dystrophy had significant increases in both serum GPT and GOT, but not of ornithine transcarbamylase (OTC). The increases occurred prior to the onset of clinical signs, and regression followed successful treatment (Orstadius *et al.*, 1959).

Progressive herditary muscular dystrophies have occurred in hamsters, mice, chickens, and ducks (Weyer, 1966). In hamsters, mice, and chickens the disease was related to an autosomal recessive factor, and increases in serum aldolase and CPK occurred in the clinical disease of the first three species (Asmundson *et al.*, 1966; Cornelius *et al.*, 1959a; Holliday, 1963; Homburger *et al.*, 1966; Hansenfeld *et al.* 1962; Wrogemann and Blanchaer, 1968). Some controversy has arisen concerning the CPK content in sera of dystrophic mice. Hansenfeld *et al.* (1962) reported serum CPK elevations during both preclinical and clinical stages of mouse dystrophy but not at any time in the carriers of the syndrome; however, Schapira and Dreyfus (1963) did not find increases in serum CPK but did report increases of serum aldolase. In muscularly dystrophic chickens, serum values of GOT were increased; the elevations occurred prior to the onset of clinical signs. Homburger *et al.* (1966) reported that serum enzyme increases in dystrophic hamsters developed prior to histopathologic changes or clinical signs. Hazlewood and Ginski (1968) demonstrated differences in membrane potential between normal and muscular dystrophic mice; there is some evidence of pathologic changes in hamsters at the level of the redox systems (Lochner and Brink, 1967).

2. Osteopathies

Bone contains a considerable amount of extracellular alkaline phosphatase (AP). Growing bone has a much greater content of AP than does mature bone. A considerable amount of this bone AP enters the bloodstream during an animal's period of maturation; the result is higher serum values among immature animals than among mature animals. Serum AP values become elevated in nutritional osteopathies such as "rickets" and osteomalacia of dogs (Campbell, 1962; Hime, 1968), secondary hyperparathyroidism of horses (Krook and Love, 1964), and ostrodystrophia fibrosa of "New World" primates as the result of vitamin D deficiency (Hunt *et al.*, 1967). Elevation is associated with a generalized increase of osteocytic activity. Campbell (1962) reported normal serum AP, calcium, and phosphorus values in puppies with osteoporosis produced experimentally by feeding a low-calcium high vitamin D diet.

Both serum calcium and phosphorus may be normal, and only a slight elevation of serum AP may occur in osteopathies. Generally, the elevations occurring in osteopathies of mature animals are no greater than those of normal immature animals. These elevations are relatively small compared to those occurring in obstructive hepatic disorders where serum AP may be increased tenfold or more.

3. PANCREAS

Experimental studies and clinical case reports of pancreatitis have generally dealt with dogs. Knowledge of serum and fecal enzymic activity, in both acute and chronic forms of pancreatitis of dogs, is of value in establishing both diagnoses and prognoses. While increases in serum activity of amylase and lipase are of particular diagnostic value in the acute form, increases of these enzymes are not necessarily specific for pancreatitis or indicative of its severity (Challis *et al.*, 1957; Geokas *et al.*, 1968; Loeb and Edge, 1962; Nemir *et al.*, 1963). Challis *et al.* (1957) have reported that serum amylase activity may be elevated by parenteral injections of ACTH in both intact and pancreatectomized dogs, indicating that the source of the increases may not necessarily be the pancreas, and that increases may occur in other conditions resulting from stress. Fasting, trauma, and renal insufficiency also result in increased serum amylase activity. In persons with renal insufficiency, there is association between increases of blood urea nitrogen values and increased serum amylase and lipase activities. Serum amylase normally passes through the glomeruli of some species. In the serum of dogs with acute pancreatitis, amylase activity increases within the first 12 hours after the insult and generally attains its peak within 24 hours (Rapp, 1962). If the insult does not persist, serum values return to normal in 2 to 6 days. Serum lipase activity reaches its peak a few hours after serum amylase does. Lipase activity may remain elevated for considerably longer periods than does amylase activity which may make the former more satisfactory for diagnostic purposes, because the clinician frequently may not observe the patient until some time after the onset of the disease (Cornelius, 1960; Cornelius and Kaneko, 1963; Geokas *et al.*, 1968).

Freezing does not affect the activity of either serum lipase or amylase. Determination of amylase activity is generally carried out by either an amyloclastic technique, in which rate of starch disappearance is measured or by a saccharogenic test method which measures the rate of appearance of reducing sugars. Maltase present in normal dog serum is sufficient in quantity to cause discrepancies between the two basic methods for the determination of amylase. While the discrepancy may not be great from the clinical standpoint, the amyloclastic technique yields more exact values. Maltase was found in serum of normal lambs, calves, horses, and rabbits (Rapp, 1962); pig serum contained the highest amount of maltase activity and that of cats, the lowest. Measurable amounts of amylase were not found in normal serum of monkeys or man (Persky *et al.*, 1934). Olive oil is the substrate generally used for determining lipase activity and formerly the period of incubation for lipase determination was 12 hours or longer, but techniques requiring shorter periods of incubation, i.e., an hour, are now available (Brobst and Brester, 1967; Dirstine *et al.*, 1968).

Serum leucine amino peptidase content has been reported to be of value for the diagnosis of pancreatitis in man; however, as Wilkinson (1962) has noted, it is of no additional diagnostic value over serum lipase or amylase determinations. Reports of similar work with animals were not encountered. Investigators have shown the part played in pancreatitis by elastase and collaginase, but there is no known work demonstrating their value in diagnosis of the disease (Geokas *et al.*, 1968). Primary pancreatic neoplasms generally do not result in increases of pancreatic enzymes in serum, but they may result in obstruction of the duct system. These neoplasms may obstruct the flow of the common bile duct, producing a clinical picture and serum enzyme profile similar to that of obstructive jaundice.

4. BLOOD CELLULAR ELEMENTS

Enzymopathies of cellular elements of human blood are recognized (Kitchen, 1968; Valentine, 1968), but they have not been reported in lower animals. The erythrocytic enzymes of glycolysis and the pentose phosphate pathway differ quantitatively among the various species of animals (Smith *et al.*, 1965). Tada *et al.* (1961) demonstrated higher levels of LDH, glucose 6-phosphate dehydrogenase, aldolase, and reduced values of glutathione (GSH) in reticulocytes then in mature erythrocytes of rabbits. Smith and Osburn (1967) and Smith (1968) have reported sheep with remarkably low values of erythrocytic glutathione but without hemolytic disorder. Erythrocytes of horses have less reducing capacity for methemoglobin than those of man (Robin and Harley, 1967); Kaneko *et al.* (1969) reported no change in glutathione or pyruvate kinase activity in the sera of experimentally produced cases of equine infectious anemia, but they did record increases in lactate dehydrogenase and of glucose 6-phosphate dehydrogenase (G6PD) of erythrocytes; they believed these resulted from the younger population of circulating erythrocytes. In cases of bovine erythropoietic porphyria, and of carriers of it, erythrocyte GSH was significantly less stable than normal and G6PD was unchanged (Kaneko and Mills, 1970). Transketolase enzymic activity of the pentose phosphate pathway of erythrocytes has been used as a means of conducting a functional evaluation of thiamine (Brin, 1964).

5. CENTRAL NERVOUS SYSTEM

The content of creatine phosphokinase in the central nervous system (CNS) tissue of sheep is second in quantity only to that found in striated muscle (J. M. M. Brown and Wagner, 1968). In an attempt to use serum CPK values as a means for detecting degenerative CNS disturbances of sheep, Smith and Healy (1968) determined levels of activity of both serum GOT and CPK in a limited number of cases of muscular dystrophy, polioencephalomalacia, and focal symmetrical encephalomalacia. They reported that both serum GOT and CPK were increased significantly in muscular dystrophy, but only serum CPK was increased appreciably in the CNS diseases. Workers concerned with CNS disorders in human beings have reported increases of cerebral spinal fluid CPK, GOT, and LDH activity in cases of degenerative CNS disorders (Castello et al., 1967; Cunningham et al., 1965; Freck, 1967; Veery, 1962). These increases of activity in CNS disorders were not correlated with increases in protein concentration or serum enzyme values.

6. THYROID

Functional thyroid disorders of man produce significant inverse correlations in serum CPK activity and protein-bound iodine values (Graig and Smith, 1965; Graig and Ross, 1963; Fleisher and McConahey, 1964; Griffiths, 1963). Fleisher and McConahey (1964) reported some increase in serum LDH and GOT in hypothyroidism, but they were not nearly as great as was the CPK increase.

7. LIVER

Liver dysfunction produces a variety of serum enzyme profiles. Hepatocellular degeneration such as cloudy swelling and lipidosis may be preceded by enzyme loss to the serum, and probably in no other organ is there a greater degree of species variation. Hepatic glutamic pyruvate transaminase (GPT) activity is high in the liver of rats, cats, and dogs, but it is considerably lower in other tissues. In contrast, however, there are relatively small quantities of hepatic GPT in pigs, cattle, sheep, and horses, making its presence of little significance in these species when considering enzymes of hepatic specificity (Cornelius et al., 1958; Boyd, 1962a; Nagode et al., 1966; Gerber, 1965). Increased concentrations of serum alkaline phosphatase (AP) in the dog may be indicative of obstruction of the biliary system; however, in the cat, which has only a quarter of the hepatic alkaline phosphatase activity that the dog has, AP determination is of little value (Kritzler and Beaubien, 1949; Kramer and Sleight, 1968). Some apparently morphologically homogeneous single cell populations, such as those of erythrocytes and hepatocytes, have different enzymic systems, which are associated with the age of the cells or their topographical location within the tissue mass. This age or topographical difference may result in a different serum enzyme profile depending on the selectivity of the degenerative process (Boyd, 1962a; Freedland et al., 1963).

Selection of serum enzymes which will reflect the liver's condition involves consideration of more than their specificity. Other desirable parameters are the ease with which the enzyme determination can be carried out in the clinic, and the significant proportional increases in activity which could occur in both low grade cellular degenerations and massive acute insults. No single enzyme of all species has met these requirements completely. The urea cycle enzymes, ornithine transcarbamylase (OTC) and arginase (ARG), are liver specific in ureotelic animals. However, these enzymes have relatively short half-lives in serum, and thus some difficulty arises in detecting cases in which a single acute hepatic insult has occurred 3 to 4 days earlier and the serum OTC and arginase activities have returned to normal (Cornelius et al., 1962). Glutamic dehydrogenase (GD) and sorbitol dehydrogenase (SD) are relatively hepatic specific for domestic animals, but they too have short serum half-lives (Boyd, 1962a; Ford, 1965, 1967; Healy, 1968; Freedland et al., 1965).

Experimental hepatocellular degeneration is frequently produced by giving CCl_4 orally. When this substance is used, the experimenter must be careful in interpreting alterations of the serum enzyme profile as other tissue, such as muscle and kidney, are affected and, in turn, contribute to the alteration of profile (Ford and Lawrence, 1965). For this reason, less hepatocellular specific enzymes, such as GOT and NADP-ICD, may also be contributed to serum by the nonhepatic tissues damaged.

a. Dogs and Cats

Serum glutamic-pyruvate transaminase (GPT) is the enzyme most frequently used for detecting acute hepatic necrosis in dogs and cats. Cornelius et al. (1959b) and Cornelius and Kaneko (1960) reported that both serum GOT and GPT were significantly increased in dogs and cats with hepatocellular degeneration, and that GPT was significantly specific for hepatic damage. When experimental CCl_4 hepatotoxicity is produced in dogs and cats, values of serum GOT and GPT were increased within 24 hours to their peak levels of 300 times those of normal serum. Serum GOT and GPT returned to normal in approximately 7 and 10 days, respectively; hence, serum levels are dependent on the degree of damage done and length of time of the inuslt. In the case of acute hepatocellular damage in cats and dogs, serum GPT is specific enough to confirm a diagnosis, and repeated determinations should assist in establishing a prognosis. A combination of both serum GPT and sorbitol dehydrogenase would increase the specificity and be appropriate in confirming a diagnosis and establishing a prognosis (Cornelius *et al.*, 1959b; Cornelius and Kaneko, 1960; Hoe and Harvey, 1961; Hoe and O'Shea, 1965; Beckett *et al.*, 1964; Hoe and Jabara, 1967). With the exception of cases of acute poisonings, serum enzyme concentrations seldom reach the peaks reported for experimental CCl_4 poisoning, and for clinical cases, serum GPT values 10 times normal and greater may be regarded as severe, and two- to eightfold increases as mild. Mild increases in serum GPT and AP may result from passive cogestion and lipidosis, which are reversible disturbances and generally reflect a primary disease process in some organ other than liver (Hoe and Jabara, 1967). Other enzymes increased in serum when hepatocellular degeneration occurs are isocitrate dehydrogenase (ICD) (Cornelius, 1961) ; α-hydroxybutyrate dehydrogenase (Hoe and Jabara, 1967) ; malate dehydrogenase (MD) (Lettow, 1960) ; ornithine transcarbamylase (OTC) (R. W. Brown and Grisolia, 1959; Carper and Roesler, 1968) ; sorbitol dehydrogenase (SD), quinine oxidase (Lettow *et al.*, 1962) ; alkaline phosphatase (AP) (Carlsten *et al.*, 1961; Van Vleet and Alberts, 1968) ; 5′-nucleotidase (Housset *et al.*, 1967) ; arginase (Cornelius and Freedland, 1962) ; and lactate dehydrogenase (LDH) (Hoe and Jabara, 1967). Following an acute hepatic insult, the more liver-specific enzymes arginase, OTC, and SD return to their normal serum values in 3 to 4 days.

In chronic and low-grade progressive forms of hepatic dysfunctions of cats and dogs, such as those resulting from chronic poisoning and neoplastic infiltration, the more liver-specific enzymes such as OCT, arginase, and SD may not be signicantly elevated in serum, and GTP only mildly if at all elevated. If the disease process is sufficient to cause bile stasis, either intra- or extrahepatic, such as would a neoplasm in the head of the pancreas or fatty degeneration, serum AP may become significantly elevated only in the dog (Roberts, 1930; Carlsten *et al.*, 1961; Hoe and Jabara, 1967; Kramer and Sleight, 1968). The liver appears to be the primary source of the increase in serum enzymic activity in obstructive disorders, but it must be noted that bone and intestinal mucosa are also major contributors to normal serum. Recently, Kaplan and Righetti (1969) have presented some convincing evidence that the source of the increased serum alkaline phosphatase, in rats with ligated bile ducts, is the result of *de novo* synthesis of hepatic enzyme.

Their evidence included the use of radioisotope label and cyclohexamide. Although the experimental animals were rats, there is every indication by electrophoretic mobility studies that the same will be true in other species. The activities of selected enzymes in normal dog serum are compiled in Table III.

Cat liver alkaline phosphatase has approximately a quarter the activity of that of dog liver, and when obstruction of the biliary duct occurs, the AP of hepatic lymph increases more significantly in the dog than in the cat. It has been suggested that serum AP is passed in the urine of cats. However, it has been demonstrated that, in contrast to most other animals, the renal glomeruli of cats normally contain high levels of AP (Gomori, 1941), and AP activity of urine probably derives from the nephron. Kramer and Sleight (1968) reported that the iso-enzymes of serum AP of cats with ligated common bile ducts were found in association with α_3- and β_1-globulins, and that no significant change in their total serum activity occurred. In normal cats only the β_1-globulin form was located in the serum. The probable reason for low serum AP activity in normal cats and lack of significant change in total AP activity of cats with experimentally obstructed bile duct is the low hepatic AP content (Kritzler and Beaubien, 1949; Carlsten et al., 1961; Kramer and Sleight, 1968).

Serum AP is increased above normal adult values in such physiologic conditions as pregnancy and immaturity; it is the result of higher serum levels of placental and bone AP, respectively (Dalgaard, 1948; Gutman, 1959; Yong, 1967). In dogs with malignant lymphoma, the liver is the most common nonreticulocytic organ to be infiltrated (Van Pelt and Conner, 1968), and in cases in which it is involved, serum AP, LDH, and GPT are frequently moderately elevated (Hoe and Jabara, 1967). The source of the elevated serum LDH may be some tissues in addition to liver. In bovine lymphoma the neoplastic cells are relatively rich in LDH, and this may be the same in canine malignant lymphoma (Freedland et al., 1963). Serum AP may also be elevated in hyperadrenal-corticosteroidism and hyperparathyroidism.

b. Pigs

Orstadius et al. (1959) reported enzymic changes in the serum of pigs with nutritional hepatic dystrophy. Significant increases occured in serum MD, LDH, OCT, GPT, and GOT prior to the onset of clinical signs, but frequently there was concurrent nutritional muscular dystrophy as well as hepatic dystrophy, and the source of some of these increases was other than hepatic. Michel et al. (1969) observed increases in serum OTC in pigs with nutritional hepatic necrosis, but noted that the increase is

TABLE III

ACTIVITIES OF SERUM ENZYMES OF DOGS[a]

Enzyme	No. animals	Mean S.D.	Unit	Source
Arginase (plasma)	23	0.5 ± 0.16^b (range 0.0–4.6)	IU/liter	Cornelius et al. (1962)
Lipase		<1.0	Sigma Tietz	Cornelius (1960)
Sorbitol dehydrogenase	64	0.82 ± 0.09	IU/liter	Lettow et al. (1962)
Creatine phosphokinase	177	adult female <2 adult male <3	IU/liter	Cardinet (in preparation)
Alkaline phosphatase		100	IU/liter (phenylphosphate)[c]	Freeman et al. (1938)
		44.4	IU/liter (β-glycerophosphate)[d]	Svirbely et al. (1946)

[a] See also Table I for additional enzyme data.
[b] Converted from original units of reference to International Units (IU) per liter.
[c] 4 King Armstrong units/100 ml. serum.
[d] 5 Bodansky units/100 mg. serum.

frequently within the reported normal range. Only a moderate amount of GPT is located in pig liver, and no marked increase in serum GPT occurs following experimentally produced CCl$_4$ hepatotoxicity (Cornelius *et al.*, 1959b; Wretlind *et al.*, 1959). When ascaris larvae migrate parenterally in pigs, serum GPT, GOT, and aldolase do increase significantly (Andrews *et al.*, 1961).

c. Horses

Serum enzymes which are relatively specific for hepatocellular damage in horses are arginase (Cornelius *et al.*, 1963b), SD, glutamic dehydrogenase (GD), and ICD (Cornelius, 1961; Sova and Jicha, 1963a,b; Freedland *et al.*, 1965). Because of tissue specificity, subcellular localization, greater than the proportional increases in serum activity, and the ease of determinations of serum, sorbitol dehydrogenase (SD) would appear to be the enzyme of the choice for detecting cases of hepatocellular degeneration in horses. However, the values of the above-mentioned enzymes, including SD, generally return to normal within 4 to 5 days after a single acute insult. Serum GOT and GPT increase in the same conditions and remain elevated for 7 days and longer but are not specific for hepatic tissue. Serum GPT does not become elevated to nearly so high a degree in horses as it does in dogs and cats and, thus, is of little real use as an indicator of hepatic damage in the horse. By repeated determinations of both serum SD and GOT, a diagnosis could be confirmed and a prognosis established. The SD could give the necessary specificity, and the GOT should indicate the progression or retardation of the disease. The activities of selected enzymes in normal horse are recorded in Table IV.

TABLE IV
ACTIVITIES OF SERUM ENZYMES OF HORSES[a]

Enzyme	No. animals	Mean ± S.D. (IU/liter)	Source
Arginase (plasma)	22	10.6 ± 18.0[b] (range 0.0–70.0)	Cornelius *et al.* (1962)
Sorbitol dehydrogenase	12	0.67 ± 0.58[b] (range 0.0–1.83)	Freedland *et al.* (1965)
Creatine phosphokinase	96	1.0 ± 0.9 (range 0.0–3.0)	Gerber (1965)
	43	1.3 ± 0.9 (range 0.0–3.6)	Cardinet *et al.* (1967)

[a] Table I gives additional enzyme data.
[b] Converted from original units of reference to International Units (IU) per liter.

d. Cattle and Sheep

Serum enzyme profiles of cattle and sheep with hepatocellular degeneration are similar to those of horses. Serum GOT is elevated and remains elevated for longer periods of time than do the more liver-specific serum enzymes (Cornelius et al., 1959b; Cornelius, 1961) arginase (Cornelius et al., 1963b), glutamic dehydrogenase (GD) (Ford and Boyd, 1962), sorbitol dehydrogenase (SD) (Ford, 1965; Ford and Lawrence, 1965; Healy, 1968), which are also sensitive indicators of acute hepatocellular degeneration. Hepatic lipidosis, acetonemia, hypocalcemia and coliform mastitis are associated with significant increases in serum GOT, ICD and LDH (Cornelius et al., 1958; Ford and Boyd, 1960; Gould and Grames, 1960).

In serum of sheep and cattle with experimentally produced CCl_4, dimidium bromide, sporidesmin and ragwort hepatotoxicities, significant increases in serum OTC, GD, and SD occur. The latter three agents do not produce these changes in the serum until 3 to 30 days after their administration (Ford, 1965, 1967). With the continuous administration of a constant amount of CCl_4 to sheep, a population of resistant hepatocytes develops. However, if the treatment is interrupted for a few days the cells again become sensitive (Ford and Lawrence, 1965), indicating the possibility of either an acquired resistance to the CCl_4 or of the cell becoming sensitive as it ages.

Serum AP has wide normal ranges in both sheep and cattle, and it is of little or no clinical diagnostic significance when hepatocellular necrosis occurs (Boyd, 1962a); Ford and Boyd, 1962). However, the values in the individual animal remain constant for weeks and, thus, may be of experimental value. Significantly higher values are found in immature and pregnant animals than occur in normal adult nonpregnant animals (Allcroft and Folly, 1941; Garner, 1952).

e. Miscellaneous Species

The serum enzyme profile of rats with hepatocellular degeneration appears to be similar to that of dogs and cats. Serum GOT, GPT, fumarase, ICD, and GD are elevated in experimentally produced hepatotoxic conditions (Friedman and Lapan, 1964; Boyd, 1961).

Wisecup et al. (1969) have reported wide normal variations of serum GOT and GPT values within individual chimpanzees. In a report concerning infectious hepatitis of chimpanzees, Hartwell et al. (1968) observed serum GOT and GPT levels above normal in acutely affected individual animals, but they noted that the mean values for the acutely affected groups were not significantly greater than normal. However, as the authors have pointed out the specimens were taken only once a week, and this accounts for the absence of increased activities as they may have not been obtained during their peak activity.

V. Concluding Remarks

Serum enzymes are valuable diagnostic aids and continued development of commercially prepared, simplified kits will increase their employment and lower their cost to the point where they can be used in the smallest of veterinary clinics. Their use permits the clinician to make a more specific diagnosis and accurate surveillance of a disease process.

The search for serum enzymes with clinical significance remains active and as new reports are evaluated and become routinely utilized, simplified determination techniques will follow. Because this form of diagnostic aid is rapidly expanding, the clinician must be prepared to evaluate reports of their employment and implement them where possible. It is hoped that this review has not only presented the position as it is now but will enable the reader to evaluate the further developments of serum enzymes as diagnostic aids.

REFERENCES

Allcroft, W. M., and Folley, S. V. (1941). Observations on the serum phosphatase of cattle and sheep. *Biochemical Journal* **35**, 254–266.

Amelung, D. (1960). Untersuchungen zur Grösse der Eliminationsgeschwindigkeit von Fermenten aus dem Kaninchen-Serum. *Zeitschrift für physiologische Chemie* **318**, 219–228.

Andrews, M. F., McIlwain, P. K., and Eveleth, D. F. (1961). Serum transaminase and aldolase during migration of larval ascaris serum in swine. *American Journal of Veterinary Research* **22**, 1026–1029.

Apella, E., and Markert, C. L. (1961). Dissociation of lactate dehydrogenase into subunits with guanidine hydrochloride. *Biochemical and Biophysical Research Communications* **6**, 171–176.

Asmundson, V. S., Kratzer, F. H., and Julian, L. M. (1966). Inherited myopathy in the chicken. *Annals of the New York Academy of Sciences* **138**, 49–58.

Augustinsson, K-B. (1958). Electrophoretic separation and classification of blood plasma esterases. *Nature* **181**, 1786–1789.

Augustinsson, K-B. (1959a). Electrophoresis studies on blood plasma esterases. I. Mammalian plasmata. *Acta Chemica Scandinavica* **13**, 571–592.

Augustinsson, K-B. (1959b). Electrophoresis studies on blood plasma esterases. II. Avian, reptilian, amphibian and piscene plasmata. *Acta Chemica Scandinavica* **13**, 1081–1096.

Augustinsson, K-B. (1959c). Electrophoresis studies on blood plasma esterases. III. Conclusions. *Acta Chemica Scandinavica* **13**, 1097–1105.

Augustinsson, K-B. (1961). Multiple forms of esterase in vertebrate blood plasma. *Annals of the New York Academy of Sciences* **94**, 844–860.

Beckett. A. D., Burns, M. J., and Clark. C. H. (1964). A study of the blood glucose. serum transaminase and electrophoretic patterns of dogs with infectious canine hepatitis. *American Journal of Veterinary Research* **25**, 1186–1190.

Bergmeyer, H. U. (1963). "Methods of Enzymatic Analysis." Academic Press, New York.

Bjorsell, K. A., Holtenius, P., and Jacobsson, S. A. (1969). Studies on parturient paresis with special reference to the downer cow syndrome. *Acta Veterinaria Scandinavia* **10**, 36–43.

Blincoe, C., and Dye, W. B. (1958). Serum transaminase in white muscle disease. *Journal of Animal Science* **17**, 224–226.

Blincoe, C., and Marble, D. W. (1960). Blood enzyme interrelationships in white muscle disease. *American Journal of Veterinary Research* **21**, 866–869.

Boyd, J. W. (1961). The intracellular distribution, latency and electrophoretic mobility of L-glutamate-oxaloacetate transaminase from rat liver. *Biochemical Journal* **81**, 834–841.

Boyd, J. W. (1962a). The comparative activity of some enzymes in sheep, cattle and rats—Normal serum and tissue levels and changes during experimental liver necrosis. *Research in Veterinary Science* **3**, 256–268.

Boyd, J. W. (1962b). Glutamate-oxaloacetate transaminase isoenzymes in rat serum. *Clinica Chimica Acta* **7**, 424–431.

Brin, M. (1964). Erythrocyte as a biopsy tissue for functional evaluation of thiamine adequacy. *Journal of the American Medical Association* **187**, 762–766.

Brobst, D., and Brester, J. E. (1967). Serum lipase determination in the dog using a one-hour test. *Journal of the American Veterinary Medical Association* **150**, 767–771.

Brown, J. M. M., and Wagner, A. M. (1968). A note on the distribution of creatine phosphokinase (CPK) activity in sheep. *Journal of the South African Veterinary Medical Association* **39**, 13–15.

Brown, R. W., and Grisolia, S. (1959). Ornithine transcarbamylase activity in serum. *Journal of Laboratory and Clinical Medicine* **54**, 617–620.

Bruns, F. H., and Neuhaus, J. (1955). Die Aktivität einiger Serum- und Leberenzyme beim experimentallen Tetrachlorkohlenstoffschaden der Maus. *Biochemische Zeitschrift* **326**, 242–251.

Campbell, J. R. (1962). II. Bone dystrophy in puppies. *Veterinary Record* **74**, 1340–1348.

Cardinet, G. H., Fowler, M. E., and Tyler, W. S. (1963). The effects of training exercise and tying-up on serum transaminase activity in the horse. *American Journal of Veterinary Research* **24L**, 980–984.

Cardinet, G. H., Litterell, J. F., and Freedland, R. A. (1967). Comparative investigations of serum creatine phosphokinase and glutamic-oxaloacetic transaminase activities in equine paralytic myoglobinuria. *Research in Veterinary Science* **8**, 219–226.

Cardinet, G. H., Litterell, J. F., Holliday, T. A., and Freedland, R. A. Investigations of serum creatine phosphokinase activities in the dog. (In Preparation.)

Carlsten, A., Edland, Y., and Thulesius, O. (1961). Biliruin, alkaline phosphatase and transaminases in blood and lymph during biliary obstruction in the cat. *Acta Physiologica Scandanavica* **53**, 58–67.

Carper, H. A., and Hanson, J. B. (1967). Lactic dehydrogenase isoenzymes in the horse. *American Journal of Veterinary Clinical Pathology* **1**, 18–19.

Carper, H. A., and Roesler, A. R. (1968). A sensitive method for the determination of serum ornathine carbamyl transferase (OCT) in domestic animals. *American Journal of Veterinary Clinical Pathology* **2**, 15–20.

Castello, J. C., Sastre, F. G., and Lopez, H. U. (1967). Creatine-phosphokinase in cerebrospinal fluid from subjects with nontumorous neurological diseases. *Revista clínica española* **106**, 12–14.

Challis, T. W., Reid, C., and Hinton, J. W. (1957). Study of some factors which influence the level of serum amylase in dogs and humans. *Gastroenterology* **33**, 818–822.

Cleeve, H. (1962). Biochemical experiences in partial hepatectomy. *Journal of Clinical Pathology* **15**, 93.

Cook, V. P. (1967). Serum creatine phosphokinase in myocardial damage. *American Journal of Medical Technology* **33**, 275–280.

Cornelius, C. E. (1960). Pancreatic disease. *California Veterinarian* **14**, 24.

Cornelius, C. E. (1961). Serum isocitric dehydrogenase (SIC-D) activities in domestic animals with experimental hepatic necrosis and in equine hepatopathy. *Cornell Veterinarian* **51**, 559–568.

Cornelius, C. E., and Freedland, R. A. (1962). The determination of arginase activity in serum by means of gel filtration. *Cornell Veterinarian* **52**, 344–350.

Cornelius, C. E., and Kaneko, J. J. (1960). Serum transaminase activity in cats with hepatic necrosis. *Journal of American Veterinary Medical Association* **137**, 62–66.

Cornelius, C. E., and Kaneko, J. J., eds. (1963). "Clinical Biochemistry of Domestic Animals," p. 309. Academic Press, New York.

Cornelius, C. E., Theilen, G. S., and Rhode, E. A. (1958). Quantitative assessment of bovine liver function, using the sulfobromophthallin sodium clearance technique. *American Journal of Veterinary Research* **19**, 560–566.

Cornelius, C. E., Law, G. R., Julian, L. M., and Asmundson, V. S. (1959a). Plasma aldolase and glutamic oxaloacetic transaminase activity in inherited muscular dystrophy of domestic chickens. *Proceedings of the Society for Experimental Biology and Medicine* **101**, 41–44.

Cornelius, C. E., Bishop, J., Switzer, J., and Rhode, E. A. (1959b). Serum and tissue transaminase activities in domestic animals. *Cornell Veterinarian* **49**, 116–126.

Cornelius, C. E., Douglas, G. M., Gronwall, R. R., and Freedland, R. A. (1962). Comparative studies on plasma arginase and transaminases in hepatic necrosis. *Cornell Veterinarian* **53**, 181–191.

Cornelius, C. E., Burnham, L. G., and Hill, H. E. (1963a). Serum transaminase activities of thoroughbred horses in training. *Journal of the American Veterinary Medical Association* **142**, 639–642.

Cornelius, C. E., Douglas, G. M., Gronwall, R. R., and Freedland, R. A. (1963b). Comparative studies on plasma arginase and transaminases in hepatic necrosis. *Cornell Veterinarian* **53**, 181–191.

Crawley, G. J., and Sevenson, M. J. (1963). Blood serum enzymes as diagnostic aid in canine heart disease. *American Journal of Veterinary Research* **24**, 1271–1270.

Cunningham, V. R., Phillips, J., and Field, J. (1965). Lactic dehydrogenase isoenzymes in normal and pathological spinal fluids. *Journal of Clinical Pathology* **18**, 765–770.

Dalgaard, J. B. (1948). Phosphatase in cats with obstructive jaundice. *Acta Physiologica Scandanavica* **15**, 290–303.

Dirstine, P. H., Sorbel, C., and Henry, R. J. (1968). A new rapid method for the determination of serum lipase. *Clinical Chemistry* **14**, 1097–1106.

Dreyfus, J. C., and Shapira, G. (1954). Biochemical study of muscle in progressive muscular dystrophy. *Journal of Clinical Investigation* **33**, 794–797.

Dreyfus, J. C., Shapira, G., Shapira, F., and Demos, J. (1956). Activités enzymatiques de muscle humain. *Clinica Chimica Acta* 1, 434–449.

Dreyfus, J. C., Shapira, G., and Shapira, F. (1958). Serum enzymes in the physiopathology of muscle. *Annals of the New York Academy of Sciences* 75, 235–249.

Eshchar, J., and Zimmerman, H. J. (1967). Creatine phosphokinase in disease. *American Journal of Medical Science* 253, 272–282.

Fleisher, G. A., and McConahey, W. M. (1964). Serum creatine kinase, lactic dehydrogenase, and glutamic-oxalacetic transaminase in thyroid diseases and pregnancy. *Journal of Laboratory and Clinical Medicine* 64, 857.

Fleisher, G. A., and Wakim, K. G. (1956). Transaminase in canine serum and cerebrospinal fluid after carbon tetrachloride poisoning and injection of transaminase concentrates. *Proceedings of the Staff Meetings of the Mayo Clinic* 31, 640–648.

Ford, E. J. H. (1965). Changes in the activity of ornathine carbamyl transferase (OCT) in the serum of cattle and sheep with hepatic lesions. *Journal of Comparative Pathology* 75, 299–308.

Ford, E. J. H. (1967). Activity of sorbitol dehydrogenase in the serum of sheep and cattle with liver damage. *Journal of Comparative Pathology* 77, 405–411.

Ford, E. J. H., and Boyd, J. W. (1960). Some observations of bovine acetonaemia. *Research in Veterinary Science* 1, 232–241.

Ford, E. J. H., and Boyd, J. W. (1962). Cellular damage and changes in biliary excretion in a liver lesion of cattle. *Journal of Pathology and Bacteriology* 83, 39.

Ford, E. J. H., and Lawrence, J. A. (1965). Hepatic and serum changes following repeated administration of small amounts of carbon tetrachloride to sheep. *Journal of Comparative Pathology* 75, 185–202.

Freck, E. (1967). Uber die Kreatin-Kinase in Liquor Cerebrospinalis. *Klinische Wochenschrift* 45, 973–977.

Freedland, R. A., Theis, J. H., and Cornelius, C. E. (1963). Blood enzymes in bovine lymphosarcoma. *Annals of the New York Academy of Sciences* 108, 1313–1320.

Freedland, R. A., Hjerpe, C. A., and Cornelius, C. E. (1965). Comparative studies on plasma enzyme activities in experimental hepatic necrosis in the horse. *Research in Veterinary Science* 6, 18–23.

Freedland, R. A., Martin, K. D., and McFarland, L. Z. (1966). A survey of glutamic dehydrogenase activity in four tissues of normal and starved Coturnix. *Poultry Science* 45, 986–991.

Freeman, S., Chen, Y. P., and Ivy, A. C. (1938). On the cause of the elevation of serum phosphatase in jaundice. *Journal of Biological Chemistry* 124, 79–87.

Friedman, M. M., and Lapan, B. (1964). Enzyme activities during hepatic injury caused by carbon tetrachloride. *Clinical Chemistry* 10, 335–345.

Friend, C., Wroblewski, F., and LaDue, J. S. (1955). Glutamic-oxaloacetic transaminase activity of serum in mice with viral hepatis. *Journal of Experimental Medicine* 102, 699–704.

Garner, R. J. (1952). Serum alkaline phosphatase in cattle in health and disease. *Journal of Comparative Pathology and Therapeutics* 62, 287–291.

Geokas, M. C., Murphy, D. R., and McKenna, R. D. (1968). The role of elastase in acute pancreatitis. I. Intrapancreatic elastolytic activity in bile-induced acute pancreatitis in dogs. *Archives of Pathology* 86, 117–142.

Gerber, H. (1964a). Aktivitätsbestimmungen von Serumenzymen in der Veterinarmedizin. III. B. Bestimmung der GOT-, GPT- und CPK-Aktivität in engen Organen des Pferdes als Grundlage für die klinische Verwendung von Serum-

Enzymaktivitätsbestimmung en. *Schweizer Archiv für Tierheilkunde* 107, 410–413.

Gerber, H. (1964b). Aktivitätsbestimmungen von Serumenzymen in der Veterinarmedizin. III. C. Bestimmung der SGOT-, SGPT- und SCPK-Activität bei Myoathien und Cardiopathien des Pferdes. *Schweizer Archiv für Tierheilkunde* 107, 478–491.

Gerber, H. (1964c). Aktivitätsbestimmungen von Serumenzymen in der Veterina armedizin. III. E. Serum-enzymmuster bei paralytischer Myoglobinamie der Pferdes. *Schweizer Archiv für Tierheilkunde* 107, 685–697.

Gerber, H. (1965). Aktivitätsbestimmungen von Serumenzymen in der Veterinarmedizin. III. D. Bestimmung der LDH, MDH, SHD, SLDH, ALD und der alphaamylase Aktivität in einigen Organen des Pferdes. *Schweizer Archiv für Tierheilkunde* 107, 626–631.

Gerber, H. (1966). Aktivitätsbestimmungen von Serumenzymen in der Veterinarmedizin. III. G. LDH-isoenzyme in einigen Organen und im Serumkranken und gesunder Pferde. *Schweizer Archiv für Tierheilkunde* 108, 33–46.

Gomori, G. (1941). The distribution of phosphatase in normal organs and tissues. *Journal of Cellular and Comparative Physiology* 17, 71–83.

Gould, C. M., and Grames, F. C. (1960). Milk fever. *Veterinary Record* 72, 338–340.

Graig, F. A., and Ross, G. (1963). Serum creatine phosphokinase in thyroid disease. *Metabolism, Clinical and Experimental* 12, 57–59.

Graig, F. A., and Smith, J. C. (1965). Serum creatine phosphokinase activity in altered thyroid states. *Journal of Clinical Endocrinology and Metabolism* 25, 723–731.

Griffiths, P. D. (1963). Creatinephosphokinase levels in hypothyroidism. *Lancet* I, 894.

Grimm, F. C., and Doherty, D. G. (1961). Properties of the two forms of malic dehydrogenase from beef heart. *Journal of Biological Chemistry* 236, 1980–1985.

Gutman, A. B. (1959). Serum alkaline phosphatase activity in diseases of the skeletal and hepatobiliary systems. A consideration of the current status. *American Journal of Medicine* 27, 875–901.

Hansenfeld, D. J., Wiesmann, U., and Richtinch, R. (1962). Plasma creatine kinase activity in mice with hereditary muscular dystrophy. *Enzymologia biologica et clinica* 2, 246–249.

Hartwell, W. V., Kimbrough, R. D., and Love, G. J. (1968). Serum transaminase activity related to pathologic changes of liver in chimpanzees. *American Journal of Veterinary Research* 29, 1449–1452.

Hazlewood, C. F., and Ginski, J. M. (1968). Muscular dystrophy: *In vivo* resting membrane potential and potassium distribution in strain 129 mice. *American Journal of Physical Medicine* 47, 87–91.

Healy, P. J. (1968). Serum ornathine carbamyl transferase activity in sheep and cattle. *Clinical Chimica Acta* 22, 603–609.

Henley, K. S., Schmidt, E., and Schmidt, F. W. (1966). "Enzymes in Serum, Their Use in Diagnosis." Bannerstone House, 301–327 East Lawrence Avenue, Springfield, Illinois.

Hess, B., and Raftopoulo, R. (1957). Uber die Apfelsauredehydrogenase in menschlichen Serum, in Liquor Cerebrospinalis und anderen Korperflussigkeiten. *Deutsches Archiv für Klinische Medizin* 204, 97–106.

Hime, J. M. (1968). Some aspects of nutritional bone disease in domestic dog. A short review. *Symposia of the Zoological Society of London* 21, 2–9.

Hirschberg, E., and Osnos, M. (1962). Differential effects of inhibitors on the glutamic dehydrogenases of mouse liver, brain, and glioma. *Proceedings of the American Association of Cancer Research* **3**, 329.

Hoe, C. M., and Harvey, D. H. (1961). An investigation into liver function tests in dogs. Part I. Serum transaminase. *Journal of Small Animal Practice* **2**, 22–31.

Hoe, C. M., and Jabara, A. G. (1967). The use of serum enzymes as diagnostic aids in the dog. *Journal of Comparative Pathology* **77**, 245–254.

Hoe, C. M., and O'Shea, J. D. (1965). The correlation of biochemistry and histopathology in liver disease of the dog. *Veterinary Record* **77**, 210–218.

Holliday, T. A. (1963). Muscular hypertrophy following reinnervation of denervated muscle in normal and muscular dystrophic chickens. *Anatomical Record* **145**, 241.

Holliday, T. A. (1969). Personal communication.

Homburger, F., Nixon, C. W., Eppenberger, M., and Baker, J. R. (1966). Heriditary myopathy in the Syrian hampster: Studies on pathogenesis. *Annals of the New York Academy of Sciences* **138**, 14–27.

Housset, E., Etienne, J. P., and Petite, J. P. (1967). Alkaline phosphatase and 5'-nucleitidase activity in serum. *Revue internationale d'hépatologie* **17**, 519–536.

Hunt, R. D., Garcia, F. G., and Hegsted, D. M. (1967). A comparison of vitamin D_2 and D_3 in new world primates. I. Production and regression of osteodystrophia fibrosa. *Laboratory Animal Care* **17**, 222–234.

Hunter, R. L., and Burstone, M. S. (1960). The zymogram as a tool for the characterization of enzyme substrate specificity. *Journal of Histochemistry and Cytochemistry* **8**, 58–61.

Hunter, R. L., and Markert, C. L. (1957). Histochemical demonstration of enzymes separated by zone electrophoresis in starch gels. *Science* **125**, 1294–1295.

Kaneko, J. J., and Mills, R. (1969). Concentrations, osmotic fragility and glutathione stability in bovine porphyria erythropoeitica and its carrier state. *American Journal of Veterinary Research* **30**, 1805–1810.

Kaneko, J. J., Tanaka, S., Nakajima, N., and Ushimi, C. (1969). Some enzymes of the horse erythrocyte and their changes during experimental equine infectious anemia. *American Journal of Veterinary Research* **30**, 543–549.

Kaplan, M. M., and Righetti, A. (1969). Induction of liver alkaline phosphatase by bile duct ligation. *Biochimica et Biophysica Acta* **184**, 667–669.

Kitchen, K. (1968). Comparative biology: Animal models of human hematologic disease. *Pediatric Research* **2**, 215–229.

Kramer, J. W., and Sleight, S. D. (1968). The isoenzymes of serum alkaline phosphatase in cats. *American Journal of Veterinary Clinical Pathology* **2**, 87–91.

Kritzler, R. A., and Beaubien, J. (1949). Microchemical variation of alkaline phosphatase activity of liver in obstructive and hepatocellular jaundice. *American Journal of Pathology* **25**, 1079–1097.

Krook, L., and Love, J. E. (1964). Nutritional secondary hyperparathyroidism in the horse. *Pathologia Veterinaria (Basel)* **1**, 1–98.

Kuttler, K. L., and Marble, D. W. (1958). Relationship of serum transaminase to naturally occurring and artificially induced white muscle disease in calves and lambs. *American Journal of Veterinary Research* **19**, 632–636.

Lagace, A., Hamdy, A. H., Trapp, A. L., Bell, D. S., and Pounden, W. A. (1964). Serum transaminase in selenium treated and hysterectomy-derived lambs. *American Journal of Veterinary Research* **25**, 483–486.

Lettow, E. (1960). Transaminasen-und milchsaure Dehydrogenase-bestimmungen bein Hund. *Zentralblatt für Veterinärmedizin* **7**, 188–191.

Lettow, E., Jaeger, C., and Holm, U. (1962). Sorbitdehydrogenase und chininoxydase in Serum klinisch gesunder und liberkranker Hunde. *Zentralblatt für Veterinärmedizin* **9**, 978–988.

Lochner, A., and Brink, A. J. (1967). Oxidative phosphorylation and glycolysis in the hereditary muscular dystrophy of the Syrian hamster. *Clinical Science* **33**, 409–423.

Loeb, W. E., and Edge, L. I. (1962). A method for the determination of serum amylase in the dog. *American Journal of Veterinary Research* **23**, 1117–1118.

Markert, C. L. (1963). Lactate dehydrogenase isozymes: Dissociation and recombination of subunits. *Science* **140**, 1329–1330.

Markert, C. L., and Moller, F. (1959). Multiple forms of enzymes: Tissue ontogenetic and species specific patterns. *Proceedings of the National Academy of Sciences of the United States* **45**, 753–763.

Massarrat, S. (1965). Enzyme kinetics, half-life, and immunological properties of iodine-131-labeled transaminases in pig blood. *Nature* **206**, 508–509, 1965.

Merrill, J. M., Lemley-Stone, J., Grace, J. T., and Meneely, G. R. (1956). Recent clinical experiences with serum aminopherase (transaminase) determination. *Journal of the American Medical Association* **160**, 1454–1456.

Michel, R. L., Whitehair, C. K., and Keahey, K. K. (1969). Dietary hepatic necrosis associated with selenium—vitamin E deficiency in swine. *Journal of the American Veterinary Medical Association* **155**, 50–59.

Molander, D. W., Wroblewski, F., and LaDue, J. S. (1955). Serum glutamic oxalacetic transaminase as index of hepatocellular integrity. *Journal of Laboratory and Clinical Medicine* **46**, 831–839.

Nagode, L. A., Frajola, W. J., and Loeb, W. F. (1966). Enzyme activities of canine tissues. *American Journal of Veterinary Research* **27**, 1385–1893.

Nemir, P., Hofichter, J., and Drabkin, D. L. (1963). The protective effect of proteinasis inhibitor in acute necrotizing pancreatitis: An experimental study. *Annals of Surgery* **158**, 655–665.

Nydick, J., Ruegsegger, P., Wroblewski, F., and LaDue, J. S. (1957). Variations in serum glutamic oxaloacetic transaminase activity in experimental and clinical coronary insufficiency, pericarditis, and pulmonary infarction. *Circulation* **15**, 324–334.

Orstadius, K., Wretlind, B., Lindberg, P., Nordstrom, G., and Lannek, N. (1959). Plasma-transaminase and transferase activity in pigs affected with muscular and liver dystrophy. *Zentralblatt für Veterinärmedizin* **6**, 971–980.

Owen, L. N., and Stevenson, D. E. (1961). Observations on canine osteosoacoma. *Veterinary Science* **2**, 117–129.

Paul, J., and Fortrill, P. F. (1961). Molecular variation in similar enzymes from different species. *Annals of the New York Academy of Sciences* **94**, 668–677.

Pearson, C. M. (1957). Serum enzymes in muscular dystrophy and certain other muscular and neuromuscular diseases. *New England Journal of Medicine* **256**, 1069–1075.

Persky, L., Ravin, H., Jacob, S., and Seligman, A. M. (1934). Serum lipase activity in experimental acute hemorragic pancreatitis. *A. M. A. Archives of Surgery* **23**, 232.

Rapp, J. P. (1962). Normal values for serum amylase and maltase in dogs and the effect of maltase on the saccharogenic method for determining amylase in serum. *American Journal of Veterinary Research* **23**, 343–350.

Redman, C. M. (1968). The synthesis of serum proteins on attached rather than free ribosomes of rat liver. *Biochemical and Biophysical Research Communications* **31**, 845–850.

Reichard, H. (1959). Ornithine carbamyl transferase in dog serum on intravenous injection of enzyme, choledochus ligation, and carbon tetrachloride poisoning. *Journal of Laboratory and Clinical Medicine* **53**, 417–425.

Roberts, W. M. (1930). Variations in the phosphatase activity of blood in disease. *British Journal of Experimental Pathology* **11**, 90–95.

Robin, H., and Harley, J. D. (1967). Regulation of methemoglobinaemia in horse and human erythrocytes. *Australian Journal of Experimental Biology and Medical Science* **45**, 77–88.

Rosalki, S. B. (1963). α-Hydroxybutyrate dehydrogenase activity of human tissue homogenates. *Clinica Chimica Acta* **8**, 415–417.

Rosalki, S. B., and Wilkinson, J. H. (1959). Urinary lactic dehydrogenase in renal disease. *Lancet* **II**, 327–328.

Ruegsegger, P., Nyrick, I., Freiman, A., and LaDue, J. (1959). Serum activity patterns of glutamic oxaloacetic transaminase, glutamic pyruvic transaminase and lactic dehydrogenase following graded myocardial infarctions in dogs. *Circulation Research* **7**, 4–10.

Schapira, J., and Dreyfus, J. C. (1963). Serum creatine kinase in mice with muscular dystrophy. *Enzymologia Biologica et Clinica* **3**, 53–57.

Schmidt, E., and Schmidt, F. W. (1967). Release of enzymes from the liver. *Nature* **213**, 1125–1126.

Schmidt, E., Schmidt, F. W., and Wildhirt, E. (1958). Aktivitäts Bestimmungen von Enzymen des energieliefernden Stoffwechsels im menschlichen Serum und in Leberpunktaten bei Leburerkrankungen; ferment-aktivität-Lustimmungen in der menschlichen Leber. III. *Klinsche Wochenschrift* **36**, 280–287.

Schmidt, E., Schmidt, F. W., Herfarth, C., Optiz, K., and Vogell, W. (1966). Studien zum Austritt von zelt Enzymen an madell der isolierten, perfundierten Rattenleber. III. Analyse des bei Perfusion under hypoxie Intstehenden extracellularen enzym-musters. *Enzymologia Biologica et Clinica* **7**, 185–202.

Sibley, J. A. (1958). Significance of serum aldolase levels. *Annals of the New York Academy of Sciences* **75**, 339–348.

Siegel, S., and Bing, R. J. (1956). Plasma enzyme activity in myocardial infarction in dog and man. *Proceedings of the Society for Experimental Biology and Medicine* **91**, 604–607.

Siekert, R. G., and Fleisher, G. A. (1956). Serum glutamic oxalacetic transaminase in certain neurologic and neuromuscular diseases. *Proceedings of the Staff Meetings of the Mayo Clinic* **31**, 459–464.

Smith, J. B. (1968). Low erythrocyte glucose-6-phosphate dehydrogenase activity and primaquine insensitivity in sheep. *Journal of Laboratory and Clinical Medicine* **71**, 826–833.

Smith, J. B., and Healy, P. J. (1968). Elevated serum creatine phosphokinase activity in diseases of the central nervous system in sheep. *Clinica Chimica Acta* **21**, 295–296.

Smith, J. B., and Osborn, B. E. (1967). Glutathione deficiency in sheep erythrocytes. *Science* **158**, 374–375.

Smith, J. B., Barnes, J. K., Kaneko, J. J., and Freedland, R. A. (1965). Erythrocytic enzymes of various animal species. *Nature* **205**, 298–299.

Sova, Z., and Jicha, J. (1963a). Serum glutamic-oxalacetic acid and serum glutamic-pyruvic acid transaminase in the diagnosis of liver disease in horses. *Zentralblatt für Veterinärmedizin* **10A**, 293–304.

Sova, Z., and Jicha, J. (1936b). The activity of malic, lactic and sorbic dehydrogenases in the serum of health horses and those with liver disease. *Zentralblatt für Veterinärmedizin* **10A,** 305–313.

Stevenson, D. E. (1961). Demonstration of alkaline phosphatase activity following agar-gel electrophoresis. *Clinica Chimica Acta* **6,** 142–143.

Strandjord, P. E., Thomas, K. E., and White, L. P. (1959). Studies on isocitric and lactic dehydrogenases in experimental myocardial infarction. *Journal of Clinical Investigation* **38,** 2111–2118.

Svirbely, J. L., Monaco, A. R., and Alford, W. C. (1946). The comparative efficiency of various liver function tests in detecting hepatic damage produced in dogs by xylidine. *Journal of Laboratory and Clinical Medicine* **31,** 1133.

Swingle, K. F., and Young, S. (1959). The relationship of serum glutamic oxaloacetic transaminase to nutritional muscular dystrophy in lambs. *American Journal of Veterinary Research* **20,** 75–77.

Tada, K., Watanabe, Y., and Fujiwara, T. (1961). The enzyme activities and coenzyme contents in the reticulocyte of rabbits. *Tohoku Journal of Experimental Medicine* **75,** 384–392.

Thorne, C. J. R. (1960). Characterization of two malic dehydrogenase from rat liver. *Biochimica et Biophysica Acta* **42,** 175–176.

Valentine, W. N. (1968). Hereditary hemolytic anemias associated with specific erythrocyte enzymopathies. *California Medicine* **108,** 280–294.

Van Pelt, R. W., and Conner, G. H. (1968). Clinicopathologic survey of malignant lymphoma in the dog. *Journal of the American Medical Association* **152,** 976–989.

Van Vleet, J. F., and Alberts, J. (1968). Evaluation of liver function tests and liver biopsy in experimental carbon tetrachloride intoxication and extrahepatic bile duct obstruction in the dog. *American Journal of Veterinary Research* **29,** 2119–2131.

Veery, F. (1962). Diagnostic significance of cerebrospinal fluid enzymes in children (glutamatic-oxaloacetate transaminase, glutamate-pyruvate transaminase, lactic dehydrogenase and sorbitol dehydrogenase). *Enzymologia Biologica et Clinica* **2,** 233–245.

Vessell, E. S., and Bearn, A. G. (1961). Isozymes of lactic dehydrogenase in human tissues. *Journal of Clinical Investigation* **40,** 586–591.

Weyer, E. D. (1966). Experimental primary myopathies and their relationship to human muscle disease. *Annals of the New York Academy of Sciences* **138,** No. 1.

White, L. P. (1958). Some enigmas in the comparison of multiple serum enzyme levels. *Annals of the New York Academy of Sciences* **75,** 349–356.

Wieland, T., Pfleiderer, G., Haupt. I., and Worner, W. (1959). Über die Verschiedenheit der Milchsäuredrogenasen. IV. Quantitative Ermittlung einiger Enzymuerteilungmuster. Vergleichende betrachtung bei verschienden wirbeltierklassen. *Biochemische Zeitschrift* **332,** 1–10.

Wilkinson, J. H. (1962). "An Introduction to Diagnostic Enzymology." Spottiswoode, Ballantyne & Co. Ltd., London and Colchester, Great Britain.

Wisecup, W. G., Hodson, H. H., Jr., Hamly, W. C., and Felts, P. E. (1969). Baseline blood levels of the chimpanzee (*Pan troglodytes*): Liver function tests. *American Journal of Veterinary Research* **30,** 955–962.

Wretlind, B., Orstadius, K., and Lindberg, P. (1959). Transaminase and transferase activities in blood plasma and tissues of normal pigs. *Zentralblatt für Veterinärmedizin* **6,** 963–970.

Wroblewski, F. (1958). The mechanisms of alteration in lactic dehydrogenase activity of body fluids. *Annals of the New York Academy of Sciences* **75**, 322–338.

Wroblewski, F., and LaDue, J. S. (1955). Serum glutamic oxalacetic transaminase activity as index of liver all injury: Preliminary report. *Annals of Internal Medicine* [N. S.] **43**, 345–360.

Wrogemann, K., and Blanchaer, M. C. (1968). Respiration and oxidative phosphorylation by muscle and heart mitochondria of hamsters with hereditary and myocardispathy and polymyopathy. *Canadian Journal of Biochemistry* **46**, 323–329.

Wurzner, P. (1964). Einblicke in die neuev Enzymeiagnostik der Veterinarmedizin. *Tierärztliche Umschau* **19**, 511–516.

Yong, J. M. (1967). Origins of serum alkaline phosphatase. *Journal of Clinical Pathology* **20**, 647–653.

Zelman, S., Wang, C., and Appelhanz, J. (1959). Transaminases in serum and liver correlated with liver cell necrosis in needle aspiration biopsies. *American Journal of the Medical Sciences* **237**, 323–334.

Zierler, K. L. (1958a). Increased muscle permeability to aldolase produced by insulin and by albumin. *American Journal of Physiology* **192**, 283–286.

Zierler, K. L. (1958b). Increased muscle permeability to aldolase produced by depolarization and by metabolic inhibitors. *American Journal of Physiology* **193**, 534–540.

Zimmerman, H. J., Schwartz, M. A., Boley, L. E., and West, M. (1965). Comparative serum enzymology. *Journal of Laboratory and Clinical Medicine* **66**, 961–972.

Zinkle, J. G., Bush, R. M., Freedland, R. A., and Cornelius, C. E. Comparative studies on plasma and tissue sorbitol, glutamic, lactic and hydrogenase in the dog. (In Preparation).

Avian Infectious Bronchitis*

CHARLES H. CUNNINGHAM†

*Department of Microbiology and Public Health College of Veterinary Medicine,
Michigan State University, East Lansing, Michigan*

* Journal Article No. 4761 from the Michigan Agricultural Experiment Station.
† The author is Professor of Microbiology and Public Health, College of Veterinary Medicine, Michigan State University, East Lansing, Michigan.

I. Introduction

Early studies of avian infectious bronchitis (AIB) were concerned primarily with clinical manifestations of the disease and, later, with methods for the isolation and identification of the etiologic agent—the familiar pathways of investigations of a newly described infectious disease. So, frequently, the properties of an etiologic agent are the last to receive attention and infectious bronchitis virus (IBV) was no exception.

Following the establishment of AIB as a distinct disease, the utilization of progressively developing research techniques in multidisciplinary areas yielded a considerable body of information on the morphologic and biologic properties of the virus. The realization prevails today that certain properties of IBV are shared by several viruses of man and animals for which IBV is considered the prototype (Section IV,1). This emphasizes starkly the magnitude of possible interrelationships of viral etiologic agents. It is evident, too, that approaches to basic and comparative virology are seldom separable on a host species basis and that they cannot be resolved promptly and strictly into spheres of human or veterinary virology.

Research events of the past few years, a period that might be considered the maturation or "modern" period of IBV research, have now placed IBV, "IBV-like," and related viruses on common view for examination. It is as though IBV and its previously described properties were awaiting discovery.

Reflection upon the immediate past, and perspectives for the future, would indicate that basic information thus gained on IBV will be more than adequate to solve practical and applied problems of the disease it produces. Human counterparts of IBV and the relationship of certain respiratory diseases in birds and man suggest the possibility of another emerging or evolving group of pathogens.

This chapter is not intended to be an annotated bibliography or an exhaustive review of all the literature on AIB and the virus, but rather a broad overview of the relevance and relationship of some of the important early and recent findings as concepts of advances in the subject. The reader is referred to the cited references for review of specific areas of interest. Any errors of omission or commission in this chapter are unintentional by the author and should not be interpreted as minimizing or emphasizing the importance of subject matter areas or of contributions by individuals or groups.

1. DEFINITION

Avian infectious bronchitis is an acute, highly contagious, viral respiratory disease of chickens characterized by generalized respiratory distress, tracheal rales, coughing associated with the accumulation of excess mucus in the bronchii, and sneezing. In young chicks, there is also a nasal discharge. A precipitous drop of egg production occurs in laying flocks.

2. SYNONYMS

Infectious bronchitis, infektiösen bronchitis der Hühner (German), infektiöse bronchitis des Geflugels (German), la bronchite infectieuse (French), la bronchite infectieuse des gallines (French), la bronquitis infecciosa (Spanish), la bronquitie infecciosa das galinhas (Portuguese) are all synonyms.

3. ECONOMIC AND PUBLIC HEALTH SIGNIFICANCE

Avian infectious bronchitis is of considerable economic importance to the poultry industry not only as a result of high morbidity and, in some instances, mortality, but also from the debilitating nature of the disease with resulting poor utilization of feed by young chickens. The major economic loss is from ovarian damage and the precipitous and prolonged decrease in egg production in laying flocks.

Programs for immunization against the disease are costly to the poultry producer. In broiler flocks, the stress from natural infection or from vaccination may be a predisposing factor to other infections.

The virus is not presently known to be of public health significance although viruses related to it have been isolated from persons with colds (Almeida and Tyrrell, 1967; Becker et al., 1967; McIntosh et al., 1967), and neutralizing antibodies have been detected in blood from persons working with diseased birds (Miller and Yates, 1968).

II. History

The pages of history are often closed and relegated to the far corners and depths of archives to gather dust and to be ignored or forgotten. They should be opened from time to time and examined to appreciate the heritage from initial contributions, to evaluate the present status, and to give thought to perspectives. It is fitting that this be done for AIB, a disease which has emerged within the last 4 decades from the melange of the "respiratory disease complex" of poultry to a well-defined and separate entity today.

Avian infectious bronchitis, the name currently receiving preference to "infectious bronchitis" as a more definitive description, was first described and reported by Schalk and Hawn in 1931 as "an apparently new respiratory disease of baby chicks" in North Dakota in April, 1930 and throughout the North Central region of the U. S. A. The major concern was the extremely high mortality rate of infected chicks. While transmission studies were inconclusive, they did suggest the viral nature of the disease.

Although the authors were unable to find published descriptions of the identical disease, they did establish certain facts as to its nature. It is interesting to record their cautious but suggestive conclusions: "We have refrained from specifically naming the disease under discussion. It materially differs, in one phase or another, from any of the established respiratory diseases of poultry. On the other hand, it has some of the characteristics of catarrhal roup, laryngotracheitis, and perhaps more things in common with infectious bronchitis of adult fowls. Therefore, if we were pressed for a definite name we would be inclined to entitle it: infectious bronchitis of baby chicks."

Among some of the other early historic milestones of AIB were the establishment by Beach and Schalm (1936) that the etiologic agent was a virus, the first cultivation of the virus in embryonating chicken eggs by Beaudette and Hudson (1937) and modification of the virus in this medium by Delaplane and Stuart (1941), an immunization program in 1941 by Van Roekel (Van Roekel *et al.*, 1951), and identification of maternal immunity by Jungherr and Terrell (1948).

III. Incidence and Distribution

Chickens of all ages, sexes, and breeds are susceptible to natural or artificial infections with IBV. According to the review by Estola (1966), the disease is of world wide prevalence.

IV. Etiology

1. CLASSIFICATION

Classification of a virus such as IBV, which possesses some properties similar to those of a major group of viruses as well as some unique properties of its own, posed complications that could not be resolved until more adequate information was available.

Infectious bronchitis virus, at least on the basis of medium size (Section IV,2,a), ribonucleic acid (RNA) content (Section IV,3,a), and ether sensitivity (Section IV,3,b), has properties similar to the myxo- and paramyxoviruses. It has been suggested previously that IBV might be included tentatively with the myxoviruses on these bases (Cunningham, 1963; Cabasso, 1965; Estola, 1966; Estola and Weckström, 1967; Tevethia and Cunningham, 1968). The virus has been included also in a group identified as "other RNA-helical-enveloped viruses" (Wilner, 1969).

Extracellular IBV differs, however, from the myxo- and paramyxo-viruses in the shape and distribution of the surface projections (Section IV,2,a), only partial disruption of the virion by ether without the release of recognizable internal components or the formation of rosettes (Section IV,3,b), and the lack of direct hemagglutination except under special conditions (Section IV,8).

Berry *et al.* (1964) examined several properties of IBV and concluded that when its unique morphologic and biologic characteristics were compared to those of influenza virus, the proper place of IBV in classification would have to await further information. Similar caution has been expressed (Akers, 1963) with respect to the cytopathic effects (CPE) produced by IBV on chicken embryo kidney cell (CEKC) culture (Section IV,11,c) as a marker for classification.

By means of electron microscopy, Almeida and Tyrrell (1967) examined uncharacterized viruses, 229E (Hamre and Procknow, 1966), B814 (Tyrrell and Bynoe, 1965), and Lakey (Tyrrell and Bynoe, 1965) that cause human respiratory disease and reported the following: "Probably the most interesting finding from these experiments was that two human respiratory viruses, 229E and B814, are morphologically identical with avian infectious bronchitis. Their biological properties, as far as they are known, are consistent with this."

McIntosh *et al.* (1967) verified Almeida and Tyrrell's original recognition (1967) of the indistinguishable morphologic features of IBV and 229E and found that additional isolates of "IBV-like" viruses from persons with respiratory disease had the same features.

Studies of the morphogenesis of IBV and 229E by Becker *et al.* (1967) and of IBV by Nazerian and Cunningham (1968) added the further information (Section IV,5,a) that, although this group of viruses shared some properties with the myxo- and paramyxoviruses, they differed in morphologic features as intracellular and extracellular virus.

The size, RNA content, and ether sensitivity of mouse hepatitis virus (David-Ferreira and Manaker, 1965; Mallucci, 1965) are also similar to IBV.

In recognition of mutual interest in a new group of viruses emerging with some members which infect the respiratory tract of birds and man and others the liver of mice, an informal group of virologists (Tyrrell *et al.*, 1968) proposed that these avian, human, and murine viruses be named "coronaviruses" with IBV as the prototype. This name was selected because of the characteristic resemblance of the viruses to the solar corona. In addition to the previously mentioned properties, these viruses have a similar density and they replicate in cytoplasmic vesicles.

The suggestion for naming this group of viruses is now being considered by the Vertebrate Virus Committee of the International Committee for the Nomenclature of Viruses.

Although many isolates of IBV from various parts of the world have been studied, there is no uniform system of designation of members of the group such as is used for certain other groups of viruses. Frequently, identity is either designated by an accession number in a diagnostic laboratory where the particular virus was isolated, the name of the flock owner, the name of the state, the name of the original investigator, an arbitrarily designated numerical system, or other systems.

The Beaudette strain, which has been used most frequently for various studies, is the virus originally isolated by Beaudette and Hudson (1937) and passed hundreds of times in chicken embryos. It is commonly referred to as the "chicken embryo adapted" strain. Many investigators retain the proper name in honor of the late Dr. F. R. Beaudette of New Jersey who contributed so much to the early work on AIB.

Van Roekel *et al.* (1951) first isolated the strain now known as the Massachusetts virus and maintained it in chicken passage. This virus was designated the Van Roekel strain in early literature but Dr. H. Van Roekel modestly requested deletion of his name with substitution of the name of the state of origin.

An arbitrary numerical code system by the author for various isolates of the virus has resulted in references to IBV-41, IBV-42, and IBV-46 which identify the Massachusetts, Beaudette, and Connecticut strains, respectively. These codes have been retained by some investigators to whom the viruses have been supplied.

2. MORPHOLOGIC FEATURES

a. Size and Shape

Although negatively stained extracellular IBV (Fig. 1) has, in part, a superficial architectural resemblance to the myxo- and paramyxoviruses, the most characteristic morphologic feature that sets it apart from the above group of viruses, according to composite data from recent reports, is the shape of the surface projections. Further distinctive evidence is found in the unique features of the virus during replication (Section IV,5,*a*).

Early microscopy (Reagan and Brueckner, 1952) of shadow cast virus in allantoic fluid indicated the diameter of the Beaudette, Wachtel, Massachusetts, and Michigan strains to be from 60 to 100 mμ.

Berry *et al.* (1964) examined the A163 and H17 strains isolated in England and the Connecticut and Beaudette strains of the U. S. A. All 4 strains in allantoic fluid closely resembled each other and were described

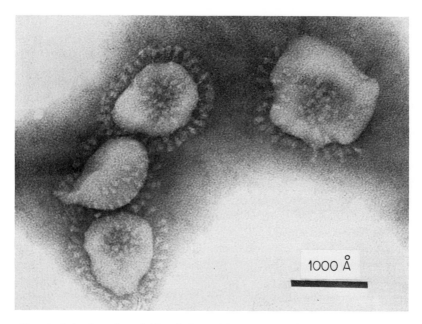

FIG. 1. Infectious bronchitis viral particles treated with unheated nonimmune rabbit serum. The particles remain unaltered and illustrate the morphologic features of the virus. ×250,000. (Berry and Almeida, 1968.)

as being considerably pleomorphic with diameters between 800 and 1200 Å. The pear-shaped or bulbous surface projections, 90 to 110 Å in diameter on the distal end, were attached to the virus by a narrow neck. It was emphasized that the surface projections of IBV differed from those of influenza virus which are rod-shaped or straight projections.

The report by Berry *et al.* (1964), and the prompt recognition by Almeida and Tyrrell (1967) that the human respiratory viruses 229E and B814 were morphologically identical to IBV, was the first clue to the individual and common properties of these viruses which defined their differences from the myxo- and paramyxoviruses.

Estola and Weckström (1967) examined a Finnish strain of IBV (IBV$_F$) in allantoic and CEKC fluids, and it was their opinion that no structural properties were found to argue distinctly against the classification of IBV among myxoviruses. The virus was between 100 and 120 mμ in diameter with a slight tendency to pleomorphism. They stated, however, that the surface projections were either straight or had a knoblike dilation at the distal end, but gave no clear impression of the pear shape described by Berry *et al.* (1964).

According to McIntosh *et al.* (1967), the Beaudette virus in allantoic fluid and 229E and B814 viruses in fluids from cell and organ cultures have an overall diameter of 160 mμ with a variation $\pm$40 mμ, all are moderately pleomorphic without filaments or tails, and the widely spaced surface projections distributed fairly uniformly on the surface of the virus are 20 mμ long, narrow at the base, but 10 mμ wide at the outer edge.

Surface projections of the Beaudette virus in CEKC fluid (Nazerian, 1965) and of the Massachusetts virus in allantoic fluid as reported by Nazerian and Cunningham (1967) were not as pronounced as those described by other authors.

The recent work by Berry and Almeida (1968) substantiates all previous microscopy of negatively stained virus in allantoic fluid (Fig. 1).

There has been no clear evidence of the internal structure of any of the IBV viruses examined.

The virus in cells of the chorioallantoic membrane (CAM) of embryonated chicken eggs was first examined by Domermuth and Edwards (1957) using the shadow cast technique. The virus appeared to be round, average diameter of 178 mμ, and was arranged in clumps, short chains, in pairs, or singly. Some particles were 200 mμ in diameter with a doughnut shape.

The Beaudette virus stained in the cytoplasm of cells of the CAM (Becker et al., 1967) (Figs. 2 and 3) and of fibroblast cultures from the chicken embryo (Nazerian and Cunningham, 1968) (Fig. 4) has an overall diameter of 67 to 110 mμ (mean 82 mμ) (Becker et al., 1967), but the surface projections so characteristic of extracellular virus are not evident. The virus does not have a distinct nucleoid, but it does possess a double membrane or shell (Becker et al., 1967; Nazerian and Cunningham, 1968) composed of a 7 to 8 mμ inner shell and a 9 to 17 mμ outer shell (Becker et al., 1967). The virus lacks an electron transport zone between the outer and inner shells. The morphologic features of IBV, in general, are shared by 229E (Becker et al., 1967) and mouse hepatitis (David-Ferreira and Manaker, 1965; Becker et al., 1967) viruses.

The virus passes readily through Berkefeld V, N, and W filters (Beach and Schalm, 1936; Beaudette and Hudson, 1937) and Seitz EK filters. From the data with filters of graded porosity, the size of the virus is about 100 mμ (Muldoon and Cunningham, 1961; Estola, 1966; Tevethia and Cunningham, 1968) which agrees closely with the results from centrifugation and electron microscopy.

b. Density and Sedimentation Coefficient

The density of the Beaudette virus from allantoic fluid is 1.23 (Cunningham, 1966b; Tevethia and Cunningham, 1968) and from CEKC it is 1.24 (Ellis, 1965; Cunningham, 1966b), as determined by isopycnic density gradient centrifugation with CsCl which has an inactivating effect on the virus. Linear sucrose density gradients for both zonal and isopycnic gradient centrifugation markedly improve the recovery of infectious virus as compared to CsCl, and the density is 1.19. The sedimentation constant is 334 S, from which the virus is calculated to be spherical with dimensions between 80 to 100 mμ (Ellis, 1965; Cunningham, 1966b) which agrees closely with those obtained by filtration and electron microscopy.

In terms of infectivity as plaque forming units (PFU), a 868-fold purification of the Beaudette virus is obtainable after 2 cycles of centrifugation at 109,000 $\times$ g with a reduction of greater than 99% protein (Tevethia and Cunningham, 1968).

3. Viral Components

a. Nucleic Acid

Infectious bronchitis virus contains RNA as determined by fluorescence microscopy with acridine orange and susceptibility of the virus to RNase (Akers, 1963; Cunningham, 1963; Akers and Cunningham, 1968) and to coriphosphine (Berry, 1967).

Further evidence that IBV is an RNA-containing virus is the suppression of viral replication by DL-parafluorophenylalanine, an inhibitor of synthesis of RNA, and the lack of effect by aminopterin (4-aminopteroyl-L-glutamic acid) (Akers, 1963; Cunningham, 1963; Akers and Cunningham, 1968), 5-bromouracil and 6-azauracil (Akers, 1963), and by halogenated deoxyuridine derivatives such as 5-iodo-2'-deoxyuridine, 5-bromo-2'-deoxyuridine, and 5-fluoro-2'-deoxyuridine which are inhibitors of synthesis of deoxyribonucleic acid (DNA) (Estola, 1966).

b. Lipid

The presence of essential lipids in the virus is evidenced by its sensitivity to ether (Petek and Corazzola, 1958; Akers, 1963; Mohanty and Chang, 1963; Berry et al., 1964; Biswal et al., 1966; Cunningham, 1966b; Estola, 1966; Nazerian and Cunningham, 1967; Akers and Cunningham, 1968; Tevethia and Cunningham, 1968), chloroform (Estola, 1966; von Bülow, 1967a), sodium dodecyl sulfate (Berry et al., 1964), and sodium deoxycholate (Estola, 1966; Tevethia and Cunningham, 1968).

Ether (Berry et al. 1964; Nazerian and Cunningham, 1967) and sodium dodecyl sulfate (Berry et al., 1964) remove the surface projections from the virus and split the coat with the release of the internal components, but their structure has not been determined. Virus thus treated does not form rosettes as do the myxo- and paramyxoviruses treated in the same fashion.

c. Enzyme

Neuraminidase-like activity is associated with the hemagglutinin of the Massachusetts virus which linearly liberates N-acetylneuraminic acid from N-acetylneuraminic acid–lactose in 30 minutes with the optimum at 37°C., pH 6.5. The neuraminidase activity of the hemagglutinin is destroyed in 45 minutes at 56°C. (Biswal, 1965; Biswal et al., 1966) (Section IV,8).

According to Berry et al. (1964) neuraminidase is not detectable by direct chemical analysis of their viruses concentrated by centrifugation for electron microscopy.

d. Protein

The surface projections of the virus are not only morphologically unique but their possible chemical composition is of interest. The presence of sulfhydryl-containing components, or thiols, of the viral protein is indicated by inactivation of the virus by p-hydroxymercuribenzoate as a first-order reaction and the arresting or reversal of the reaction by L-cysteine. L-Cysteine in itself has no deleterious effect on the virus. Virus inactivated by it can be reactivated by dialysis to remove the L-cysteine (Powers, 1965; Cunningham, 1966b; Lukert, 1967). Thiol groups are involved in both viral and cellular receptors (Lukert, 1967) (Section IV,5,b).

4. RESISTANCE TO PHYSICAL AND CHEMICAL AGENTS

a. Heat

Most strains of IBV in allantoic fluid as tested in chicken embryos are inactivated at 56°C. in 15 minutes (Hofstad, 1956; Quiroz and Hanson, 1958; Estola, 1966), but some survive for 30 to 45 minutes (Hofstad, 1956), 60 to 75 minutes (Singh, 1960), and others for up to 160 minutes (von Bülow, 1967a).

Survival curves reflect quantitative thermal sensitivity differences between strains of the virus (Singh, 1960; von Bülow, 1967a). Thermal sensitivity appears to be related to the number of passages of a strain of virus in chicken embryos. The Beaudette virus, which is sensitive (S) to 56°C. for about 10 minutes, has been included in most studies of the parameters of sensitivity at various temperatures because of its extensive use as the antigen in neutralization tests (Section IV,9).

Strains of IBV in low numbers of passages in chicken embryos have been reported to have characteristic 2-component survival curves of first-order kinetics for each (Singh, 1960) indicative of S and thermal resistant particles (R) in the same population. After selective inactivation of S particles, the specific reaction rate (k) for the recovered R particles is similar to that for R in the mixed population. The R particles can be maintained as a single component in successive passages in chicken embryos with a paralleling increase in k. At the 13th passage, k approaches, but does not equal, k for the S particles in the original SR population. Two-component survival curves can be reproduced with a mixture of recovered R particles and S particles (Beaudette virus).

Inactivation of the Beaudette virus in allantoic fluid as tested in chicken embryos (Page and Cunningham, 1962) and in cell culture fluid as tested by PFU in CEKC (Cunningham and Spring, 1965) follows first-order kinetics. The energy of activation for inactivation of the virus is of the approximate order of 23,000 calories per mole with chicken embryos and 29,500 calories per mole with CEKC.

The Massachusetts virus in allantoic fluid as tested in chickens maintains its pathogenicity for at least 24 hours in water buffered at pH 6.39 to 7.85 (Raggi, 1958).

Lyophilized Iowa 33 and 97 viruses sealed *in vacuo* are inactive in about 6 months at 37°C. with 2-component survival curves (Hofstad and Yoder, 1963).

Virus can be stored for long periods at low temperatures, preferably —60°C. or lower, as infective allantoic or cell culture fluids.

b. Ionic Stabilization against Heat

The effect of salt solutions on the thermal stability of IBV in allantoic fluid and tested quantitatively in chicken embryos is of interest (Hopkins, 1967). The Beaudette virus is more stable in $1\,M$ $MgSO_4$, Na_2SO_4, Na_2HPO_4, or K_2SO_4 than in $1\,M$ NaCl, KCl, $CaCl_2$, or $MgCl_2$, especially at 50°C. for up to 80 minutes. The Massachusetts, Connecticut, and Iowa 97 viruses are stabilized in $1\,M$ $MgSO_4$ at 50°C. for at least 40 minutes. Results with all 4 strains in distilled water are similar on inactivation of the virus to those previously described. The inactivation rates are dependent on the type and concentration of the salt, as well as time and temperature. The stabilizing activity of the salts appears to be related to their anions and their valence.

c. pH

The Beaudette virus in allantoic fluid at 4°C. is stable at pH 3.0 for 14 days, labile at pH 10.6 in 2 days, with maximal stability at pH 7.8

for 170 days as tested qualitatively in chicken embryos (Cunningham and Stuart, 1947). At room temperature, the virus is stable at pH 2.0 for an hour (Quiroz and Hanson, 1958).

In cell culture fluid, the Beaudette virus assayed by PFU in CEKC is stable at 4°C. when tested at 30 minutes at pH 3.0 but labile at pH 11.0 (Stinski and Cunningham, 1969).

The IBV_F in cell culture fluid is labile at pH 2.9 to 3.1 in 4 hours at room temperature and stable at pH 7.1 to 7.3, based on CPE in CEKC (Estola, 1966).

d. Chemical Agents

The Beaudette virus is inactivated in 3 minutes at room temperature by many agents commonly employed for disinfection among which are 1% liquor cresolis saponatus, 1% phenol, 1/10,000 $KMnO_4$, 70% ethyl alcohol, and 1% formalin as tested qualitatively in chicken embryos (Cunningham and Stuart, 1946). Another report indicates that 1% phenol has no effect on the virus in an hour at room temperature (Quiroz and Hanson, 1958).

Inactivation of the Beaudette virus by formalin (1/2,000 and 1/4,000), pH 7.5, at 37°C. is linear, whereas inactivation of 4 strains of IBV in low numbers of chicken embryo passages is curvilinear (Singh, 1960). Recovered R particles (Section IV,4,a) of 2 of the viruses were more resistant to formalin than their SR population.

Virus in the liquid state and virus dried over anhydrous $CaCl_2$ is inactivated in 16 hours by 10% ethylene dioxide gas, but virus previously dehydrated by sublimation is not inactivated under the same conditions (Mathews and Hofstad, 1953).

There are several reports of the effect of trypsin on IBV, but the results are not uniform. This may be due to differences among the strains and the methods employed. Further investigations should be made to ascertain the reasons for the discrepancies.

One group of workers (Corbo and Cunningham, 1959; Muldoon, 1960; Nazerian, 1960; Muldoon and Cunningham, 1961; Cunningham, 1963; Nazerian and Cunningham, 1967) has presented evidence that trypsin inactivates several strains of IBV from the U.S.A.

In an early study using the shadow cast technique for electron microscopy (Nazerian, 1960), it was reported that trypsin removed a 17 to 22 mμ thick outer coat of the virus. With the negative staining technique (Nazerian, 1965; Nazerian and Cunningham, 1967), the reduction in size of the virus was found to be due to the removal of the surface projections by trypsin.

On the basis of the above results, and those with sulfhydryl reagents and lipid solvents (Section IV,3,b,d), it may be concluded that lipoproteins are associated with at least the surface projections of IBV.

Other authors report that certain strains of IBV remain morphologically normal (Berry et al., 1964) and infectious (Steele and Luginbuhl, 1964; Estola, 1966; von Bülow, 1967a) after treatment with trypsin.

5. REPLICATION

Recent advances in some of the physical and biologic aspects of the intracytoplasmic replication of IBV permit a more definite interpretation of the sequential events.

a. Physical

According to electron microscopy (Becker et al., 1967), the time of first appearance of viral particles in the endoplasmic reticulum of cells lining the CAM following intra-allantoic inoculation is related to the concentration of virus in the inoculum: 12 hours with high concentrations

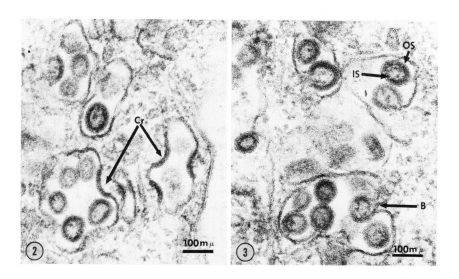

FIG. 2. Infectious bronchitis virus in the chorioallantoic membrane. Crescents (Cr) are formed by the bulging of cisternal membranes and the close apposition of a dense underlying layer. × 69,000. (Becker et al., 1967.)

FIG. 3. Infectious bronchitis viral particles in the chorioallantoic membrane. The complete viral particle has a double outer shell (OS) and a dense inner shell (IS) surrounded by a core of amorphous material. There is continuity of the vesicular membrane with the OS of a budding particle (B). ×69,000. (Becker et al., 1967.)

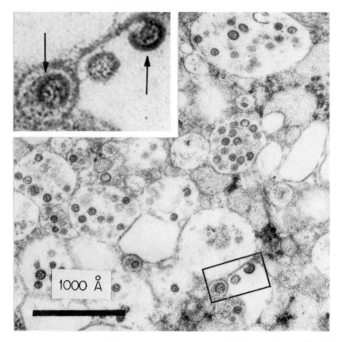

1000 Å

Fɪɢ. 4. Infectious bronchitis viral particles in chicken embryo fibroblasts in advanced stage of infection. × 30,000. Cellular organelles cannot be distinguished but viral particles are within numerous vesicles. The inset is a higher magnification (× 100,000) of viral particles in the outlined area. The nucleoid is not distinct and the shell is poorly defined. (Nazerian and Cunningham, 1968.)

of the Beaudette 66579 virus and death of the embryo in 24 hours, and 18 hours with low concentrations of the Beaudette (IBV-42) virus but with death of the embryo delayed for 6 to 12 hours later than with the 66579 virus.

The developing viral particles appear first in the form of a crescent of the vesicular membrane bulging from the cytoplasm into the vesicular lumen with incorporation of the membrane into the outer coat of the virus (Figs. 2 and 3). As the crescent continues to bulge, the inner shell is completed and the outer double membrane is pinched off. Although it is possible that some of the cytoplasm communicated directly with the extracellular space, budding was not seen to occur at the cell membrane.

Replication of the CEKC-propagated Beaudette virus in chicken embryo fibroblast cultures is entirely cytoplasmic by budding into cytoplasmic vesicles (Fig. 4) but not at the cell membrane (Nazerian and Cunningham, 1968). The vesicles appeared, however, to open to the surface of the cell for release of the virus.

b. Biologic

(1) *Embryonated chicken eggs.* The time of the beginning and end of the log phase of the virus in allantoic fluid from chicken embryos inoculated intra-allantoically, and measured by the quantal dose-response in chicken embryos as the median embryo infective dose$_{50}$ (EID$_{50}$), is related to the concentration and embryo passage level of the virus.

With a high concentration of low embryo passage virus as the inoculum, the log phase begins at about 6 hours. When lesser amounts of virus are used, the log phase is delayed for 12 or 18 hours. In all cases, the end of the log phase occurs bewteen 24 and 30 hours followed by a gradual decline during the next 12 to 20 hours (Hitchner and White, 1955; Muldoon, 1960; Singh, 1960; Yates *et al.*, 1968).

High embryo passage virus may be in the log phase as early as 4 hours with the maximum at 18 hours (Hitchner and White, 1955).

The chicken embryo is approximately 1.0 log unit more sensitive than CEKC to IBV (Lukert, 1965; von Bülow, 1966a) and approximately 3.0 log units more sensitive than chicken embryo liver cells (CELiC) (Lukert, 1965).

(2) *Cell culture.* Cultures of CEKC (Section IV,11,c) are the most sensitive to IBV (Lukert, 1965; von Bülow, 1966a,b). Although initial adsorption of IBV to CEKC is inefficient, this cell system has been used as the model for studies of replication of the virus.

Adsorption of virus is relatively temperature independent but the efficiency at 4°C. ranges from about 10% (Lukert, 1967) to 30% (Stinski, 1969), and at 37°C. it is about 40% (Lukert, 1967; Stinski, 1969) based on infectivity tests as PFU. Entry of the virus into the cell is temperature dependent.

Beaudette virus labeled with ^{32}P adsorbs to but does not enter the cell at 4°C. for an hour (Stinski, 1969). Virus thus adsorbed is not dissociated from the cell when treated with buffer at pH 2.0 for 10 seconds, and the cell is unaffected. At 25°C. or 37°C., the rate constants of entry of the virus into the cell are linear and related directly to temperature. After 2 hours at 37°C., there is a significant intracellular degradation of the virus with the ^{32}P activity related to acid-soluble, RNase-sensitive material.

In addition to temperature, the complexity of initial adsorption of the Beaudette virus is influenced not only by the heterogeneity of the cell types in CEKC which differ in their susceptibility, but also by thiol groups, a macromolecular inhibitor associated with γ-globulins ranging from 7 to 19 S in bovine, swine, chicken, and rabbit serum reversible by a number of simple sugars (Lukert, 1967), and by neuraminidase (Biswal *et al.*, 1966). All these substances have an effect on and are related to the receptor sites of virus and host cells.

Syncytia (Akers, 1963; Lukert, 1966a; Akers and Cunningham, 1968) are sequentially and directly related to the various stages of the replication and release of the virus and provide a unique microscopic marker of the CPE of the virus. Subsequent necrosis of the syncytia is reflected as plaques demonstrable by the agar overlay method (Section IV,11,*c*).

It has been established (Lukert, 1965) from one-step growth curves of cell-associated and released virus that the eclipse phase of the virus in CEKC is about 4 to 5 hours followed by the log phase with maximum infectivity in about 12 to 16 hours. In CELiC, the eclipse phase is about 6 to 7 hours followed by the log phase with maximal infectivity in about 24 hours. The median cell culture infective dose$_{50}$ (CCID$_{50}$), based on CPE in both cell systems, is equivalent to the homologous PFU titers when corrected for the Poisson distribution (Section IV,11,*c*).

Similar growth curves have been reported based on CCID$_{50}$ (Akers, 1963; Estola, 1966; von Bülow, 1966a,b; Akers and Cunningham, 1968).

(3) *Cytochemistry.* Fluorescence microscopy with acridine orange (AO) (Akers, 1963; Akers and Cunningham, 1968) and coriphosphine (Berry, 1967) stains is useful for identification of the RNA of IBV, but it is not as sensitive as infectivity tests, CPE, or immunofluorescence for early detection of the developing virus. Viral RNA is not detected by AO prior to 24 hours after inoculation of CEKC with the Beaudette virus (Akers, 1963; Akers and Cunningham, 1968), although viral replication is exponential at this time. During maturation of the virus, progressive aggregation and coalescing of RNA granules is quite evident. Prior to disruption of the cell, almost the entire cytoplasm may be filled with the RNA.

Distribution of acid phosphatase activity during early infection of cells with IBV is the same as that in control cells, and release of this enzyme does not occur until the latter stages of infection. Lysosomes apparently play no part in the CPE induced by IBV (Lukert, 1967).

(4) *Immunofluorescence.* The earliest visible fluorescence in CEKC and chicken embryo lung cell (CELuC) cultures infected with the Beaudette virus (Lukert, 1966a) occurs at 4 hours, which corresponds to the end of the eclipse phase of the one-step growth curve (Lukert, 1965). Initially, the fluorescence is primarily in the perinuclear region, but it spreads peripherally until the entire cytoplasm is intensely and diffusely stained. Granular fluorescence is present in the latter stages of infection. The development of fluorescence parallels replication of the virus and the accompanying CPE. These findings are in agreement with other reports (Stultz, 1962; J. L. Brown, 1969) but disagree with one (Mohanty *et al.*,

1964) on intranuclear development of fluorescence of the same strain of virus.

6. STRAIN CLASSIFICATION

Immunologic differences by neutralization and chicken immunity tests have resulted in the presently recognized major serotypes of IBV: Massachusetts, Connecticut, Iowa 97, Iowa 69, Gray, and Holte (Jungherr et al., 1956; Hofstad, 1958; Winterfield et al., 1964a,b; Hitchner et al., 1966; Purchase et al., 1966a; von Bülow, 1967a; Berry and Stokes, 1968). Isolates which have been considered serologically different from the previously recognized types are JMK (Winterfield et al., 1964a), Cuxhaven (Germany) (von Bülow, 1967a), and Australian "T" (Cumming, 1963; von Bülow, 1967a) viruses.

Other serotypes may exist, and there is some uncertainty as to the exact relationship of one type to another as there are some weak and variable cross reactions. Also, flocks may experience a series of exposures to the several serotypes (Hitchner et al., 1964, 1966).

The Beaudette virus is antigenically related to the Massachusetts serotype, and it has been used extensively as the reference virus for neutralization tests. Some serologic differences between these viruses have been reported (von Bülow, 1966c) based especially on cross-neutralization tests with the Beaudette virus antiserum and the respective viruses (Chomiak et al., 1963).

7. ANTIGENS

At least 3 antigenically distinct, noninfectious, soluble antigens extracted by ether from the Massachusetts and Beaudette viruses in allantoic fluid and the CAM and demonstrable by immunodiffusion have been described (Tevethia, 1964; Tevethia and Cunningham, 1968). The antigens are smaller than the virion and are not sedimentated with it at $109,000 \times g$. The antigens may be differentially identified on the basis of size by filtration, bouyant density in CsCl, thermal sensitivity, sensitivity to trypsin, pepsin, and RNase. Antigen 2 may reside in the virion with antigens 1 and 3 distributed over the surface of the virion.

The Beaudette virus partially purified and concentrated from allantoic fluid by centrifugation has been described (Steele and Luginbuhl, 1964) as an antigen possessing complement-fixing activity stable to trypsin, 50°C. and 100°C. for 30 minutes, and ultraviolet irradiation for 50 seconds. Under similar conditions, viral infectivity was inactivated.

8. HEMAGGLUTINATION

One of the problems encountered with IBV is that the virus in allantoic fluid from chicken embryos does not cause direct hemagglutination

(HA) unless, as reported by one group of workers, it is treated with trypsin (Section IV,4,*d*) (Corbo and Cunningham, 1959; Muldoon, 1960; Muldoon and Cunningham, 1961; Cunningham, 1963; Biswal *et al.*, 1966; Purchase *et al.*, 1966a) or ether (Biswal, 1965; Biswal *et al.*, 1966) or unless a noninfectious hemagglutinin is isolated by diethylaminoethyl (DEAE) chromatography (Biswal *et al.*, 1966). The treated virus is reported to react only with chicken or turkey erthrocytes. Virus of low numbers of chicken embryo passages agglutinates erthrocytes to a greater extent than the Beaudette virus which causes little or no agglutination.

Trypsin-treated IBV reduces the electrophoretic mobility of chicken and turkey erythrocytes but to a lesser degree than that produced by PR8 influenza virus, Newcastle disease virus (NDV), or neuraminidase. The effect of trypsin on the erythrocyte can largely be excluded as a major influence, since the enzyme does not destroy receptors on the erythrocyte for subsequent adsorption by trypsin-treated IBV, PR8, or NDV. Neuraminidase removes the receptors for these viruses (Biswal, 1963; Cunningham, 1963).

That a trypsin-sensitive HA inhibitor is in allantoic fluid is evidenced by the fact that HA by trypsin-treated virus is eliminated upon the addition of normal allantoic fluid (NAF) or allantoic fluid containing the virus (Nazerian, 1965; Nazerian and Cunningham, 1967). The inhibitor is either competitive with the virus for receptors on the erythrocyte or adsorbs to the virus and prevents its reaction with the erythrocyte.

Specific inhibition of HA by anti-IBV chicken serum has not been demonstrated even with serum treated with a number of reagents to remove naturally occurring nonspecific inhibitors (Muldoon, 1960; Muldoon and Cunningham, 1961), and the reaction is not presently applicable as a serologic test. Trypsin-treated virus will, however, stimulate the production of neutralizing antibody (Muldoon and Cunningham, 1961).

The noninfectious hemagglutinin of the Massachusetts virus, 60 to 70 mμ in diameter, is selectively separable from infectious viruses by elution from DEAE with NaCl gradients (Biswal *et al.*, 1966). Neither the Beaudette virus nor NAF yield the hemagglutinin under the same procedures. The hemagglutinin does not sediment at $136,000 \times g$ for 2 hours. On a dry weight basis, the hemagglutinin is a lipoprotein (34.2% lipid, 51.2% protein) with trace amounts of carbohydrate and RNA but no detectable DNA.

The noninfectious hemagglutinin causes direct HA and elutes from the erythrocyte after destroying the receptors on the erythrocyte for itself or for trypsin- or ether-treated IBV but not for PR8 or NDV. Neuraminidase destroys the receptors for the hemagglutinin on the erythrocyte and affects those of the ectoderm of the CAM to inhibit replication of infectious virus.

Rabbit anti-IBV hemagglutinin serum inhibits HA to a slight degree and produces a single immunodiffusion line with the hemagglutinin (Biswal, 1965; Biswal *et al.*, 1966).

9. NEUTRALIZATION

Neutralization of the Beaudette virus by heated, anti-IBV chicken serum is a first-order reaction dependent on time, concentration of antibody, and temperature as assayed in chicken embryos (Page and Cunningham, 1962; Lukert, 1966b) and in CEKC by PFU (Cunningham and Spring, 1965; Lukert, 1966b; Stinski and Cunningham, 1967, 1969). On the basis of antibody equivalents and neutralization constants, antigenic differences between the Massachusetts and Connecticut viruses can be detected by the plaque method (Cunningham and Spring, 1965).

Recent research described below has provided much meaningful information on the virus–antibody complex and certain parameters of the neutralization reaction.

The enhancing effect of guinea pig complement and the C′1 fraction of chicken serum on the neutralizing potential of heated anti-IBV homotypic (chicken) and heterotypic (rabbit) serum as tested in chicken embryos has been demonstrated quite conclusively (Berry and Almeida, 1968).

Electron microscopy reveals clear distinctions between the effects of the antisera. Antibody in heated homotypic antiserum attaches only to the surface projections of the virus (Fig. 5). With unheated homotypic antiserum, the heat-labile components form a halo around the virus (Fig. 6).

Heterotypic antiserum contains antibodies against both the surface projections and the envelope of the virus and attaches to these sites. In addition, the unheated heterotypic antiserum produces holes approximately 100 Å in diameter in the virus membrane, suggesting a form of lysis of the virus (Fig. 7). Anti-chicken embryo fibroblast heterotypic serum also produces similar holes which suggest that the envelope of IBV is closely related to the host material.

A neutral complex of the Beaudette virus and antibody in anti-Massachusetts chicken serum is readily dissociated at pH 1.7 (Stinski and Cunningham, 1967, 1969). The 2 components can be reassociated at pH 7.3 with a neutralization rate similar to that of the original reaction. The neutral complex adsorbs to CEKC and can be dissociated by acid with subsequent infection of the cell by the virus.

Further work (Stinski, 1969) with ³²P labeled virus illustrated that virus without and with 7 S (IgG) homotypic antibody adsorbs to but does not enter CEKC at 4°C. At 25°C. or 37°C., the rate constants of entry into the cell are linear but faster for virus without antibody, and

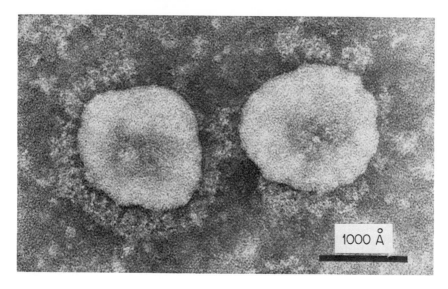

Fig. 5. Infectious bronchitis viral particles treated with heated homotypic chicken antiserum. The particles are clumped and the surface projections are obscured. × 300,000. (Berry and Almeida, 1968.)

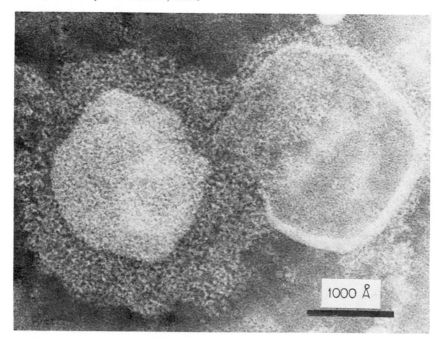

Fig. 6. The overall appearance of infectious bronchitis viral particles treated with unheated homotypic chicken antiserum. × 300,000. (Berry and Almeida, 1968.)

related directly to temperature. The rate of degradation within the cell is the same for virus without and with antibody. Little, if any, of the intracellular acid-soluble, RNase-sensitive material associated with degraded virus (Section IV,5,b) is detected in cells containing neutralized virus. On the basis of the report (Berry and Almeida, 1968) that antibody in homotypic antiserum attaches to the viral projections and not with the envelope, it is hypothesized (Stinski, 1969) that the attached 7 S (IgG) antibody has a role in determining degradation of the virus to the point where replication does not occur.

10. INTERFERENCE AND SYNERGISM

Interference with the production of NDV by IBV has been reported as occurring in chickens (Hanson *et al.*, 1956; Bankowski *et al.*, 1957; Hanson and Alberts, 1959; Raggi and Lee, 1964), chicken embryos (Luginbuhl and Jungherr, 1953; Raggi *et al.*, 1963; Lacey, 1968), chicken kidney cells (Beard, 1968), and CEKC (J. L. Brown, 1969). Avian encephalomyelitis (AE) virus interferes with IBV in chicken embryos (Yates *et al.*, 1968).

The mechanism of interference has not been clearly defined, but it has been suggested that the interfering virus blocks the attachment sites for the superinfecting virus.

Coexistence but not synergism has been reported for IBV and laryngo-

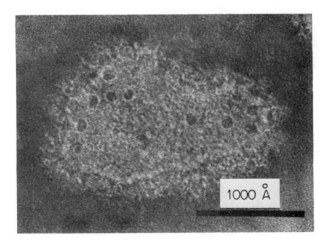

FIG. 7. Infectious bronchitis virus and unheated heterotypic rabbit antiserum. The particles appear flattened and distinct holes, approximately 100 Å across, in the viral membrane have a definite wall around them. × 300,000. (Berry and Almeida, 1968.)

tracheitis (Raggi *et al.*, 1967b). Synergism exists between IBV and *Mycoplasma gallisepticum* (Adler *et al.*, 1962) and *Hemophilus gallinarum* (Raggi *et al.*, 1967a) in chickens.

11. LABORATORY HOST SYSTEMS

a. *Embryonated Avian Eggs*

The allantoic chamber of 9- to 12-day-old chicken embryos is the route of choice for inoculation because of the simplicity of operation and sensitivity to IBV (Cunningham, 1947, 1952; Estola, 1966), but other routes may be used (Cunningham and Jones, 1953; Cunningham, 1966a). The possible presence of maternal antibody precludes the use of the yolk sac route, although embryos from immune flocks may be used for other routes of inoculation. The genetic influence of the embryo in response to IBV is probably more important than the effect of maternal antibody (Purchase *et al.*, 1966b).

On initial isolation, and for the first few passages, the predominating features of infection of the embryo are gross lesions among which are curling and dwarfing of the embryo, thickening and fibrosis of the amniotic membrane, and urates in the mesonephros (Loomis *et al.*, 1950; Estola, 1966). Embryo mortality is variable and generally low for the first few passages, although different strains of the virus vary in this respect (Sato *et al.*, 1955; Estola, 1966). Temperature of incubation also has an effect on replication of the virus (Simpson and Groupé, 1959).

Successive passage of the virus in embryos is accompanied by a paralleling decrease in pathogenicity, antigenicity, and immunogenicity for the natural host with an increase in lethality for the embryo. Embryo mortality is the major criterion of infection by "embryo-adapted" virus of which the Beaudette virus is the classic example. After inoculation via the allantoic chamber, the virus is widely distributed throughout the embryo except for the yolk sac (Cunningham and El Dardiry, 1948) as determined by infectivity tests. Distribution of the virus can also be determined with ^{35}S and ^{32}P labeled virus (Levine, 1957).

When gross lesions and death of the embryo are indicative of infection (Hitchner and White, 1955) both should be scored as responses for quantitative assay of infectivity.

It has been reported (Steele and Luginbuhl, 1964) that the Beaudette virus at the 245th passage in chicken embryos is capable of stimulating the production of neutralizing antibody in chickens. At the 300th passage (Larose and Van Roekel, 1961) the Massachusetts virus can infect chickens.

The possible presence of adeno-like (Burke *et al.*, 1968), AE (Calneck *et al.*, 1960), chicken embryo lethal orphan (CELO) (Ablashi *et al.*,

1965), and ND (Fontaine *et al.*, 1965; Lacey, 1968) viruses, and perhaps others, as contaminants of chicken embryos and cell cultures derived from them must be considered in the use of these cultural systems for IBV.

The turkey embryo supports replication of the Beaudette and Massachusetts viruses, but only after the latter has been adapted by alternating chicken and turkey embryo passages. Turkey "embryo-adapted" virus after 17 passages in turkey embryos is not markedly modified in its pathogenicity, antigenicity, or immunogenicity for chickens (DuBose, 1967).

b. *Animals*

The Beaudette (Simpson and Groupé, 1959; Estola, 1966, 1967), and Massachusetts, Iowa 97, Gray, and IBV_F (Estola, 1966, 1967) viruses may be successfully propagated intracerebrally, but not intraperitoneally or intranasally, in serial passage in suckling mice up to 12 days of age using either virus in allantoic or CEKC fluids (Estola, 1966) as inoculum. Signs of infection are hypersensitivity, locomotor ataxia, and ascending paralysis followed by death 3 to 4 days after inoculation. Histologically, there is a nonpurulent encephalitis or encephalitis with infiltration of various cell types (Estola, 1966). Mice older than the above ages are refractory (Simpson and Groupé, 1959; Estola, 1966). Virus in low chicken embryo passage (Simpson and Groupé, 1959) and the Connecticut, Iowa 609, and Holte viruses (Estola, 1967) are not adaptable to mice.

The mouse-adapted virus is not infective for chickens by the intracerebral route, but it can be titrated in mice, chicken embryos, or CEKC and neutralized by anti-IBV_F guinea pig or anti-Beaudette rabbit sera (Estola, 1966).

Two-day-old suckling rabbits, but not adult rabbits or 2-day-old suckling guinea pigs, are susceptible to intracerebral inoculation with IBV_F (Estola, 1966).

After 25 serial passages in the brains of mice, the Beaudette mouse-adapted virus is lethal for chicken embryos incubated at 34°C. but not at 38°C., whereas the parent virus is lethal at both temperatures. Cultivation of the mouse-adapted virus in chicken embryos at 38°C. results in a subline which kills chicken embryos more slowly at 34°C. and more rapidly at 38°C. than the parent virus, but it is less virulent for suckling mice. This result is considered to be a selection of variants from the original population (Simpson and Groupé, 1959).

c. *Cell Cultures*

One of the most rewarding areas of investigation of IBV has been the use of cell and tissue cultures. Different isolates of IBV have been cultivated with varying degrees of success in avian cell and tissue culture systems such as adult chicken kidney cells, the de-embryonated chicken egg, the isolated CAM, chicken embryo heart, trachea, whole chicken embryo fibroblasts (CEFiC), CEKC, CELuC, and CELiC. The reader is referred to several articles for general information (Cunningham, 1960; Mallmann and Cunningham, 1963; Cunningham and Spring, 1965; Lukert, 1965, 1966a,b, 1967; Estola, 1966; von Bülow, 1966a,b).

Mammalian cell line systems such as the PK-15 swine kidney (Lukert, 1967), human epidermoid carcinoma of the larynx (H. Ep. #2), human epidermoid carcinoma of the pharynx (KB), normal human amnion (FL, AV-3), mouse fibroblasts (L-929), human embryonic kidney (HEK), and African green monkey kidney (BS-C-1) (Lacey, 1968), mouse liver (Earle's L strain) (Fahey and Crawley, 1956), and baby hamster kidney (BHK-21) cells (J. L. Brown, 1969) are reported not to support growth of IBV. Monkey kidney cells are reported to support growth of the virus without CPE (Fahey and Crawley, 1956; Steele and Luginbuhl, 1964).

Strains of IBV vary in their adaptability to cell cultures including CEKC. Initial isolation of the virus is best accomplished with embryonated chicken eggs. Isolates of the virus in low chicken embryo passage usually adapt less well to cell cultures than virus of high embryo passage, but exceptions have been reported (Kawamura et al., 1961; Estola, 1966; von Bülow, 1966a,b).

A "cell-attachment-and-growth factor" (CAGF) in allantoic fluid containing Massachusetts virus enhances the attachment and rapid formation of CEFiC on glass surface (Mallmann and Cunningham, 1963). The CAGF is not present in NAF or in CEFiC and tissues of chickens infected with the virus. The CPE by the CAGF can be assayed quantitatively, but it is not serologically or cytopathically identical to the virus. Virus separated from the CAGF by anion exchange resin and by the limiting dilution technique adapts more readily to CEFiC than virus not treated with resin.

The main criterion of infection of CEKC are the syncytia which increase in size and number of nuclei simultaneously and sequentially and are directly related to the development of the virus (Akers, 1963; Akers and Cunningham, 1968). Plaques are the result of necrosis of the infected cells and syncytia. Syncytia are inconspicuous in CELuC (Lukert, 1966a).

The PFU of the virus follows a linear relationship with the dose of virus and is inhibited by specific antiserum (Cunningham and Spring, 1965; Lukert, 1966b); the frequency distribution is according to the Poisson distribution, thus indicating single-cell infection; the coefficient of variation is near the value statistically expected from the total number of plaques counted; and repeated assays are within statistical practicability (Cunningham and Spring, 1965). Similar results have been reported on the basis of $CCID_{50}$ (von Bülow, 1966a,b).

The first report on PFU by the Beaudette virus in CEKC (Wright and Sagik, 1958) indicated that PFU titers are 4 times as high as EID_{63} (conversion from EID_{50} quantal unit equivalent to one enumerative PFU unit) titers. The chicken embryo has since been found to be more sensitive to IBV than CEKC, and $CCID_{63}$ titers in CEKC and CELiC are equivalent to homologous PFU titers (Lukert, 1965).

Tracheal organ explant cultures from 4-week-old chickens have been used for cultivation of the Massachusetts, Beaudette, Connecticut, Boney, Iowa 97, and the Regional Poultry Research Laboratory (RPL, Purchase et al., 1966a) viruses contained in allantoic fluid (Colwell and Lukert, 1969). Rounding and sloughing of ciliated epithelial cells and complete cessation of ciliary movement as a specific CPE confirmed by immunofluorescence has been compared to natural infection in chickens.

V. Pathogenesis and Epizootiology

1. Natural Hosts

The chicken is the natural host for IBV and all ages, sexes, and breeds are susceptible. Other avian species are not known to be naturally infected (Cunningham, 1966c; Hofstad, 1969).

2. Transmission

The virus in secretions from the respiratory tract of infected chickens spreads rapidly throughout a flock under natural conditions with chickens developing respiratory signs as early as 36 hours. Airborne transmission among cohabitating birds is considered to be the natural route of infection (Levine and Hofstad, 1947), but the optimal environmental conditions are not known.

Following aerosol exposure of chickens to several isolates representing the different serotypes of IBV (Hofstad and Yoder, 1966), virus may be recovered from the trachea and lungs by 24 hours and through 8 days. Virus also multiplies in nonrespiratory tissue such as the kidney, pancreas, spleen, liver, and bursa of Fabricius, and can be detected occasionally in the blood. There is essentially no difference between serotypic distribution of the virus in tissues. Virus of the 85th embryo passage multiplies primarily in the trachea and lungs.

Contaminated feed, water, clothing, utensils, and equipment, as well as the movement of personnel from house to house or flock to flock may serve for indirect transmission of the virus (Purchase et al., 1966a).

3. Carriers

Vectors do not appear to be a factor in the transmission of IBV.

Recurrence of IBV in certain areas or on the same premises year after year indicates that recovered chickens may possibly serve as "carriers" of the virus as an inapparent infection (Purchase *et al.*, 1966a) or that there is a continual cross infection rather than a true carrier state (Cook, 1968). This aspect of the epizootiology of AIB is not clearly understood.

Virus can be isolated from lung and tracheal specimens during the incubative and throughout the respiratory phases of the disease which may vary from 24 hours to as long as 4 weeks after infection (Hofstad, 1947; Fabricant and Levine, 1951; Cunningham, 1957) and from cloacal contents up to 24 days after oral infection (Pette, 1959) and eggs as long as 43 days after infection (Fabricant and Levine, 1951).

More recently, IBV has been isolated from the trachea or cloaca of chickens in strict isolation up to 49 days after intratracheal inoculation and for over 4 months when isolation was less effective. In the latter circumstance, virus was isolated from chickens with a significant titer of neutralizing antibody (Cook, 1968).

4. Clinical Features

The most characteristic signs in chicks less than 5 or 6 weeks old are respiratory distress, tracheal rales, coughing, sneezing, and nasal discharge with generalized weakness and depression as the disease progresses. Swollen sinuses and excessive lachrymation may be present. The morbidity rate is high, and the mortality rate may be as high as 25% or more. Feed consumption and weight gains (Prince *et al.*, 1962) are markedly reduced. Permanent damage to the ovary and oviduct resulting later in false or "internal" layers may occur if chicks are infected under 2 weeks of age.

In chickens over 6 weeks of age and in adult birds, the signs are similar to those in chicks, but nasal discharge does not occur as frequently. There is generally temporary retardation of feed consumption and growth. The disease may be unnoticed unless the flock is examined carefully. Environmental temperatures from 12.6°C. to 23.8°C. do not adversely affect 4- to 8-week-old infected chickens (Prince *et al.*, 1967).

In growing stock and adult birds, the morbidity rate may be high but the mortality rate is usually low. There is usually a precipitous drop in egg production in laying flocks varying with the period of lay. In some instances, the production may cease within a week. Some 6 to 8 weeks or more may elapse before production returns to the preinfection level, but in most cases this is never attained.

The reduction in egg production, increase in the number of unsettable hatching eggs, and reduced hatchability of those eggs set (Broadfoot and Smith, 1954) is reflected in the small, soft-shelled, malformed, and abnormal quality (McDougall, 1968) of the first eggs when a flock starts to return to production. If pullets are in good condition there may be only a slight drop in egg production, with a return to normal within a few weeks after recovery from respiratory signs. Some flocks may be so severely affected that, even after clinical recovery, the flock is not an economic unit and must be replaced.

It has been found possible to hatch and raise chicks free from AIB from previously infected parent stock which was apparently reinfected naturally during the time of collection of the eggs as determined by viral neutralization tests. There were no clinical signs other than lowered quality of the eggs. The chicks remained free of the disease for 12 months (Cook and Garside, 1967).

5. Gross Lesions

Serous or catarrhal exudate in the nasal passages, sinuses, lower trachea and bronchii, congestion and edema of the lungs, fibrinous inflammation or cloudiness of the air sac membranes with possible yellow, caseous exudate are the commonly encountered gross lesions at necropsy. Yellow, caseous plugs may be in the lower trachea and bronchii of chicks that die. Catarrhal inflammation of the nasal passages and sinuses is seldom encountered in chickens over 2 months of age.

Fluid yolk material may be present in the abdominal cavity of layers, but this abnormality is not specifically related to AIB. The length and weight of the oviduct are markedly reduced, and about 21 days is required for return to normal (Sevoian and Levine, 1957). There may be permanent damage to the oviduct (Broadfoot et al., 1956).

6. Histopathologic Changes

The tracheal mucosa undergoes cyclic changes in 3 main phases for 18 to 21 days following intratracheal instillation of the virus: (a) acute phase (1 to 3 days), epithelial hypertrophy and marked edema; (b) reparative phase (6 to 9 days), epithelial hyperplasia and marked cellularity of the propria; and (c) immune phase (12 to 18 days), restoration of the epithelium and either follicular or mild, focal, diffuse lymphoid infiltration of the propria (Jungherr et al., 1956; Oshel, 1961).

Significant histologic changes are not present in the liver, spleen, and kidney. Inclusion bodies are not formed (Hofstad, 1945).

Histologic changes in the oviduct are reduction of the height of the cellular epithelium lining the oviduct, the cells become cuboidal with some loss of cilia, dilatation of the glands, and lymphocytic foci and cellular infiltration in the lamina propria and intertubular stroma (Sevoian and Levine, 1957).

Nephrosis associated with AIB is reflected in swollen, pale tubules and ureters often distended with urate crystals (Cumming, 1963).

7. Immunity

a. Active

Active immunity results from natural or artificial infection with immunogenic strains of IBV. The primary antigenic stimulus is accompanied by a marked but transient increase of total globulin and γ-globulin (Dimopoullos and Cunningham, 1956).

About 3 weeks are required before neutralizing antibody is of significantly high titer for diagnostic purposes (Section VI,3,a). Immunity may persist for periods to perhaps a year but may decline sufficiently for reinfection to occur, especially with an overwhelming challenge dose of virus or experience with severe natural infection. The plurality of serotypes complicates clinical interpretation of the immune status, particularly with reinfection as cross immunity is not always effective for subsequent infections.

Local tracheal immunity has an important role in immunity. Chickens recovered from aerosol infection with a high embryo passage virus may be resistant for relatively short periods of time to subsequent challenge with low embryo passage virus even though the neutralizing antibody level is low or not demonstrable (Hofstad, 1967).

b. Passive

Naturally acquired passive immunity results from maternal antibodies in the yolk of eggs laid by hens recovered from natural or artificial infection. Antibodies are demonstrable in the blood of embryos from about 15 days of incubation (Jungherr and Terrell, 1948). The antibody titer of the yolk is high for the first 2 weeks after the chick hatches but then declines to negligible levels at about 4 weeks and the chick is then susceptible to IBV. Passive immunity does not prevent respiratory infection but does serve to reduce the severity of the disease.

VI. Diagnosis

Diagnosis of AIB may embrace one or more of the following: (1) clinical features, (2) isolation of the virus, and (3) serologic tests.

1. CLINICAL FEATURES

Similarities of the respiratory signs of AIB, Newcastle disease, and laryngotracheitis make differential diagnosis difficult in the early stages of disease. When neurologic disturbances associated with Newcastle disease and the forced expiration associated with laryngotracheitis are present as the disease develops, a presumptive diagnosis may be possible on the basis of clinical signs, morbidity and mortality, and duration of the disease.

2. ISOLATION OF VIRUS

Infectious bronchitis virus may be readily isolated from lungs, trachea, and bronchii collected from chickens during the incubation period and throughout the respiratory phase of the disease (Cunningham, 1952). Suspensions of these specimens can be used as inoculum for chickens or for embryonated chicken eggs.

a. Infectivity and Cross-Immunity Tests in Chickens

Infectivity and cross-immunity tests in chickens may be employed for diagnostic purposes, but they are generally not performed because of the usual limitations of isolation facilities and constant sources of suitable birds. The most important use of chickens would be for mainte-nance of the virus in the natural host by serial passage and for the pro-duction of antiserum for serologic studies.

b. Embryonated Chicken Eggs

Isolation of IBV is most frequently done by inoculating 9- to 12-day-old chicken embryos via the allantoic chamber with a properly prepared suspension of lung, trachea, and bronchii from infected chickens (Cun-ningham, 1952, 1966c). Identity of the virus is based on the gross patho-logic alterations. Since it is frequently necessary to make additional passages of the virus before typical alterations are produced, one or two of the living embryos should be examined 3 days postinoculation and the allantoic fluid collected for further passage in embryos or for inoculation of chickens. The remaining embryos should be examined 6 or 7 days post-inoculation. In some instances, 3 or 4 passages of the virus in embryos become necessary for the production of typical lesions. Further passages are not feasible and probably would not offer additional information.

3. SEROLOGIC TESTS

Several serologic tests are available either individually or in combina-tion for identification of antigen or antibody. Each has its own advantages for specific basic and applied use under optimal conditions. The tests employ either the decreasing virus (DV)–constant serum or constant virus–decreasing serum (DS) methods (Cunningham, 1966a).

a. Neutralization

Blood should be collected during the acute phase and the convalescent phase, at least 3 weeks postinfection (Dimopoullos and Cunningham, 1956), of the disease for comparison of neutralization indices (Cunningham, 1966a). Serum can be inactivated or not inactivated at 56°C. for 30 minutes (Berry and Almeida, 1968), but for comparative studies all sera should receive the same treatment.

(1) *Embryonated chicken eggs.* The DV method of quantal assay uses appropriate dilutions of virus with equal quantities of antiserum for inoculating 5 chicken embryos, 9- to 12-days old, per mixture via the allantoic chamber.

The neutralization index (NI), the difference between the EID_{50} of the virus alone and of the virus–serum mixture, should not exceed 1.5 log units with normal serum, although this value might be somewhat high in view of more refined techniques developed since this norm was first established (Cunningham, 1951). An NI of 2 log units or greater is considered positive for AIB antibody.

A DS method has been described (Fontaine *et al.*, 1963; Purchase *et al.*, 1966a) as being advantageous for screening large numbers of sera for epizootiologic surveys. Using only one dilution of serum with virus to inoculate 4 to 6 embryos, the results are reported to correlate well with those by the DV method as to positive, negative, or equivocal with respect to neutralizing antibody.

A newly described method (Berry and Almeida, 1968) has been reported whereby a mixture of virus and serum is incubated for an hour at 37°C., overnight at 4°C., and then diluted 10-fold and titrated for viral infectivity in chicken embryos. Differences in neutralization of virus by heated and nonheated homotypic and heterotypic antisera (Section IV,9) are clearly evident.

(2) *Cell cultures.* Plaque reduction for the detection of neutralizing antibody by the DV method has been reported to be a practical test (Lukert, 1966b). Results are comparable to the classic DV method with chicken embryos, but the NI based on PFU is lower. It has been suggested that with the plaque reduction method, an NI of 0.0 to 1.0 log units be considered as negative, 1.0 to 1.5 as equivocal or suspect, and 1.5 and above as positive.

The DS method by plaque assay is especially applicable for identification of antibody by neutralization rate constants, study of the virus–

host cell interaction, and the kinetics of infection (Cunningham and Spring, 1965; Stinski, 1969) (Section IV,9).

A test described as an interference serologic test (Beard, 1968) has been used to demonstrate the antigen–antibody relationships between serotypes of IBV. The basis of the test is that chicken kidney cells not infected by a neutral mixture of IBV and antibody are susceptible to NDV as determined by the CPE in stained cells. The test can be performed by either the DV or DS method.

The DV and DS methods can be used with the CPE in CEKC being the criterion of the response. There is the necessity, however, for a CEKC-adapted virus. Possible difficulties in scoring the CPE either as a graded or an "all-or-nothing" response (Cunningham, 1966a) must be considered.

On the basis of variable quantitative relationships between the DV and DS methods of assay in chicken embryos or by CPE in CEKC, the DS method has been recommended for testing for neutralizing antibody. The slope of the neutralization line depends on the pathogenicity of the virus and the susceptibility of the host system, but not on the character of the antiserum. Curves for the DS method follow the Poisson distribution (von Bülow, 1967b).

b. Immunodiffusion

The immunodiffusion (agar-gel diffusion, agar-gel precipitation) test is particularly useful for the rapid, routine differential identification of IBV, NDV, fowl plague, chicken embryo lethal orphan, infectious laryngotracheitis, fowl pox and pigeon pox antigen and precipitating antibody in addition to the normally accepted virus isolation and neutralization tests (Woernle, 1966), appraisal of antibody response to vaccination (Maire et al., 1967), and for study of the antigens of IBV (Tevethia, 1964; Tevethia and Cunningham, 1968) (Section IV,7). Antigens can be prepared from the CAM or from the allantoic fluid of infected chicken embryos. Precipitating antibody for IBV is transient in chickens and antiserum should be collected from 7 to 23 days after infection with the optimum being at about 15 days. Defatted antiserum and agar containing 8% NaCl are suggested for maximal results.

c. Immunofluorescence

This procedure has been employed with considerable success for the identification and study of IBV in infected cell cultures (Mohanty et al., 1964; Braune and Gentry, 1965; Lukert, 1966a, 1969; J. L. Brown, 1969), tracheal organ explants (Colwell and Lukert, 1969), and for differentiation between the Massachusetts, Connecticut, Iowa 97, and RPL serotypes (Lukert, 1969). Cross fluorescence between serotypes is considered to correspond more closely to cross-protection tests in chickens than to cross-neutralization tests by the DS plaque reduction method in CEKC (Lukert, 1969). The use of divalent or polyvalent antisera and either frozen sections or impression smears of the tracheal explants has been suggested for routine diagnosis of IBV.

d. Complement-Fixation

Direct (Brumfield and Pomeroy, 1957; Steele and Luginbuhl, 1964) and indirect (Steele and Luginbuhl, 1964) complement-fixation (CF) tests have been applied to IBV. The direct test (Steele and Luginbuhl, 1964) employs the Beaudette virus as antigen concentrated from allantoic fluid by centrifugation and guinea pig antiserum prepared against the virus in chicken kidney cells. The indirect test, based on the inhibition of the direct CF test system, has been used for titration of anti-Beaudette chicken serum. Anti-Massachusetts and Connecticut chicken sera with neutralizing antibody against the homologous viruses do not react with the Beaudette virus in the indirect CF test (Steele and Luginbuhl, 1964).

e. Hemagglutination

Although IBV does not cause direct HA of chicken or turkey erythrocytes and hemagglutination-inhibition (HI) is not applicable, induction of HA by trypsin-treated virus has been used as a supplementary test for identification of IBV (Section IV,8).

An indirect HA test has been described whereby anti-IBV chicken serum agglutinates tannic acid-treated horse erythrocytes to which virus in either low or high chicken embryo passage has been previously adsorbed. There is good correlation between indirect HA and the NI in chicken embryos (W. E. Brown et al., 1962).

4. Differential Diagnosis

A presumptive diagnosis differentiating AIB from Newcastle disease and laryngotracheitis, two of the most commonly encountered viral respiratory diseases of chickens resembling AIB, may be made if typical clinical signs of infection are present (Section VI,1).

Isolation of IBV in embryonated chicken eggs and the several available serologic tests have been described (Section VI,2,3). The following are presented as the basic laboratory procedures initially used for differentiation of NDV and laryngotracheitis virus (LTV) from IBV. Newcastle disease virus is lethal for embryonated chicken eggs inoculated via the allantoic chamber and HA and HI tests can be performed with the allantoic fluid from the infected embryos. Laryngotracheitis virus produces gross lesions on the CAM inoculated via this route, but HA and HI tests are not applicable.

Serologic tests such as virus neutralization, immunodiffusion, and immunofluorescence are applicable for differentiation of NDV and LTV from IBV using properly prepared antigen and antibody.

It has been suggested that the thermolability of IBV differentiates it from quail bronchitis virus (DuBose and Grumbles, 1959) and that the acid stability of IBV differentiates it from NDV, LTV, and fowl pox virus (Quiroz and Hanson, 1958).

VII. Treatment

There is no specific treatment for AIB. Proper husbandry should be practiced to alleviate environmental stress and to maintain feed consumption.

VIII. Prevention and Control

1. MANAGEMENT

Avian infectious bronchitis is one of the most contagious of the respiratory diseases of chickens. Prevention of spread of the disease is best accomplished by isolation of the flock, adding day-old chicks as replacements and rearing them in isolation, and sound management and husbandry. Even with the most strict precautions, AIB may occur, and this has necessitated the use of vaccines in a control program.

2. IMMUNIZATION

Immunization against AIB was first practiced about 1941 in the New England states (Van Roekel et al., 1951) by inoculating a few chickens of a flock 8- to 16-weeks old with virulent IBV which allowed natural spread of the virus throughout the flock. This was a deliberately produced infection at an age of the chicken when the disease would produce the least economic loss. Recovered chickens were then immune to AIB through the laying year in contrast to the disastrous results that might occur with natural infection of the layers.

With the increasing interest in AIB, the virus, and the development of more suitable vaccines, the original method of immunization was discontinued.

a. Types of Vaccines

The success of a vaccination program depends on the purity and potency of the vaccine and its application under the conditions for which it is specifically intended. Directions for use of a vaccine as supplied by the producer should be followed explicitly.

Vaccines containing active and inactive IBV have received extensive research attention, and advocates affirm the respective advantages and disadvantages of each type.

(1) *Inactivated virus vaccines*. Although possessing the advantage of being noninfectious, these vaccines have not proved to be entirely satisfactory and are not used extensively in the U. S. A. β-Propiolactone-inactivated virus has been reported to be efficacious (Berry, 1965) and not efficacious (Winterfield, 1967; McDougall, 1968; Brion et al., 1969). Some success has been reported with formalin-inactivated virus (Woernle, 1961).

(2) *Active virus vaccine*. Virus for these vaccines is modified by serial passage in embryonated chicken eggs, generally 25 or more passages, for reduction of the pathogenicity but retention of the immunogenicity of the virus (Section IV,11,a). Modified viruses are capable of being transmitted from chicken to chicken.

The embryo passage at which a particular strain of virus is sufficiently modified for use as a vaccine is difficult to ascertain and probably varies between the strain of virus and the method of modification. Virus for vaccines for broilers should be of low pathogenicity but still capable of inducing the desired short-term immunity. Long-term immunity is desired for laying flocks and breeders, and the virus for the vaccine does not need to be as highly modified as that for broilers.

The Massachusetts and Connecticut virus serotypes are used as monovalent vaccines, with the former being reported to induce better immunity against heterologous strains of IBV (Hofstad, 1961). In view of the diversity of naturally occurring serotypes of IBV (Hitchner et al., 1964, 1966; Winterfield et al., 1964a,b), bivalent IBV vaccines containing the Massachusetts and Connecticut serotypes have been used but the former is reported to interfere with the development of antibodies against the latter (Winterfield, 1968).

Vaccines may be applied by aerosols or by dusting, but the common procedure is to place the vaccine in the drinking water (Hofstad, 1969). All these methods are based on economy of administration of the vaccine. Placing the vaccine in the drinking water is not without disadvantages due to the effect of environmental influences on the virus.

Chickens possessing maternal antibodies can be vaccinated against AIB (Raggi and Lee, 1965). Broilers are commonly vaccinated when they are 4 to 5 days old and then again at 4 weeks. A better response is attained when the chickens are 6 weeks old or older, as they are immunologically more mature. Replacement flocks should be vaccinated at 2 to 4 months.

Vaccines containing NDV and IBV have been used without apparent interference with the immune response to each (Markham et al., 1956). On the basis of additional evidence that interference may occur with certain combinations of the viruses (Hanson *et al.*, 1956; Raggi and Lee, 1964), it is advisable that IBV vaccines be administered separately whenever possible and practical.

IX. Commentary

As attested to by the literature cited in this chapter, there is presently a wealth of omnifarious information about AIB. For this the contributors deserve accolades, but it is clearly evident that much additional specific information is needed.

Further investigation is required on the pathogenesis of strains of the virus and epizootiology, residence of the virus and its possible lysogenic state within infected chickens, and the public health aspects of the relationship of IBV to those viruses causing human respiratory disease.

Answers are needed on the genetics and chemical composition of the virus, the influence of the host cell and its physiologic response to the virus, reasons for the relative restriction of the virus to replication within avian cell systems, and the extra- and intracellular biophysical events of the virus–host cell relationship.

Of prime importance is means for prompt recognition and categorization of new isolates as to serotype and their relationship, one to another, to reduce the confusion in terminology due to the many designations in current use. From this could evolve selection of strains of the virus for use as immunizing agents. A central reference laboratory properly financed, staffed, and equipped could contribute immeasurably to solving many of the problems of IBV and also serve as a center for continuing education and training.

ACKNOWLEDGMENTS

Permission to use copyright material was granted by the Cambridge University Press for Figs. 1, 4, 5, 6, and 7 and by the American Society for Microbiology for Figs. 2 and 3.

Photomicrographs for Figs. 1, 5, 6, and 7 were kindly supplied by Dr. J. D. Almeida; Fig. 4 by Dr. K. Nazerian; and Figs. 2 and 3 by Dr. K. McIntosh.

The author expresses his appreciation to the above, to those who very generously responded and supplied reprints, to those who voluntarily supplied preprints, to his colleagues and students for their contributions on AIB and the virus, and to all others who have assisted in any way in the preparation of this chapter.

Appreciation is extended to the editors, Drs. C. A. Brandly and C. E. Cornelius, for the privilege of attempting a general survey of the past and a focus on the present status of AIB and the virus with thoughts and perspectives for the future.

REFERENCES

Ablashi, D. V., Chang, P. W., and Yates, V. J. (1965). The effect of a latent CELO virus infection in the chicken embryo, on the propagation of Newcastle disease and influenza viruses. *Avian Diseases* **9**, 407–417.

Adler, H. E., McMartin, D. A., and Ortmayer, H. (1962). The effect of infectious bronchitis virus on chickens infected with Mycoplasma gallisepticum. *Avian Diseases* **6**, 267–274.

Akers, T. G. (1963). Some cytochemical studies of the multiplication of infectious bronchitis virus in chicken embryo kidney cells. Ph.D. Thesis, Michigan State University, East Lansing, Michigan. Cited by Cunningham (1963).

Akers, T. G., and Cunningham, C. H. (1968). Replication and cytopathogenicity of avian infectious bronchitis virus in chicken embryo kidney cells. *Archiv für die gesamte Virusforschung* **25**, 30–37.

Almeida, J. D., and Tyrrell, D. A. J. (1967). The morphology of three previously uncharacterized human respiratory viruses that grow in organ culture. *Journal of General Virology* **1**, 175–178.

Bankowski, R. A., Hill, R. W., and Raggi, L. G. (1957). Response of eight week old susceptible chickens to Newcastle disease (B-1) and infectious bronchitis viruses. *Avian Diseases* **1**, 195–206.

Beach, J. R., and Schalm, O. W. (1936). A filterable virus, distinct from that of laryngotracheitis, the cause of a respiratory disease of chicks. *Poultry Science* **15**, 199–206.

Beard, C. W. (1968). An interference type of serological test for infectious bronchitis virus using Newcastle disease virus. *Avian Diseases* **12**, 658–665.

Beaudette, F. R., and Hudson, C. B. (1937). Cultivation of the virus of infectious bronchitis. *Journal of the American Veterinary Medical Association* **90**, 51–60.

Becker, W. B., McIntosh, K., Dees, J. H., and Chanock, R. M. (1967). Morphogenesis of avian infectious bronchitis virus and a related human virus (229E). *Journal of Virology* **1**, 1019–1027.

Berry, D. M. (1965). Inactivated infectious bronchitis vaccine. *Journal of Comparative Pathology* **75**, 409–415.

Berry, D. M. (1967). Intracellular development of infectious bronchitis virus. *Nature* **216**, 393–394.

Berry, D. M., and Almeida, J. D. (1968). The morphological and biological effects of various antisera on avian infectious bronchitis virus. *Journal of General Virology* **3**, 97–102.

Berry, D. M., and Stokes, K. J. (1968). Antigenic variations in isolates of infectious bronchitis virus. *Veterinary Record* **82**, 157–160.

Berry, D. M., Cruickshank, J. G., Chu, H. P., and Wells, R. J. H. (1964). The structure of infectious bronchitis virus. *Virology* **23**, 403–407.

Biswal, N. (1963). Electrokinetic studies on erythrocytes treated with modified infectious bronchitis virus. M.S. Thesis, Michigan State University, East Lansing. Cited by Cunningham (1963).

Biswal, N. (1965). The hemagglutinin of infectious bronchitis virus. Ph.D. Thesis, Michigan State University, East Lansing, Michigan. Cited by Cunningham (1966b).

Biswal, N., Nazerian, K., and Cunningham, C. H. (1966). A hemagglutinating fraction of infectious bronchitis virus. *American Journal of Veterinary Research* **27**, 1157–1167.

Braune, M. O., and Gentry, R. F. (1965). Standardization of the fluorescent antibody technique for the detection of avian respiratory viruses. *Avian Diseases* **9**, 535–545.

Brion, A., Moraillon, A., and Cakala, A. (1969). Valeur de la vaccination contre la bronchite infectieuse par virus inactive a la beta-propiolactone. Personal communication. *Recherches Vétérinaires* (in press).

Broadfoot, D. I., and Smith, W. M., Jr. (1954). Effects of infectious bronchitis in laying hens on egg production, percent unsettable eggs and hatchability. *Poultry Science* 33, 653–654.

Broadfoot, D. I., Pomeroy, B. S., and Smith, W. M., Jr. (1956). Effects of infectious bronchitis in baby chicks. *Poultry Science* 35, 757–762.

Brown, J. L. (1969). Immunofluorescence of avian infectious bronchitis virus and Newcastle disease virus in singly and dually infected cell cultures. M.S. Thesis, Michigan State University, East Lansing, Michigan.

Brown, W. E., Schmittle, S. C., and Foster, J. W. (1962). A tannic acid modified hemagglutination test for infectious bronchitis of chickens. *Avian Diseases* 6, 99–106.

Brumfield, H. P., and Pomeroy, B. S. (1957). Direct complement fixation by turkey and chicken serum in viral systems. *Proceedings of the Society for Experimental Biology and Medicine* 94, 146–149.

Burke, C. N., Luginbuhl, R. E., and Williams, L. F. (1968). Avian adeno-like viruses —characterization and comparison of seven isolates. *Avian Diseases* 12, 483–505.

Cabasso, V. J. (1965). The emerging classification of animal viruses—a review. *Avian Diseases* 9, 471–489.

Calnek, B. W., Taylor, P. J., and Sevoian, M. (1960). Studies on avian encephalomyelitis. IV. Epizootiology. *Avian Diseases* 4, 325–347.

Chomiak, T. W., Luginbuhl, R. E., and Steele, F. M. (1963). Serologic differences between the Beaudette and Massachusetts strains of infectious bronchitis virus. *Avian Diseases* 7, 325–331.

Colwell, W. M., and Lukert, P. D. (1969). Effects of avian infectious bronchitis virus (IBV) on tracheal organ cultures. *Avian Diseases* 13, 888–894.

Cook, J. K. A. (1968). Duration of experimental infectious bronchitis in chickens. *Research in Veterinary Science* 9, 506–514.

Cook, J. K. A., and Garside, J. S. (1967). A study of the infectious bronchitis status of a group of chicks hatched from infectious bronchitis infected hens. *Research in Veterinary Science* 8, 74–82.

Corbo, L. J., and Cunningham, C. H. (1959). Hemagglutination by trypsin-modified infectious bronchitis virus. *American Journal of Veterinary Research* 20, 876–883.

Cumming, R. B. (1963). Infectious avian nephroses (uraemia) in Australia. *Australian Veterinary Journal* 39, 115–147.

Cunningham, C. H. (1947). Cultivation of the virus of infectious bronchitis of chickens in embryonated chicken eggs. *American Journal of Veterinary Research* 8, 209–212.

Cunningham, C. H. (1951). Newcastle disease and infectious bronchitis neutralizing antibody indexes of normal chicken serum. *American Journal of Veterinary Research* 12, 129–133.

Cunningham, C. H. (1952). Methods employed in the diagnosis and investigation of infectious bronchitis and Newcastle disease. *Proceedings Book of the 89th Annual Meeting of the American Veterinary Medical Association, Atlantic City, New Jersey* pp. 251–257.

Cunningham, C. H. (1957). Symposium on immunization against infectious bronchitis virus. I. Some basic properties of infectious bronchitis virus. *American Journal of Veterinary Research* 18, 648–654.

Cunningham, C. H. (1960). Recent studies on the virus of infectious bronchitis. *American Journal of Veterinary Research* 21, 498–503.

Cunningham, C. H. (1963). Newer knowledge of infectious bronchitis virus. *Proceed-

ings of the XVIIth World Veterinary Congress, Hannover, Germany, 1963 Vol. 1, pp. 607–610.

Cunningham, C. H. (1966a). "A Laboratory Guide in Virology," 6th ed. Burgess, Minneapolis, Minnesota.

Cunningham, C. H. (1966b). Newer information on the properties of infectious bronchitis virus. *Proceedings of the 13th World's Poultry Congress, Kiev, Russia, 1966* pp. 416–418.

Cunningham, C. H. (1966c). Infectious bronchitis of poultry. *In* "International Encyclopedia of Veterinary Medicine" (T. Dalling and A. Robertson, eds.), Vol. I, pp. 477–483. I. W. Green & Son, Ltd., Edinburgh.

Cunningham, C. H., and El Dardiry, A. H. (1948). Distribution of the virus of infectious bronchitis of chickens in embryonated chicken eggs. *Cornell Veterinarian* **38**, 381–388.

Cunningham, C. H., and Jones, M. H. (1953). The effect of different routes of inoculation on the adaptation of infectious bronchitis virus to embryonating chicken eggs. *Proceedings Book of the 90th Annual Meeting of the American Veterinary Medical Association, Toronto, Canada.* pp. 337–342.

Cunningham, C. H., and Spring, M. P. (1965). Some studies of infectious bronchitis virus in cell culture. *Avian Diseases* **9**, 182–193.

Cunningham, C. H., and Stuart, H. O. (1946). The effect of certain chemical agents on the virus of infectious bronchitis of chickens. *American Journal of Veterinary Research* **7**, 466–469.

Cunningham, C. H., and Stuart, H. O. (1947). The pH stability of the virus of infectious bronchitis of chickens. *Cornell Veterinarian* **37**, 99–103.

David-Ferreira, J. F., and Manaker, R. A. (1965). An electron microscope study of the development of a mouse hepatitis virus in tissue culture cells. *Journal of Cell Biology* **24**, 57–78.

Delaplane, J. P., and Stuart, H. O. (1941). The modification of infectious bronchitis virus of chickens as the result of propagation in embryonated chicken eggs. *Rhode Island Agricultural Experiment Station, Bulletin* **284**, 1–20.

Dimopoullos, G. T., and Cunningham, C. H. (1956). Electrophoretic and serum neutralization studies of infectious bronchitis of chickens. *American Journal of Veterinary Research* **17**, 755–762.

Domermuth, C. H., and Edwards, O. F. (1957). An electron microscope study of chorioallantoic membrane infected with virus of avian infectious bronchitis. *Journal of Infectious Diseases* **100**, 74–81.

DuBose, R. T. (1967). Adaptation of the Massachusetts strain of infectious bronchitis virus to turkey embryos. *Avian Diseases* **11**, 28–38.

DuBose, R. T., and Grumbles, L. C. (1959). The relationship between quail bronchitis virus and chicken embryo lethal orphan virus. *Avian Diseases* **3**, 321–344.

Ellis, L. F. (1965). Centrifugation studies of infectious bronchitis virus. Ph.D. Thesis, Michigan State University, East Lansing, Michigan. Cited by Cunningham (1966b).

Estola, T. (1966). Studies on the infectious bronchitis virus of chickens isolated in Finland with reference to the serological survey of its occurrence. *Acta Veterinaria Scandinavica* Supplementum **18**, 1–111.

Estola, T. (1967). Sensitivity of suckling mice to various strains of infectious bronchitis virus. *Acta Veterinaria Scandinavica* **8**, 86–87.

Estola, T., and Weckström, P. (1967). Electron microscopy of infectious bronchitis virus. *Annales Medicinae Experimentalis Fenniae (Helsinki)* **45**, 30–31.

Fabricant, J., and Levine, P. P. (1951). The persistence of infectious bronchitis in eggs and tracheal exudates of infected chickens. *Cornell Veterinarian* **41**, 240–246.

Fahey, J. E., and Crawley, J. F. (1956). Propagation of infectious bronchitis virus in tissue culture. *Canadian Journal of Microbiology* **2**, 503–510.

Fontaine, M. P., Chabas, D., Fontaine, M., and Brion, A. J. (1963). A simplified technique for the serum-neutralization test in infectious bronchitis. *Avian Diseases* **7**, 203–206.

Fontaine, M. P., Fontaine, M., Chabas, D., and Brion, A. J. (1965). Presence of a Newcastle disease-like agent in chicken embryo cells. *Avian Diseases* **9**, 1–7.

Hamre, D., and Procknow, J. J. (1966). A new virus isolated from the human respiratory tract. *Proceedings of the Society for Experimental Biology and Medicine* **121**, 190–193.

Hanson, L. E., and Alberts, J. O. (1959). Factors affecting interference with Newcastle disease. *American Journal of Veterinary Research* **20**, 352–356.

Hanson, L. E., White, F. H., and Alberts, J. O. (1956). Interference between Newcastle disease and infectious bronchitis viruses. *American Journal of Veterinary Research* **17**, 294–298.

Hitchner, S. B., and White, P. G. (1955). Growth-curve studies of chick embryo-propagated infectious bronchitis virus. *Poultry Science* **34**, 590–594.

Hitchner, S. B., Appleton, G. S., and Winterfield, R. W. (1964). Evaluation of the immunity response to infectious bronchitis virus. *Avian Diseases* **8**, 153–162.

Hitchner, S. B., Winterfield, R. W., and Appleton, G. S. (1966). Infectious bronchitis virus types—incidence in the United States. *Avian Diseases* **10**, 98–102.

Hofstad, M. S. (1945). A study of infectious bronchitis in chickens. I. The pathology of infectious bronchitis. *Cornell Veterinarian* **35**, 22–31.

Hofstad, M. S. (1947). A study of infectious bronchitis in chickens. IV. Further observations on the carrier status of chickens recovered from infectious bronchitis. *Cornell Veterinarian* **37**, 29–34.

Hofstad, M. S. (1956). Stability of avian infectious bronchitis virus at 56°C. *Cornell Veterinarian* **46**, 122–128.

Hofstad, M. S. (1958). Antigenic differences among isolates of avian infectious bronchitis virus. *American Journal of Veterinary Research* **19**, 740–743.

Hofstad, M. S. (1961). Antigenic and immunological studies on several isolates of avian infectious bronchitis virus. *Avian Diseases* **5**, 102–107.

Hofstad, M. S. (1967). Immunity following aerosol exposure to high-embryo-passage avian infectious bronchitis virus. *Avian Diseases* **11**, 452–458.

Hofstad, M. S. (1969). Avian infectious bronchitis. Personal communication. *In* "Diseases of Poultry" (Editorial Committee of the American Association of Avian Pathologists, eds.), 6th ed. Iowa State Univ. Press, Ames, Iowa (in press).

Hofstad, M. S., and Yoder, H. W., Jr. (1963). Inactivation rates of some lyophilized poultry viruses at 37 and 3°C. *Avian Diseases* **7**, 170–177.

Hofstad, M. S., and Yoder, H. W., Jr. (1966). Avian infectious bronchitis—virus distribution in tissues of chicks. *Avian Diseases* **10**, 230–239.

Hopkins, S. R. (1967). Thermal stability of infectious bronchitis virus in the presence of salt solutions. *Avian Diseases* **10**, 261–267.

Jungherr, E. L., and Terrell, N. L. (1948). Naturally acquired passive immunity to infectious bronchitis in chicks. *American Journal of Veterinary Research* **9**, 201–205.

Jungherr, E. L., Chomiak, T. W., and Luginbuhl, R. E. (1956). Immunologic differences in strains of infectious bronchitis virus. *Proceedings of the 60th Annual*

Meeting of the United States Livestock Sanitary Association, Chicago, Illinois pp. 203–209.

Kawamura, H., Isogai, S., and Tsubahara, H. (1961). Propagation of avian infectious bronchitis virus in chicken kidney tissue culture. *National Institute of Animal Health Quarterly* 1, 190–198.

Lacey, R. B. (1968). The use of serially propagated African green monkey kidney cells in the detection of a latent Newcastle disease virus in chicken embryos. Ph.D. Thesis, Michigan State University, East Lansing, Michigan.

Larose, R. N., and Van Roekel, H. (1961). The effects of rapid embryo passage upon the infectious bronchitis virus. *Avian Diseases* 5, 157–168.

Levine, P. P. (1957). The distribution of P^{32} and S^{35} in bronchitis infected embryos. *Avian Diseases* 1, 110–114.

Levine, P. P., and Hofstad, M. S. (1947). Attempts to control airborne infectious bronchitis and Newcastle disease of fowls with sterilamps. *Cornell Veterinarian* 37, 204–210.

Loomis, L. N., Cunningham, C. H., Gray, M. L., and Thorpe, F., Jr. (1950). Pathology of the chicken embryo infected with infectious bronchitis virus. *American Journal of Veterinary Research* 11, 245–251.

Luginbuhl, R. E., and Jungherr, E. L. (1953). Simultaneous titration of Newcastle disease and infectious bronchitis viruses in embryonating eggs. *Poultry Science* 32, 911–912.

Lukert, P. D. (1965). Comparative sensitivities of embryonated chicken's eggs and primary chicken embryo kidney and liver cell cultures to infectious bronchitis virus. *Avian Diseases* 9, 308–316.

Lukert, P. D. (1966a). Immunofluorescence of avian infectious bronchitis virus in primary chicken embryo kidney, liver, lung, and fibroblast cultures. *Archiv für die gesamte Virusforschung* 19, 265–272.

Lukert, P. D. (1966b). A plaque reduction method for the detection of neutralizing antibodies for infectious bronchitis virus. *Avian Diseases* 10, 305–313.

Lukert, P. D. (1967). Characterization of receptors and lysosomes of cells susceptible to infectious bronchitis virus. Ph.D. Thesis, Iowa State University, Ames, Iowa.

Lukert, P. D. (1969). Differentiation of avian infectious bronchitis virus serotypes by immunofluorescence. *Avian Diseases* 13, 847–852.

McDougall, J. S. (1968). Infectious bronchitis in laying fowls. Its effect upon egg production and subsequent egg quality. *Veterinary Record* 83, 84–86.

McIntosh, K., Dees, J. H., Becker, W. B., Kapikian, A. Z., and Chanock, R. M. (1967). Recovery in tracheal organ cultures of novel viruses from patients with respiratory disease. *Proceedings of the National Academy of Sciences of the United States* 57, 933–940.

Maire, C., Renault, L., Woernle, H., Perrault, C., Stucky, B., Lelievre, J., and Toumeyragues, J. (1967). Bronchite infectieuse aviaire. Intérêt de la recherche des anticorps neutralisants et des anticorps précipitants. *Recueil de Médicine Vétérinaire* 143, 411–426.

Mallmann, V. H., and Cunningham, C. H. (1963). A study of infectious bronchitis virus before and after resin treatment for separation from a cell-attachment-and-growth factor. *American Journal of Veterinary Research* 24, 359–366.

Mallucci, L. (1965). Observations on the growth of mouse hepatitis virus (MHV-3) in mouse macrophages. *Virology* 25, 30–37.

Markham, F. S., Hammar, A. H., Perry, E. B., and Tesar, W. C. (1956). Combined

Newcastle disease-infectious bronchitis vaccine and the absence of interference phenomena. *Cornell Veterinarian* **46**, 538–548.

Mathews, J., and Hofstad, M. S. (1953). The inactivation of certain animal viruses by ethylene oxide (carboxide). *Cornell Veterinarian* **43**, 452–461.

Miller, L. T., and Yates, V. J. (1968). Neutralization of infectious bronchitis virus by human sera. *American Journal of Epidemiology* **88**, 406–409.

Mohanty, S. B., and Chang, S. C. (1963). Development and ether sensitivity of infectious bronchitis virus of chickens in cell cultures. *American Journal of Veterinary Research* **24**, 822–826.

Mohanty, S. B., DeVolt, H. M., and Faber, J. E. (1964). A fluorescent antibody study of infectious bronchitis virus. *Poultry Science* **43**, 179–182.

Muldoon, R. L. (1960). Some characteristics of the hemagglutinating activity of infectious bronchitis virus. Ph.D. Thesis, Michigan State University, East Lansing, Michigan. Cited by Cunningham (1963).

Muldoon, R. L., and Cunningham, C. H. (1961). Some characteristics of the hemagglutinating activity of infectious bronchitis virus. *Bacteriological Proceedings (Society of American Bacteriologists)* **61**, 157.

Nazerian, K. (1960). Electron microscopy studies of the virus of infectious bronchitis and erythrocytes agglutinated by trypsin modified virus. M.S. Thesis, Michigan State University, East Lansing, Michigan. Cited by Cunningham (1963).

Nazerian, K. (1965). Electron microscopic studies of infectious bronchitis virus. Ph.D. Thesis, Michigan State University, East Lansing, Michigan. Cited by Cunningham (1966b).

Nazerian, K., and Cunningham, C. H. (1967). Electron microscopy of the hemagglutinin of infectious bronchitis virus. *Proceedings of the 25th Annual Electron Microscopy Society of America, Chicago, Illinois* pp. 94–95.

Nazerian, K., and Cunningham, C. H. (1968). Morphogenesis of avian infectious bronchitis virus in chicken embryo fibroblasts. *Journal of General Virology* **3**, 469–470.

Oshel, D. D. (1961). A study of some variables in the neutralization test as used for potency testing commercially available infectious bronchitis vaccines. M.S. Thesis, Michigan State University, East Lansing, Michigan.

Page, C. A., and Cunningham, C. H. (1962). The neutralization test for infectious bronchitis virus. *American Journal of Veterinary Research* **23**, 1065–1071.

Petek, M., and Corazzola, S. (1958). Azione inattivante dell'etere etilico e del siero fresco sul virus della bronchite infettiva. *Veterinaria Italiana* **9**, 515–520.

Pette, J. (1959). Zur Ausscheidung des Hühner-bronchitisvirus im Kloakeninhalt. *Monatshefte für Tierheilkunde* **11**, 296–300.

Powers, C. D. (1965). Inactivation of infectious bronchitis virus infectivity by para-chloromercuribenzoate. M.S. Thesis, Michigan State University, East Lansing, Michigan. Cited by Cunningham (1966b).

Prince, R. P., Potter, L. M., Luginbuhl, R. E., and Chomiak, T. (1962). Effect of ventilation rate on the performance of chicks inoculated with infectious bronchitis virus. *Poultry Science* **41**, 268–272.

Prince, R. P., Whitaker, J. H., Luginbuhl, R. E., and Matterson, L. D. (1967). Effect of environmental temperatures on healthy chicks and chicks inoculated with infectious bronchitis virus. *Poultry Science* **46**, 1098–1102.

Purchase, H. G., Cunningham, C. H., and Burmester, B. R. (1966a). Identification and epizootiology of infectious bronchitis in a closed flock. *Avian Diseases* **10**, 111–121.

Purchase, H. G., Cunningham, C. H., and Burmester, B. R. (1966b). Genetic differences among chicken embryos in response to inoculation with an isolate of infectious bronchitis virus. *Avian Diseases* **10**, 162–172.

Quiroz, C. A., and Hanson, R. P. (1958). Physical-chemical treatment of inocula as a means of separating and identifying avian viruses. *Avian Diseases* **2**, 94–98.

Raggi, L. G. (1958). A note on survival time of an infectious bronchitis virus at various pH in distilled water. *Poultry Science* **37**, 1464–1465.

Raggi, L. G., and Lee, G. G. (1964). Infectious bronchitis virus interference with growth of Newcastle disease virus. II. Interference in chickens. *Avian Diseases* **8**, 471–480.

Raggi, L. G., and Lee, G. G. (1965). Lack of correlation between infectivity, serologic response and challenge results in immunization with an avian infectious bronchitis vaccine. *Journal of Immunology* **94**, 538–543.

Raggi, L. G., Lee, G. G., and Sohrab-Haghighat, V. (1963). Infectious bronchitis virus interference with Newcastle disease virus. I. Study of interference in chicken embryos. *Avian Diseases* **7**, 106–122.

Raggi, L. G., Young, D. C., and Sharma, J. M. (1967a). Synergism between avian infectious bronchitis virus and Haemophilus gallinarum. *Avian Diseases* **11**, 308–321.

Raggi, L. G., Asmar, J., and Lee, G. G. (1967b). Coexistence of infectious bronchitis and laryngotracheitis. *Avian Diseases* **11**, 419–426.

Reagan, R. L., and Brueckner, A. L. (1952). Electron microscope studies of four strains of infectious bronchitis virus. *American Journal of Veterinary Research* **13**, 417–418.

Sato, T., Surgimori, T., Ishii, S., and Matumoto, M. (1955). Infectious bronchitis of chickens in Japan. II. Identification of the causative agent as the virus of infectious bronchitis of chickens. *Japanese Journal of Experimental Medicine* **25**, 143–150.

Schalk, A. F., and Hawn, M. C. (1931). An apparently new respiratory disease of baby chicks. *Journal of the American Veterinary Medical Association* **78**, 413–422.

Sevoian, M., and Levine, P. P. (1957). Effects of infectious bronchitis on the reproductive tracts, egg production, and egg quality of laying chickens. *Avian Diseases* **1**, 136–164.

Simpson, R. W., and Groupé, V. (1959). Temperature of incubation as a critical factor in the behavior of avian bronchitis virus in chicken embryos. *Virology* **8**, 456–469.

Singh, I. P. (1960). Some properties of infectious bronchitis virus as determined by thermal and formalin inactivation. Ph.D. Thesis, Michigan State University, East Lansing, Michigan.

Steele, F. M., and Luginbuhl, R. E. (1964). Direct and indirect complement-fixation tests for infectious bronchitis virus. *American Journal of Veterinary Research* **25**, 1249–1255.

Stinski, M. F. (1969). Interaction of nonneutralized and neutralized avian infectious bronchitis virus with the chicken embryo kidney cell. I. Entry into the cell. II. Viral degradation. Ph.D. Thesis, Michigan State University, East Lansing, Michigan.

Stinski, M. F., and Cunningham, C. H. (1967). The infectious bronchitis virus-neutralizing antibody complex. *Proceedings of the XVIIIth World Veterinary Congress, Paris, 1967* Vol. 2, p. 625.

Stinski, M. F., and Cunningham, C. H. (1969). Neutralizing antibody complex of infectious bronchitis virus. *Journal of Immunology* **102**, 720–727.

Stultz, W. E. (1962). Fluorescent antibody studies of infectious bronchitis virus. M.S. Thesis, Michigan State University, East Lansing, Michigan. Cited by Cunningham (1963).

Tevethia, S. S. (1964). Studies of the antigens of infectious bronchitis virus. Ph.D. Thesis, Michigan State University, East Lansing, Michigan. Cited by Cunningham (1966b).

Tevethia, S. S., and Cunningham, C. H. (1968). Antigenic characterization of infectious bronchitis virus. *Journal of Immunology* **100**, 793–798.

Tyrrell, D. A. J., and Bynoe, M. L. (1965). Cultivation of a novel type of common-cold virus in organ cultures. *British Medical Journal* **1**, 1467–1470.

Tyrrell, D. A. J., Almeida, J. D., Berry, D. M., Cunningham, C. H., Hamre, D., Hofstad, M. S., Mallucci, L., and McIntosh, K. (1968). Coronaviruses. *Nature* **220**, 650.

Van Roekel, H., Clarke, M. K., Bullis, K. L., Olesiuk, O. M., and Sperling, F. G. (1951). Infectious bronchitis. *American Journal of Veterinary Research* **12**, 140–146.

von Bülow, V. (1966a). Infektiöse Bronchitis der Hühner. I. Viruszüchtung in Zellkulturen aus Hühnerembryonieren. *Zentralblatt für Veterinärmedizin* **13B**, 345–363.

von Bülow, V. (1966b). Infektiöse bronchitis der Hühner. II. Änderung der Virusvirulenz nach Serienpassagen in Zellkulturen. *Zentralblatt für Veterinärmedizin* **13B**, 671–683.

von Bülow, V. (1966c). Infektiöse bronchitis der Hühner. III. Vergleichende Untersuchungen der Virulenz und Wirksamkeit von vier Lebendvakzinen. *Zentralblatt für Veterinärmedizin* **13B**, 767–781.

von Bülow, V. (1967a). Infektiöse bronchitis der Hühner. IV. Charakterisierung eines neuen Feldstammes des IB-virus (IBV-10). *Zentralblatt für Veterinärmedizin* **14B**, 151–162.

von Bülow, V. (1967b). Untersuchungen über den Neutralisationstest bei der infektiösen Bronchitis der Hühner. *Zentralblatt für Veterinärmedizin* **14B**, 321–342.

Wilner, B. I. (1969). "A Classification of the Major Groups of Human and Other Animal Viruses," 4th ed. Burgess, Minneapolis, Minnesota.

Winterfield, R. W. (1967). Immunity response from an inactivated infectious bronchitis vaccine. *Avian Diseases* **11**, 446–451.

Winterfield, R. W. (1968). Respiratory signs, immunity response, and interference from vaccination with monovalent and multivalent infectious bronchitis vaccines. *Avian Diseases* **12**, 577–584.

Winterfield, R. W., Hitchner, S. B., and Appleton, G. S. (1964a). Immunological characteristics of a variant of infectious bronchitis virus isolated from chickens. *Avian Diseases* **8**, 40–47.

Winterfield, R. W., Cumming, R. B., and Hitchner, S. B. (1964b). Serological study of Australian chickens affected with a uremia disease syndrome. *Avian Diseases* **8**, 234–244.

Woernle, H. (1961). Impfversuche mit Adsorbat-Vakzine bei der infektiösen Bronchitis des Huhnes. *Monatshefte für Tierheilkunde* **13**, 136–142.

Woernle, H. (1966). The use of the agar-gel diffusion technique in the identification of certain avian virus diseases. *Veterinarian* **4**, 17–28.

Wright, B. S., and Sagik, B. P. (1958). Plaque formation in monolayers of chicken embryo kidney cells. *Virology* **5,** 573–574.

Yates, V. J., Ablashi, D. V., and Chang, P. W. (1968). The effect of a latent avian encephalomyelitis virus infection in the chicken embryo on the propagation of Newcastle disease, influenza, and infectious bronchitis viruses. *Avian Diseases* **12,** 401–411.

Immunologic Injury to Dogs

ROBERT O. JACOBY AND RICHARD A. GRIESEMER*

Department of Veterinary Pathology, The Ohio State University, Columbus, Ohio

* Dr. Jacoby is Assistant Professor of Immunopathology in the Department of Veterinary Pathology at the Ohio State University. His current address is Department of Pathology, University of Chicago, Chicago, Illinois. Dr. Griesemer is Professor and Chairman, Department of Veterinary Pathology, The Ohio State University, Columbus, Ohio.

I. Introduction

Dramatic advances in immunologic research during the past decade have increased our understanding of the role of immune mechanisms in disease processes. The dog has played a central role in the advancement of knowledge, particularly in relation to transplantation, hypersensitivity, and autosensitivity.

This review is intended to summarize the current status of information on immunologic injury in dogs and to suggest potential directions for future research. The discussion is organized in 6 sections: development of immunity, serum proteins, hypersensitivity, autosensitivity, transplantation, and tumor immunity. Limitations of length of chapters prevent our citing all pertinent references; consequently, we have selected the most timely and comprehensive reports, whenever possible.

II. Development of Immunity

1. General Considerations

The lymphoreticular system is responsible for the development and maintenance of adaptive immune mechanisms (Good and Papermaster, 1964). The structural components of the lymphoreticular system may be separated into a tripartite developmental and functional hierarchy composed of the stem cell compartment (probably bone marrow), the so-called central lymphoid tissue composed of thymus and gut-associated lymphoid tissue (GALT), and the peripheral lymphoid tissue composed of spleen and lymph nodes. Current evidence suggests that bone marrow may seed pluripotential stem cells to both central and peripheral lymphoid tissues. Central lymphoid tissue probably directs the differentiation of stem cells to immunologically competent cells (Daniels *et al.*, 1968; Mitchell and Miller, 1968).

2. Lymphoid Tissue

In the dog, lymphoid tissues mature during the last third of fetal life. The thymus is present by day 40 of gestation, and lymphoid cells appear in the lymph nodes and spleen by day 48 and day 54, respectively. At birth, Peyer's patches are present in the small intestine, and population of the lymphoid tissues is essentially complete (Kelly, 1963; Hayes, 1968). The adult dog is reported to have about 1.5 to 2.8×10^9 mobilizable small lymphocytes per kilogram of body weight or about 7 times the number found in the peripheral blood (Schnappauf and Schnappauf, 1968). These lymphocytes originate in peripheral lymphoid tissues and probably recirculate from blood to lymph (Benninghoff *et al.*, 1968). Architecturally, mature canine lymphoid tissue resembles that found in other mammals (M. E. Miller *et al.*, 1964). Senile changes occurring in the lymphoid tissue of aging dogs include involution of the lymph nodes and thymus, nodular hyperplasia of the splenic white pulp, and intrathymic epithelial cyst formation (Mulligan, 1963; Kruvskii, 1967).

3. ACTIVE IMMUNITY

a. Humoral and Cell-Mediated Responses

Immunologic responsiveness to a series of antigens by many species appears to develop sequentially, rather than simultaneously (Sterzl and Silverstein, 1967). Recent evidence indicates that the dog follows this pattern. For example, a humoral antibody response can be detected at birth in pups that had been injected *in utero* with bacteriophage ϕX-174 on the 40th day of gestation (Jacoby *et al.*, 1969). Pups appear incapable, however, of responding to an aqueous solution of bovine serum albumin (BSA) injected at birth unless the albumin has been emulsified in complete Freund's adjuvant. Moreover, humoral responses to such antigens, as expressed by serum antibody titers, increase with age. Humoral responses by adult dogs vary with the nature and quantity of antigen used, as well as the route by which it is administered. In general, dogs are better producers of nonprecipitating than precipitating antisera and respond better to particulate than soluble antigens (Patterson *et al.*, 1963b; Jacoby *et al.*, 1969).

Similarly, cell-mediated responses in dogs appear to be age-dependent (Dennis *et al.*, 1969a). Allogeneic skin grafts placed on canine fetuses at the 40th or 48th day of gestation are rejected in a protracted fashion (mean survival time of 42 days), whereas neonatal dogs are able to reject allogeneic skin from the same donor as rapidly as adult dogs, the mean survival time of the graft being of 9.5 days.

The senile changes in canine lymphoid tissue associated with aging may portend a diminished capacity to respond to antigenic stimulation as has been demonstrated in mice (Hanna *et al.*, 1967).

b. Role of the Central Lymphoid Tissue

The thymus and GALT appear to share control of the structural and functional development of the immune system (M. D. Cooper *et al.*, 1967), the thymus governing the maturation of cell-mediated defenses and the GALT regulating humorally mediated defenses. Consequently, removal of the central lymphoid tissue prior to full immunologic development should ablate, or at least diminish, immunologic responsiveness.

Dogs thymectomized *in utero* on the 48th day of gestation and grafted with allogeneic skin at birth retain the grafts for prolonged periods, the grafts having mean survival times of 40.8 days (Dennis *et al.*, 1969b). It has been technically impossible to remove the thymuses of younger fetuses to determine when thymic influence on immunologic development begins. Predictably, thymectomy of neonatal and adult dogs does not cripple cell-mediated responsiveness (Van de Water and Katzman, 1964; Oliveras *et al.*, 1963), because this expression of immunologic competence is mature at birth. Nevertheless, thymectomized adult dogs whose lymphoid tissues have been destroyed by x-irradiation fail to regain immunologic competence following bone marrow infusions (Chertkov *et al.*, 1965), whereas their nonthymectomized counterparts recover (Samoylina and Chertkov, 1966; Epstein *et al.*, 1967). These results indicate not only that the functional capacity of the thymus remains intact in adult dogs, but also that lymphoid cell precursors subsist in the bone marrow.

The role of canine GALT in the development of humoral responsiveness is unknown. Some control over this phase of immune function by the dog has been preempted by the thymus, since thymectomy of fetal dogs diminishes humoral antibody production against bacteriophage ϕX-174 (Dennis *et al.*, 1969b). Chretein and associates (1967) showed that Peyer's patches, in contrast to peripheral lymph nodes fail to hypertrophy in dogs subjected to subtotal lymphadenectomy, thus implying that intestinal lymphoid tissue is distinct in some manner. The function of canine GALT might be clarified by comparing the immune responses of dogs who have recovered from tonsillectomy and ileocecostomy, coupled with x-irradiation, to the responses of sham-operated x-irradiated dogs. One would expect, as has been shown in rabbits (Perey and Good, 1968), that GALT is necessary for return of humoral responsiveness of animals so treated.

4. Passive Immunity

a. Prenatal Transfer

The endotheliochorial placenta of the dog acts as a selective unidirectional barrier which permits passage of specific serum proteins from dam to fetus while blocking passage of fetal antigens to the maternal circulation (Brambell, 1958; Jackson, 1967). The quantity of antibody absorbed by a fetus during pregnancy is small. Less than 300 milligrams of maternal plasma protein reaches each fetus daily (Whipple *et al.*, 1955), and immunoglobulins represent only a fraction of this total. Gillespie and co-workers (1958) reported that about 3% of a dam's neutralizing titer to canine distemper virus is transferred to the fetus. It is not known whether prenatally transferred canine antibodies are exclusively γG-globulins as reported in most species (Brambell, 1966).

b. *Postnatal Transfer*

The bulk of passive immunity is conferred on pups during the first days of life through ingestion and absorption of colostral antibodies. Carmichael and co-workers (1962) found that maximal absorption of antibodies to infectious canine hepatitis virus occurred during the 12 hours after birth and was essentially complete by 72 hours. Gillette and Filkins (1966) reported that maximal absorption of antibodies to *Salmonella pullorum* occurred if puppies were fed 8 hours after birth and absorption was completed within 15 hours. Absorption was not detectable in pups fed antibody later than 24 hours after whelping.

The mechanism of absorption is obscure, but may involve recognition of antigenic determinants on immunoglobulin molecules by specific receptors on intestinal epithelial cells (Brambell, 1966). Factors associated with cessation of absorption are also ill-defined. Filkins and Gillette (1966) and Gillette and Filkins (1966) observed that whereas ingestion of other food is not a major factor, pups from bitches treated 24 hours prepartum with hydrocortisone or adrenal corticotropic hormone had a significantly reduced capacity to absorb antibodies through the intestine. Moog (1953) produced the same response in mice and found that it coincided with an elevation of duodenal alkaline phosphatase activity.

Colostral antibody titers of immune dams may exceed their corresponding serum antibody titers at the time of whelping, but decline markedly within several days, thus the titers correlate well with cessation of antibody absorption by puppies (Mason *et al.*, 1930; Carmichael *et al.*, 1962). Quantitative relationships have been established between the antibody titers of serum and colostrum of bitches and the serum antibody titers of their progeny (J. A. Baker *et al.*, 1959). These relationships have been used to predict the optimal time for active immunization of puppies since the presence of maternal antibody interferes with this process. Recent evidence indicates that canine colostral antibodies may represent a special class of serum proteins (IgA) selectively secreted into milk (Section III).

III. Serum Proteins

1. General Considerations

Canine serum contains about 6 grams of protein per 100 milliliters (Engle and Woods, 1960; Kozma *et al.*, 1967; Irfan, 1967). Albumin constitutes about 50% of the total serum proteins and the remaining portion consists of a structurally and functionally heterogeneous group of compounds called globulins. Paper electrophoretic analysis of canine serum usually reveals a peak in the albumin region and 4 to 6 peaks among the globulins; 2 peaks in the α-region (10–20% of the total serum protein), 1 to 2 peaks in the β-region (7–20% of the total serum protein), and 1 to 3 peaks in the γ-region (7–19% of the total serum protein) (Spector, 1956; Vesselinovitch, 1959; Engle and Woods, 1960; McKelvie et al., 1966; Irfan, 1967; Kozma et al., 1967). The wide range of values results from variations in technique, interpretation, and animal populations used for study. Immunoelectrophoretic analysis of canine serum has revealed at least 20 precipitin arcs (Okoshi et al., 1967).

2. Immunoglobulins

Globulins migrating in the β- and γ-regions are immunologically active proteins with a half-life of about 8 days (Dixon et al., 1952); they are synthesized by the lymphoreticular system in response to antigenic stimulation and are known collectively as immunoglobulins. In man, 5 classes of immunoglobulins have been recognized: IgA, IgD, IgE, IgG, and IgM (alternatively, γA, γD, γE, γG, and γM)[1] (Merler and Rosen, 1966). Canine analogs for 4 of these classes have recently been proposed as indicated in the summary of Table I. This classification may change as additional information about canine immunoglobulins becomes available.

Patterson and co-workers (1963b) had difficulty producing precipitating antibodies against heterologous serum proteins in dogs. They found subsequently that 2 types of antibody were made against the same antigenic determinant; a precipitating antibody and a nonprecipitating one (Patterson et al., 1964). The latter appeared to interfere with the ability of precipitating antibody to precipitate antigen in the region of antibody excess and resulted in a delay in attainment of equilibrium which is characteristic of canine precipitin curves. Precipitating antibody migrates electrophoretically in the γ_2-region as 2 or 3 antigenically distinct proteins which are collectively designated as canine IgG (Johnson and Vaughan, 1967; Johnson et al., 1967; Patterson, 1968). Nonprecipitating antibody migrates as a fast γ (γ_1) protein and is referred to as canine IgA. Specific antisera to canine IgA do not react with canine IgM or IgG Patterson et al., 1968), but some antisera against human IgA do crossreact with IgA from canine serum and milk (Vaerman and Heremans, 1968). Canine IgM has been identified as a fast moving γ_1 (β) macro-

---

[1] Nomenclature proposed by an international committee of immunologists in 1964. Ig = immunoglobin, γ = gamma globulin. [*Bulletin of the World Health Organization* **30**, 447–450 (1964).]

TABLE I

TYPES AND CHARACTERISTICS OF CANINE IMMUNOGLOBULINS[a]

Class	Sedimentation coefficient	Electrophoretic mobility	Selected properties
IgM	19 S	γ_1	Cross-reacts with human IgM, precipitating and agglutinating activity
IgG	7 S	γ_{2a}, γ_{2b}, (γ_{2c})	Precipitating and agglutinating activity, Arthus activity, mediates passive cutaneous anaphylaxis in guinea pigs
IgA	7 S Intermediate S (7–19 S, probably polymeric form)	γ_1	Nonprecipitating, inhibits precipitation of antigen by precipitating antibodies, present in colostrum at 4 to 80 × greater concentration than in serum, present in bronchial and salivary secretions, inhibits passive anaphylaxis induced by reaginic antibody, cross-reacts with human IgA
IgE	7 S–9 S	γ_1	Reaginic activity, Prausnitz-Küstner reactions, passive transfer of local and systemic anaphylaxis
IgD (unidentified)	—	—	—

[a] Tentative classification based on reports by Johnson and Vaughan (1967), Johnson et al. (1967), Rockey and Schwartzman (1967), Patterson et al. (1968, 1969), and Vaerman and Heremans (1968).

globulin, and Vaerman and Heremans (1968) showed cross reactions between human and canine IgM in immunoprecipitation tests. Antibodies which mediate immediate type hypersensitivity reactions (i.e., allergic rhinitis, anaphylaxis) are known as reagins. A canine immunoglobulin with reaginic properties, but antigenically distinct from IgG, IgA and IgM, has recently been identified and is provisionally designated as canine IgE (Patterson et al., 1968, 1969). Whether all reaginic activity in canine serum is restricted to IgE is not known.

3. OTHER IMMUNOLOGICALLY ACTIVE SERUM PROTEINS

Complement activity resides in an integrated system of at least 9 serum components. The components interact in sequence after antibody has bound to antigen and mediate a variety of immunologic reactions *in vitro* and *in vivo* including immune cytolysis, phagocytosis, and immune complex phenomena (Müller-Eberhard, 1968). The individual components of canine complement have not been studied, but Larin and co-workers (1957) showed that canine and guinea pig complement possess similar levels of hemolytic activity. They also used canine complement successfully in place of guinea pig complement for determining complement-fixing antibody titers in immune sera against infectious canine hepatitis virus. Normal canine serum complement levels based on hemolytic potency have been reported by several groups of investigators and generally range from 17 to 55 C'H$_{50}$ units per millileter (Baltch *et al.*, 1962, 1966; Gewurz *et al.*, 1966).

C-reactive protein is a nonantibody serum component which is found in man particularly during the acute stages of rheumatic disease and which forms a precipitate with the somatic C-polysaccharide of the pneumococcus. Dillman and Coles (1966) have isolated a protein from the serum of dogs subjected to several inflammatory stimuli that was agglutinated by an antiserum specific for C-reactive protein in man. The function of this serum fraction remains obscure.

Properdin, another physiochemically distinct normal serum protein which may participate in several immunologic reactions such as virus neutralization and bacteriostasis, has also been identified in canine serum (Baltch *et al.*, 1962; Michaelson *et al.*, 1966).

4. SERUM PROTEIN ALTERATIONS IN DISEASE

Increased quantities of serum α_2-globulins have been reported in the dog in canine distemper (Gibson *et al.*, 1965; Snow *et al.*, 1966), infectious canine hepatitis (Beckett *et al.*, 1964), renal disease (Moegle *et al.*, 1956), miscellaneous inflammatory conditions (Boguth, 1953), tumors (de Wael, 1956), allograft rejection (West *et al.*, 1960), and following cortisone administration (Bossak *et al.*, 1955). This rise seems to be nonspecific, although Howard and Kenyon (1965) were able to produce elevated α_2-globulins in normal dogs by administering histamine.

Seemingly nonspecific elevations of β-globulin in the dog have been found in chronic skin disease, endometritis, eosinophilic myositis, liver necrosis, and nephritis (Boguth, 1953; Moegle *et al.*, 1956). De Wael (1956) has claimed that β-globulins may be elevated in certain malignant, but not benign tumors. Some of these reported elevations of canine serum β-globulin may be due to specific antibody production since γM is known to migrate to this region of an electrophoretic field.

Serum gamma globulins may be elevated in almost any infectious, neoplastic, or nonspecific inflammatory disease (Boguth, 1953; de Wael,

1956; Beckett *et al.*, 1964; Snow *et al.*, 1966). They may also be increased in association with the rejection of transplanted organs (Chiba *et al.*, 1966) and in some of the so-called autosensitivity syndromes. Most of these increases probably represent host responses to specific antigenic stimulation.

Another type of canine hypergammaglobulinemia is associated with neoplastic disease of antibody-forming cells, plasma cell myeloma. Osborne and co-workers (1968b) reviewed 22 cases of canine plasma cell myeloma from 21 published reports. Unfortunately, serum protein values were available for only 11 of these cases, but each of 8 sera in this group examined for either hypergammaglobulinemia or paraproteinemia (abnormal globulins with little or no antibody activity) were positive. Bence-Jones proteinuria was found in 4 of 8 cases. The reader is referred to the review of Osborne and collaborators for a detailed account of this interesting canine gammopathy. To our knowledge, other forms of congential or acquired canine dysgammaglobulinemias have not been reported. Reviews by Alper and associates (1966) and Rosen and Janeway (1966) provide an introduction to this problem in man.

Amyloidosis must be mentioned here because it is characterized by intracellular deposition of an amorphous material (Trautwein, 1965) which may or may not contain immunologically active serum proteins (Cohen, 1967). The condition is frequently associated with chronic inflammatory disease and plasma cell myelomas. In dogs, the renal glomerulus appears to be a predilection site for amyloid deposition, and in advanced disease amyloid deposits may interfere with renal function and lead to uremia (Osborne *et al.*, 1968a).

IV. Hypersensitivity

1. General Considerations

Hypersensitivity can be defined as heightened reactivity following repeated contact with an antigen and which elevated reactivity results in immunologically induced injury to tissues. Two basic forms of hypersensitivity are recognized: immediate and delayed. Immediate hypersensitivity reactions may occur within minutes after administration of an offending agent and are mediated by circulating antibodies which unite with antigen on or near cell surfaces to cause release of proinflammatory substances. Anaphylaxis, allergy, and immune complex reactions (Arthus reactions, serum sickness) are examples of immediate-type responses (Austen, 1965; Cochrane, 1968). Delayed hypersensitivity reactions appear 12 to 48 hours after challenge with antigen and are mediated by sensitized lymphoid cells rather than circulating antibody.

When sensitized cells contact antigen, they appear to release mediator substances which are chemotactic for leukocytes, and inflammation ensues. The tuberculin reaction, contact dermatitis, allograft rejection, and certain forms of autosensitivity disease are considered prototypes of delayed hypersensitivity (Uhr, 1966; Benacerraf and Green, 1969).

2. IMMEDIATE HYPERSENSITIVITY

a. Anaphylaxis

In 1902, Portier and Richet described a syndrome in dogs characterized by bloody diarrhea, emesis, prostration, and death following attempts to immunize the animals with an extract of sea-actinia. Dogs were injected at 3-week intervals, and the fatal reaction quickly followed the second exposure. These workers decided they had not produced immunity or *prophylaxis*, but rather hypersensitivity which they called *anaphylaxis*.

The target organ for anaphylaxis varies with each species. In the dog, the liver is the principal shock organ. Sensitizing antigen, when administered intravenously, appears to be bound by anaphylactic antibody fixed on liver mast cells (Akcasu and West, 1960; Csaba et al., 1963, 1966). The mast cells release histamine to cause plasma levels to increase markedly; the histamine induces contraction of the spirally arranged musculature of intrahepatic throttling veins (Arey, 1941). Blood is retained in the liver, venous return to the heart decreases, cardiac output falls, and hypotension and shock ensue (Chou, 1965). Vasoactive amines other than histamine have not been incriminated in canine anaphylaxis (Cirstea et al., 1966).

A variety of antigens may elicit anaphylactic reactions in dogs including homologous and heterologous serum proteins (Bliss et al., 1959; Patterson et al., 1963b; Peng and Pi, 1967), ragweed antigen (Patterson and Sparks, 1962), and endotoxin (Spink et al., 1964). The microfilariae of *Dirofilaria immitis* have recently been found to provoke anaphylactic reactions following transfusion of homologous blood to infected dogs, (Ota et al., 1962). Godfrey and co-workers (1966) observed similar reactions in 75% of dogs with, and 21% of dogs without, demonstrable microfilariasis. Mantovani and Kagan (1967) have isolated an antigenic fraction of *D. immitis* which will react in skin tests or passive hemagglutination tests on dogs infected with the homologous parasite but not in tests of dogs infected with *D. repens* or *Dipetolonema* sp. In consideration of these findings, it has been recommended that either blood donors be free of microfilariae or recipients desensitized to *D. immitis*, if time permits, so that these "transfusion reactions" can be minimized (Ota et al., 1962).

b. Allergy

The term "allergy" is used to describe a heightened predisposition, often familial, to spontaneous local anaphylactic reactions which frequently involve the skin, respiratory tract, or gastrointestinal tract. The inciting agent is known as an allergen and the mediating antibody is known as a reagin. Dogs may develop allergies to a host of environmental allergens including animal flesh, cereal grains, milk, dust, feathers, tobacco, trees, mold, and internal parasites (Brunner *et al.*, 1944; Cortez *et al.*, 1947; E. Baker, 1966; Walton, 1966, 1967).

Most significant among canine allergies, for conceptual and comparative value, is allergy to ragweed pollen, which closely resembles hay fever in man (Wittich, 1941; Patterson, 1960). Susceptible dogs in the Northern Hemisphere begin to show annually recurring signs of generalized pruritis, conjunctivitis, rhinitis and, occasionally, asthma during late summer which continue until the onset of cold weather. In succeeding years, however, multisensitivities may appear in allergic animals, thereby delaying the amelioration of clinical signs (Schwartzman, 1965; Patterson, 1968). Sex, age, or breed predilections have not been established for the condition, but a high prevalence has been reported in terriers (Schwartzman and Rockey, 1967).

Sensitive animals usually have positive skin reactions to ragweed pollen (Schwartzman, 1965), and asthmatic responses may occur in some dogs that are exposed to aerosolized ragweed antigen (Patterson, 1960). Hypersensitivity to ragweed pollen can be passively transferred from affected to normal dogs with serum (Patterson and Sparks, 1962). Passively sensitized dogs challenged with ragweed antigen may display signs ranging from skin reactivity to asthma and anaphylaxis.

Ragweed allergy in dogs closely resembles hay fever in man in that both are (1) incited by ragweed pollen, (2) of proved immunologic basis, (3) demonstrable through direct or passive (P-K reaction) skin testing, (4) ameliorated by antihistamines and epinephrine, (5) clinically similar, and (6) probably familial (Schwartzman, 1965). Patterson and associates (1963c) have reinforced the last point by establishing a breeding colony of dogs with spontaneous allergy to ragweed. A major difference between the conditions in the two species is that dermatitis of obscure etiology occurs in dogs, not in man (Schwartzman, 1965).

Allergic reactions to ingested allergens in dogs consist primarily of gastrointestinal disturbances, i.e., emesis, diarrhea, but may also include cutaneous responses such as pruritis and urticaria, which lead to self-inflicted trauma (Joshua, 1956; Walton, 1966, 1967). Skin testing has been used successfully to incriminate a variety of ingested allergens in suspected cases of canine gastrointestinal allergy (Walton, 1967), but the pathogenesis of these reactions has not been studied.

Treatment of canine allergies by desensitization has been encouraging. Success appears to depend in large measure on accurate indentification of the offending allergen and proper administration of standardized allergenic extracts (E. Baker, 1969).

c. Antibodies in Anaphylaxis and Allergy

Spontaneous canine allergy, at least to ragweed pollen, appears to be mediated by a nonprecipitating, thermolabile, skin-sensitizing reaginic antibody (Patterson et al., 1963a, 1969). In contrast, normal dogs actively immunized with ragweed pollen develop nonprecipitating, thermostable antibodies similar to those elicited by immunization against heterologous serum proteins (Patterson et al., 1965; Arkins et al., 1967; Bukosky et al., 1968). The latter seem incapable of mediating either active or passive systemic anaphylaxis, but rather inhibit the reactions of dogs passively sensitized with canine reagin to challenge with ragweed extracts (Tennenbaum et al., 1963; Patterson et al., 1965). These so-called "blocking antibodies" are also produced in man by active immunization against allergens and appear to protect individuals against allergic reactions by neutralizing the offending allergen before it can bind to reagin fixed to cell surfaces (Connell, 1969).

Anaphylactic and reaginic activities to ragweed antigen seems to be located in the same serum fraction, but whether the antibodies are immunologically identical is not known definitely (Patterson et al., 1963a). Anaphylactic reactions may occur during the course of active immunization to heterologous proteins (Patterson et al., 1963b), but antibody from immunized dogs cannot sensitize normal dogs to passive cutaneous anaphylaxis (PCA) reactions. Canine anti-hapten or anti-egg albumin antibodies can, however, mediate PCA reactions in guinea pigs (Ovary et al., 1964; Patterson et al., 1964). Hence, anaphylactic activity in canine serum does not appear to be invariably associated with reaginic activity and may represent response associated with a mixture of antibody types. The literature on anaphylactic antibodies of mammals has been reviewed recently by Bloch (1967).

d. Injury Due to Immune Complexes

When antigen unites with precipitating antibody, under conditions of moderate to great antigen excess, soluble complexes are formed. These antigen-antibody complexes can precipitate in tissues, usually beneath the capillary endothelium, and initiate the release of proinflammatory factors from bound complement. A focal suppurative inflammatory process ensues, accompanied by thrombosis, necrosis, and hemorrhage when elicited in skin (Arthus reaction). Generalized immune-complex injury, such as serum sickness, may involve any tissue, but it is most common in the kidney where renal glomerular capillaries provide vulnerable sites for deposition of immune complexes. Thus, membranous glomerulonephritis is considered to be the classic lesion of immune complex disease (Cochrane, 1968).

Arthus reactivity (Patterson et al., 1964) and serum sickness (Iwasaki et al., 1967) have been produced in dogs, but evidence of spontaneous immune complex disease is scant. Nevertheless, the growing recognition of spontaneous immune complex injury in other animal species (D. D. Porter and Larson, 1968; Oldstone and Dixon, 1969) prompts consideration of its occurrence in the dog.

Viruses. Nongranulomatous uveitis and interstitial keratitis occur in about 20% of dogs during convalescence from infectious canine hepatitis (ICH). Carmichael (1964, 1965) was able to reproduce these lesions by inoculating ICH virus–antibody complexes intraocularly or by passive or reverse passive sensitization of normal dogs. Carmichael suggested that ICH virus may persist in the uvea following viremic stages of the disease and initiate immune injury on complexing with antibody in the uvea and cornea. Similarly, ICH virus may persist for prolonged periods in the endothelium of renal glomerular and interstitial capillaries (Wright, 1967a,b); thus, virus–antibody complexes may trigger some cases of interstitial nephritis or glomerulonephritis in dogs.

ICH virus–antibody complexes may affect the progression of hepatic lesions in ICH as well. Gocke and collaborators (1967) showed that dogs that were partially immune to ICH could survive acute stages of the disease only to develop chronic liver damage in the form of chronic non-suppurative hepatitis with widespread fibrosis in 7 to 8 months. The disease was invariably progressive despite the fact that ICH virus was demonstrable in hepatic tissues by immunofluorescence for only the first 7 days. These workers reproduced the syndrome by challenging passively immunized dogs with virulent virus. They speculated that excess virus and low titers of antibody may have formed immune complexes continuously, producing chronic hepatic injury. This report awaits confirmation by other workers.

Hottendorf and Nielsen (1966, 1968) suggested an immune complex pathogenesis for glomerulonephritis that was found in 20 of 29 dogs with mastocytoma. Although they did not speculate on the antigen, the filtrable agent recently incriminated in canine mastocytoma (Rickard and Post, 1968) is a plausible candidate.

Autoantigens. A group of diseases of man and lower animals is characterized by sensitivity to antigens of normal body tissues. In at least one of these conditions, systemic lupus erythematosus (SLE), circulating nuclear antigen–antibody complexes are known to be deposited in the renal glomeruli and contribute to the glomerulonephritis invariably associated with the disease (Koffler and Kunkel, 1968). Canine SLE closely resembles its human counterpart (Lewis *et al.*, 1965a), but the demonstration of immune complexes in nephritic canine kidneys has not been reported.

3. Delayed Hypersensitivity

The following discussion is restricted to contact dermatitis, flea bite dermatitis, and brief mention of delayed hypersensitivity in infectious disease. Autosensitivity and allograft rejection are covered elsewhere (Sections V and VI).

a. Contact Dermatitis

Contact dermatitis is the result of delayed cutaneous reaction to direct repeated contact with an environmental incitant. The offending agent may be any of a multitude of natural or synthetic chemical compounds (Muller, 1967). These compounds need not be antigenic in themselves, since many have haptenic properties and elicit sensitivity after combination with carrier proteins of skin (Baer and Harber, 1965).

Contact dermatitis in dogs is accompanied by severe pruritis and erythema, particularly on sparsely haired regions of the body, which may advance to excoriative or ulcerative dermatitis when self-trauma is extensive (Walton, 1965). Histologically, it appears initially as nonsuppurative dermatitis with typical perivascular mononuclear cell infiltrations common to all delayed hypersensitivity responses, but the reaction may become suppurative upon entrance of bacteria. Hyperkeratosis, acanthosis, and dermal fibrosis with mast cell infiltration characterize the chronic lesions. The severity of disease is enhanced by repeated contact with the sensitizing agent. Suspected incitants may be identified by patch testing which may evoke local dermatitis after a delay of 12 to 96 hours. Contact dermatitis cannot be passively transferred with serum, since it is cellularly mediated, thus differentiating it from dermatitis associated with immediate hypersensitivity. Cure depends on elimination of the causative agent from the dog's environment.

b. Flea Bite Dermatitis

Summer eczema of dogs, long suspected of being a hypersensitivity dermatitis (Kissileff, 1938) is now thought to be caused by sensitivity to flea bites. The reaction is similar, symptomatically and pathologically, to contact dermatitis (Muller, 1961) and may be initiated in sensitized dogs by the bite of a single flea (Kissileff, 1962).

The pathogenesis of flea bite hypersensitivity has been examined in detail recently using guinea pigs sensitized to the bite of the cat flea, *Ctenacephalides felis felis* (Benjamini *et al.*, 1960). Initial exposure of sensitized animals to flea bites or whole flea extracts could produce a delayed skin reaction within the first 5 to 7 days, evolving into a combination of delayed and immediate reactions which could be elicited up to 7 weeks and eventually predominated by immediate hypersensitivity, to progress to a nonreactive state about a month later (Benjamini *et al.*, 1961). The initial hypersensitive state could, however, be sustained for up to 18 months following a single exposure to fleas. Histologically, skin lesions reflected the change from delayed to immediate hypersensitivity, being first characterized by mononuclear cell infiltration and later by the presence of eosinophils (Larrivee *et al.*, 1964). It was then shown that an oral secretion from cat fleas contained one or more haptens which could combine with dermal collagen components during feeding to sensitize susceptible animals (Benjamini *et al.*, 1963; J. D. Young *et al.*, 1963; Michaeli *et al.*, 1965, 1966). Thus, contact dermatitis and flea bite dermatitis appear to be initiated by similar pathogenetic mechanisms. Although this work was done in guinea pigs, there is little reason to suspect that a different mechanism is operating in dogs. Hudson and co-workers (1960) showed that sensitized guinea pigs reacted to several species of fleas other than the one inducing sensitivity, indicating that all flea saliva may contain a common allergenic hapten. Futhermore, Michaeli and Goldfarb (1968) densenitized dogs and cats to flea bite hypersensitivity by weekly injections of a hapten fraction isolated from the saliva of cat fleas.

c. Infectious Agents

This topic receives brief treatment, not to minimize its importance, but because so little is known about it in dogs. Both ocular and cutaneous delayed reactions have been elicited in dogs convalescing from leptospirosis (Torten *et al.*, 1967; Ben-Efriam and Torten, 1968). Canine histoplasmosis and coccidioidomycosis (Ditchfield, 1968) are also associated with delayed-type cutaneous reactivity, but the role of hypersensitivity in the pathogenesis of these diseases requires further study. Conversely, the relative resistance of dogs to tuberculosis has not been adequately explained (Hobson and Ellett, 1968). The recent development of *in vitro* correlates of delayed hypersensitivity (David, 1967) should allow further examination of hypersensitivity in canine infectious diseases.

V. Autosensitivity

1. General Considerations

Considerable interest has been generated among immunologists by the recognition of spontaneous diseases of man and animals in which the host appears to evoke immunologic injury against its own tissues. Collectively, these are known as autosensitivity (autoimmune, autoallergic) disorders.

From a theoretic standpoint, if one accepts the hypothesis that, during immunologic development, an individual's lymphoreticular system is programmed for nonreactivity to unsequestered autoantigens (Burnet, 1959), then autosensitivity becomes, fundamentally, the manifestation of loss of tolerance to autoantigens. Mechanisms proposed to account for breakdown of tolerance to "self" include: (1) release of sequestered antigens normally concealed by physioanatomic barriers; (2) altered antigenicity of host cells by physical or chemical modification; (3) neoantigen formation following combination of autologous and exogenous determinants, e.g., viral; (4) cross reactivity between exogenous and host tissue antigens, e.g., bacterial; and (5) genetic or neoplastic abnormalities of the lymphoreticular system (Mackay and Burnet, 1963; Paterson, 1966).

Witebsky (1959) and Mackay and Burnet (1963), in the spirit of Koch, have tendered sets of postulates as guides to the categorization of spontaneous immunopathies as truly autosensitive. Table II affords a summary. We have liberally interpreted these postulates in our discussion of canine autosensitivity to stimulate further investigation of conditions which may currently satisfy only one or two of them.

TABLE II

CRITERIA FOR AUTOSENSITIVITY

Witebsky (1959)	Mackay and Burnet (1963)
1. Demonstration of circulating or cell-bound autoantibodies in patient	1. Demonstration of autoantibody in patient
2. Isolation and characterization of the antigen against which the antibody is directed	2. Hypergammaglobulinemia
	3. Deposition of denatured γ-globulin (i.e., in renal glomerulus)
3. Production of antibodies against the same antigen in experimental animals	4. Mononuclear cell responses resembling delayed hypersensitivity in damaged tissues
4. Appearance of pathologic changes in the corresponding tissue of an actively sensitized animal that are similar to those seen in the spontaneous disease	5. Presence of multiple, seemingly unrelated, autoimmune processes
	6. Favorable response to immunosuppressive therapy

2. HEMOPOIETIC DISEASES AND SYSTEMIC LUPUS ERYTHEMATOSUS

a. Autoimmune Hemolytic Anemia

Canine autoimmune hemolytic anemia (AHA) was first reported by G. Miller and associates (1957) and later described in detail by Lewis and co-workers (1963, 1965b). The disease is marked by severe, recurring hemolytic anemia accompanied by a positive reaction to the direct antiglobulin (Coombs) test, which, in contrast to man, becomes negative during remission in dogs. Clinical signs include pallor, weakness, icterus, hemoglobinuria, anorexia, fever, and malaise. Splenomegaly, peripheral lymphadenopathy, and tachycardia may be detected during physical examination. Clinicopathologically, the anemia is macrocytic and normoblastic, with polychromatophilia, anisocytosis, poikilocytosis, spherocytosis, and hyperplasia of the bone marrow. Most importantly, eluates of erythrocytes from affected dogs can passively sensitize normal canine erythrocytes for the indirect antiglobulin test, thus supporting an autoimmune pathogenesis for the condition. Nevertheless, the etiology and pathogenesis remain largely obscure. Corticosteroid therapy and splenectomy have secured temporary remissions of AHA, but permanent cures have not been reported.

b. Idiopathic Thrombocytopenic Purpura

Canine idiopathic thrombocytopenic purpura (ITP) (Magrane et al., 1959; Waye, 1960) is often, but not invariably, associated with AHA. The combined disease has been likened to Evans' syndrome in man and may herald the appearance of canine systemic lupus erythematosus (Lewis, 1968; Lewis et al., 1965b). About a third of affected dogs are reported to show spontaneous hemorrhage, usually as melena, epistaxis, hematuria or petechiae, and ecchymoses in the skin and mucous membranes. Megakaryocytes may be plentiful in the bone marrow, but circulating platelet numbers frequently fall below 10,000 per cubic milliliter. Splenomegaly and lymphadenopathy may also occur. Canine patients with ITP do respond to corticosteroids or splenectomy, but the syndrome usually recurs. Thrombocytopenia has been produced experimentally in dogs by the administration of antiplatelet serum (Tocatins and Stewart, 1939) and by the isoimmunization of dogs with homologous platelets (Baldini, 1965). As with AHA, however, the mechanisms that evoke spontaneous disease remain open for investigation.

c. Canine Systemic Lupus Erythematosus

When canine ITP, AHA, and membranous glomerulonephritis occur simultaneously or sequentially in the same animal the syndrome is called canine systemic lupus erythematosus (SLE) (Lewis *et al.*, 1965a,b; Lewis, 1968). Polyarthritis (Lewis and Hathaway, 1967), pleurisy, and butter-fly-shaped facial eruptions and hepatic necrosis have also been observed in canine SLE (Lewis *et al.*, 1965a). The anemia and thrombocytopenia may respond to corticosteroid treatment or splenectomy, but renal impairment is usually irreversible and eventually fatal. Histologically, in addition to changes accompanying ITP and AHA, thickened glomerular basement membranes, so-called "wire loop" lesions occur. They are identical to those in human SLE. Glomeruli also contain deposits of PAS-positive material and are often adhered to Bowman's capsule. Periglomerular lymphocytic and plasmacytic infiltrations occur, and fibrinoid change can sometimes be found in small renal arteries, but perivascular fibrosis, i.e., "onion skin" lesions, of splenic arteries is not reported to occur, in contradistinction to the situation in human SLE.

Serologic aberrations variably associated with canine SLE include hypergammaglobulinemia and autoantibodies against gamma globulin (rheumatoid factor), thyroid gland, erythrocytes (positive antiglobulin test), and nuclear material (antinuclear LE factor) (Lewis *et al.*, 1965a). LE cells, i.e., lupus erythematosus cells, are usually neutrophils which contain globoid intracytoplasmic bodies presumably representing nuclear material phagocytized after contact with LE factor, and are found in nearly every patient with canine SLE, but hematoxylin bodies, i.e., nuclear material, are not seen in tissues. LE cells are occasionally found in other canine diseases such as idiopathic polyarthritis and leukemia, indicating the possible participation of autosensitivity in these syndromes (Lewis, 1965).

The cause and pathogenesis of canine SLE are unknown. Attempts to produce the disease experimentally in dogs with hydralazine, a human anti-hypertensive agent, followed recognition of a lupus-like syndrome in man which accompanied administration of the drug, but these have usually been unsuccessful (Comens, 1956; Dubois *et al.*, 1957; Alarcon-Segovia *et al.*, 1967).

Lupus glomerulonephritis of NZB mice (Mellors, 1968) and man (Koffler and Kunkel, 1968) is believed to involve deposition of antigen–antibody complexes with fixation of complement in the renal glomerulus. If the same phenomenon occurs in canine SLE, immune complexes should be demonstrable in affected kidneys either immunohistochemically or ultrastructurally (McCluskey *et al.*, 1966). One might also attempt to isolate such complexes from renal tissue or peripheral blood and determine (1) their antigenic constituents and (2) their ability to produce glomerulonephritis after intravenous injection in normal dogs (Koffler and Kunkel, 1968). Isolation of complexes from blood may first require bilateral nephrectomy, since it is likely that the kidneys act as sponges for these complexes. Lewis (1968) has found that LE cells appear in the progeny of dogs with SLE as early as 4 months of age, thus giving support for genetic influences in canine SLE. Affected mice also develop lymphoma associated with viral particles, but the role of the virus in development of this multifaceted murine syndrome is unclear (Mellors, 1968). We do not know of any reports implicating immune aberrations in canine lymphoma.

3. RENAL DISEASES

a. Glomerulonephritis

Although spontaneous canine glomerulonephritis may be related to physical entrapment of immune complexes whose antigenic components are unrelated to kidney, glomerulonephritis has been experimentally produced in dogs by injection of nephrotoxic anti-kidney antibodies produced in homologous or heterologous species against canine renal antigens (Krakower and Greenspon, 1954; Stickler et al., 1956; Steblay, 1963; Robertshaw et al., 1967; Fukuda et al., 1968). This nephrotoxic serum nephritis appears to occur in two phases. Initially, nephrotoxic serum damages the renal glomerular basement membrane; later, deposition of electron dense material takes place beneath the glomerular capillary endothelium. These deposits are thought to be immune complexes comprised of either foreign serum protein antigen-antibody or autologous glomerular antigen-antibody, antigen in the latter complex being released during initial exposure to nephrotoxic serum (Movat et al., 1961).

The antigen responsible for evoking nephrotoxic antibody appears to be a soluble component of glomerular basement membrane (Shibata et al., 1966a,b). It seems closely related to a nephrotoxic antigen of human glomerular basement membrane, since antihuman glomerular basement membrane serum produces glomerulonephritis in dogs (Steblay, 1963).

Heymann and associates (1962) attempted, unsuccessfully, to produce experimental autoallergic nephritis in dogs by the injection of homologous kidney antigen emulsified in Freund's adjuvant. Spontaneous autoallergic nephritis has not been reported in dogs. Hypothetically, immunologic injury could play a role in the pathogenesis of glomerulosclerosis, one of the common renal lesions of aged dogs. Guttman and Andersen (1968) reported that low level x-irradiation accelerates development of glomerulosclerosis and IgG was found in the mesangium and capillary basement membrane of sclerosing glomeruli.

A canine homolog for human poststreptococcal rheumatic disease (Cluff and Johnson, 1965) has not been documented. There are reports, however, of postbacteremic glomerulonephritis associated with experimental *Streptococcus mitis* infection in dogs (Highman *et al.*, 1958) and occasionally we have observed chronic membranous glomerulonephritis associated with long-standing streptococcal polyarthritis. Furthermore, the valvular lesions seen in hearts of aged dogs resemble similar lesions of rheumatic heart disease in man (Jones and Zook, 1965). It is not unreasonable to speculate that a portion of the idiopathic canine membranous glomerulonephritides and endocarditides may be rheumatic sequelae to acute bacterial disease.

b. Interstitial Nephritis

Chronic interstitial nephritis (CIN) is the most frequently occurring yet least understood renal disease of dogs. It begins as an acute nonsuppurative interstitial nephritis but progresses inexorably to the subacute and chronic stages. Glomerular lesions usually are not present early in the syndrome, but membranous thickenings, fibrosis, and adhesions are evident in many chronic cases (McIntyre and Montgomery, 1952; L. J. Anderson, 1968). The natural history suggests that immunologic injury may contribute to the pathogenesis of CIN.

The initial cause of interstitial nephritis is unknown, although leptospirae are sometimes associated with the acute and subacute phases (McIntyre and Montgomery, 1952). Recently, L. J. Anderson (1967) produced subacute interstitial nephritis in 3 of 5 dogs inoculated with *Leptospira canicola*. McIntyre and Montgomery (1952) proposed that these organisms first invade the tubules from the interstitium, since glomerular lesions do not accompany acute leptospiral nephritis. If one assumes that leptospirae or some other infectious agent produce primary damage to tubular portions of the nephron, how can one account for the chronic progressive nature of CIN?

Firstly, the offending agent may remain in the tissues of carrier state individuals and become a source of constant irritation, thus provoking a chronic inflammatory response. Leptospirae (McIntyre and Montgomery, 1952) and ICH virus (Wright, 1967a,b) are capable of establishing carrier states in dogs. Moreover, delayed type hypersensitivity against leptospiral antigens can be elicited in dogs convalescing from acute leptospirosis, and L. J. Anderson (1967) found that experimental leptospiral nephritis developed only in dogs capable of considerable immune response to the organism. Thus, immunologic injury to the kidneys in CIN may result from hypersensitivity to environmental antigens, i.e., leptospirae, lodged in renal tissues. Paterson (1968) discussed this hypothesis further.

Alternatively, the causative agent may precipitate release of kidney-specific antigens which can induce an autoimmune response against kidney by the lymphoreticular system. L. J. Anderson (1968) observed that the glomerular lesions of CIN are compatible with immunologic injury by anti-kidney antibody. In this connection, Edgington and associates (1967) isolated a renal tubular epithelial antigen from rat kidney that was capable of inducing experimental allergic glomerulonephritis in immunized rats. Dixon (1968) stated that glomerular basement membrane antigens present in the urine of normal animals are nephritogenic. He suggested that renal damage from infectious agents may expose these antigens to immunocompetent cells and result in self-perpetuating immunologic injury to the kidney. If immunologic injury is a component of CIN, it then may be possible to demonstrate nephrotoxic activity in serum or lymphoid cells of affected dogs by using *in vitro* correlates of immunologic injury in cytotoxicity testing. Hypothetically, nephrotoxic activity could also be transferred to normal dogs by sensitized cells, cell fractions, or immune serums, although if such activity were cell-mediated, histocompatible donor–recipient pairs should be used for testing.

The similarity of CIN to chronic pyelonephritis of man deserves mention. Both lesions are characterized by chronic nonsuppurative interstitial inflammation, tubular atrophy, and dilatation with intratubular casts and fibrosis. Human pyelonephritis often progresses in the absence of detectable infectious agents (Angell *et al.*, 1968), so chronic pyelonephritis and CIN may develop by similar mechanisms.

4. Endocrine Diseases

a. Thyroiditis

Musser and Graham (1968) found that more than 10% of nearly 1000 Beagle dogs in a colony had evidence of spontaneous thyroiditis. Most affected dogs descended from a female with thyroiditis, and introduction of a new stud increased the incidence more than twofold. Beierwaltes and Nishiyama (1968) studied 67 Beagles from this colony and noticed histologic similarities between canine thyroiditis and human thyroiditis (Hashimoto's struma). Lesions of the canine thyroids ranged from focal lymphocytic infiltration without acinar involvement to acinar atrophy, macrophage infiltration and Hürthle cell changes of the follicular epithelium. Dogs with severe lesions had indications of subnormal thyroid function, i.e., low PBI and 24-hour ^{131}I uptake values. Antithyroglobulin antibodies were demonstrable in the sera of affected dogs, but their titer did not correlate with the severity of thyroid lesions. In addition, control dogs, purchased independently, also had serum titers to canine thyroglobulin. The pathogenesis of this disease, other than that related to its apparent familiar component, is obscure. Attempts to produce the disease in normal dogs by passive transfer of serum or lymphoid cells from thyroiditic dogs have not been reported.

Experimental allergic thyroiditis has been produced experimentally by injecting dogs with homologous thyroid extracts emulsified in Freund's adjuvant (Terplan et al., 1960). Antithyroid antibodies appeared in the blood of affected dogs, but, as in spontaneous thyroiditis, their serum titers did not correlate well with the severity of the lesions. Attempts to transfer this "autoimmune" thyroiditis to normal dogs with serum were unsuccessful.

b. Parathyroiditis

Lupulescu and collaborators (1968) induced parathyroiditis and hypoparathyroidism including a decrease in serum calcium concentrations by inoculating dogs with homologous parathyroid tissue emulsified in Freund's adjuvant. Affected animals had delayed skin reactions to intracutaneous challenge, with parathyroid tissue and contained antiparathyroid antibodies in their serum.

5. Nervous Diseases

a. Postdistemper Demyelinating Leukoencephalopathy

Canine distemper, a spontaneous viral disease of dogs, often terminates in demyelinating leukoencephalopathy, weeks to months after clinical recovery from generalized infection (Innes and Saunders, 1962). The brain and cord lesions bear morphologic resemblance to several idiopathic and virus-associated leukoencephalopathies of man and to experimental allergic encephalomyelitis (Greenfield and Norman, 1963; Paterson, 1966). Theories proposed to account for postinfectious demyelination include the following: (1) the virus persists within central nervous tissue following recovery from systemic illness and damages or destroys the myelogenic capacity of glial cells (Waksman and Adams, 1962; Appel, 1969); (2) virus–brain cell interactions cause exposure of nervous tissue antigens to immunocompetent cells which then mount an autoallergic attack on the central nervous system (Sudduth, 1955; Pette et al., 1965; Pette, 1968); and (3) the preceding mechanisms participate either simultaneously or sequentially (Webb and Smith, 1966; Paterson, 1969).

Most current evidence supports the first theory since canine distemper virus can be detected in a substantial portion of brains from affected animals (Moulton, 1956; Appel, 1969) and can induce demyelination of myelinated explants of canine cerebellum (Storts *et al.*, 1968). Nevertheless, recent data suggest a role for immune mechanisms in postdistemper leukoencephalopathy. Alvord *et al.* (1968) demonstrated precipitins against proteins of human and guinea pig brain in the sera of dogs suspected of having distemper. Furthermore, Long and Koestner (1969) discovered that sera from certain dogs with histologically confirmed disease can demyelinate canine cerebellar explants. The myelotoxic factor present in these sera as well as the antigen(s) against which it is directed have not yet been identified.

Canine distemper virus belongs to a group of viruses, the myxo- and paramyxoviruses, which may release host antigens from concealment or alter cell antigenicity during replication (Isacson, 1967). If postdistemper demyelinating leukoencephalopathy proves to have a virus-triggered autoallergic component, mechanisms by which similar viruses could incite immunologic injury would be open to direct examination.

Experimental allergic encephalomyelitis is probably the most thoroughly investigated of the experimental autosensitivity diseases and has been produced in many species (Paterson, 1966). It can be evoked in dogs by injection of homologous central nervous tissue emulsified in Freund's adjuvant (L. Thomas *et al.*, 1950; Hughes *et al.*, 1966). Clinical signs of encephalitis usually appear in 7 to 10 days, accompanied histologically by perivascular infiltrations of mononuclear cells with demyelination in the central nervous system (Lázár *et al.*, 1966). For unknown reasons, cold weather, increased humidity, rapid changes in atmospheric pressure, or electrical discharges appear to predispose sensitized dogs to clinical and pathologic exacerbations of the disease (Maros *et al.*, 1967). This finding remains unconfirmed by other workers. Demyelinating antibodies have been found in experimental allergic encephalomyelitis of rodents, but their role in the pathogenesis of the disease is unclear, since only sensitized lymphoid cells from affected animals appear capable of transferring encephalitis to normal individuals (Paterson, 1966).

b. Coonhound Paralysis

Coonhound paralysis is a spontaneous polyradiculoneuritis which may occur in dogs 7 to 14 days after sustaining a racoon bite (Cummings and Haas, 1967). Clinically and histologically, the disease resembles the Landry-Guillain-Barre syndrome of man and experimental allergic neuritis, the peripheral nerve counterpart of experimental allergic encephalomyelitis (Waksman and Adams, 1955). Speculation that coonhound paralysis begins as a viral infection has not been substantiated. Immunologic studies of the disease have not been reported, despite its similarities to experimental allergic neuritis.

6. Gastrointestinal Autosensitivity

a. Experimental Gastritis

Gastritis, gastric atrophy, and achlorhydria have developed in dogs following injection of autologous, homologous, or heterologous gastric juice and stomach extracts, usually emulsified in Freund's adjuvant (Hennes et al., 1962; Langr et al., 1967). Autoallergic gastritis has been associated with antiparietal cell antibodies capable of reacting with autologous gastric juice as well as with delayed skin reactions to gastric antigens. Krohn (1968a,b) found that absorption of vitamin B_{12} from the gut of affected dogs was decreased and that canine anti-canine gastric juice antibody partially inhibited the action of human intrinsic factor on vitamin B_{12} absorption. Pernicious anemia however, has not been reported in connection with canine experimental autoallergic gastritis.

b. Experimental Colitis

Most attempts to induce immunologic injury to the colon of the dog as a model for ulcerative colitis in man have been unrewarding (LeVeen et al., 1961; Shean et al., 1964). Acute colitis has been produced by infusions of heterologous anti-canine colon antiserum, but chronic disease did not develop and serum injections occasionally provoked anaphylactoid reactions (Bicks and Walker, 1962).

7. Miscellaneous Conditions

Polyarthritis, resembling rheumatoid arthritis of man, occurs occasionally in dogs, usually in association with canine SLE (Lewis et al., 1965a; Lewis and Hathaway, 1967). Polyarteritis nodosa has also been reported in dogs (Lewis et al., 1965b), but its pathogenesis has not been investigated.

VI. Transplantation

1. General Considerations

The greater the antigenic similarity or histocompatibility between two individuals, the less likely the individuals will be to reject each other's tissues as foreign. Transplantation (histocompatibility) antigens exist on the surface of all cells in varying concentrations. They are expressions of closely linked histocompatibility genes which appear to behave as Mendelian dominants. The antigenic strength manifested by each gene varies, so it is common to speak of "strong" and "weak" histocompatibility barriers between individuals. Transplanting across a strong barrier is generally more difficult than transplanting across a single or even multiple weak barriers (Kahan and Reisfeld, 1969).

TABLE III
TISSUE TRANSPLANTATION TERMINOLOGY

Old term and adjective		New term and adjective		Definition
Autograft	autologous	Autograft	autologous	Graft in which the donor is also the recipient
			autochthonous	Adjective denoting a tumor arising in an original host. Transplants of such tumors to another site on the host are still called autografts
Isograft	isogeneic	Isograft	isogeneic, syngeneic	Graft between genetically similar individuals which possess identical histocompatibility antigens
Homograft	homologous	Allograft	allogeneic	Graft between genetically dissimilar members of the same species
Heterograft	heterologous	Xenograft	xenogeneic	Graft between members of different species

Should a transplanted tissue or organ be recognized as foreign by the host, rejection ensues. Rejection has been considered a cell-mediated event and, as such, a prototype of delayed hypersensitivity (D. B. Wilson and Billingham, 1967). Humoral antibodies are associated with the rejection process, but their significance is incompletely understood (McDonald, 1966). Once rejection of a graft, a first-set phenomenon, has taken place an individual is sensitized to antigens present in the graft and will reject subsequent grafts containing these antigens in an accelerated manner, a second-set phenomenon. Furthermore, the sensitized state may be transferred from one animal to another by means of lymphoid cells. A further discussion of transplantation biology is provided by Russell and Monaco's review (1965).

The dog has occupied a central position in the development of organ transplantation, particularly at the level of clinical research. Accordingly, the literature is replete with articles on canine transplanation, so we have had to be selective in organizing this review. Current transplantation nomenclature given in Table III serves as an aid to the following discussion.

2. TRANSPLANTABLE ORGANS

Virtually every organ in the dog's body, except the central nervous system, has been transplanted at one time or another. Selected examples are listed in Table IV. Canine kidney transplantation has been most

TABLE IV
Examples of Transplantable Canine Organs

Organ	Investigators	Organ	Investigators
Adrenal gland	Barac (1967)	Nerve	Hirasawa et al. (1968)
			K. Ikeda (1966)
Blood	Swisher and Young (1961)	Pancreas	Idezuki et al. (1968a,b)
Bone	Arrocha et al. (1968)		Inou et al. (1968)
	Böttger (1966)		Seddon and Howard
Bone marrow	Epstein et al. (1967)		(1966a,b)
	E. D. Thomas et al.	Parathyroid gland	Fisher et al. (1967)
	(1963a,b)		Lance (1967b)
Heart	D. K. Cooper (1968)	Skin	Dennis et al. (1969a)
	Hurley and Kosek (1968)		Than et al. (1962)
	Kondo et al. (1967)		L. Thomas et al. (1957)
	Kosek et al. (1968)	Spleen	Dammin et al. (1962)
	Rowlands et al. (1968)		Marchioro et al. (1964)
Heart valve	Cleveland et al. (1967)		Norman et al. (1968)
	S. Ikeda et al. (1967)	Stomach	Lillehei et al. (1967)
	Kwong et al. (1967)		Thompson et al. (1966)
	Mohri et al. (1967)	Testis	Attaran et al. (1966)
Intestine	Lillehei et al. (1967)	Thyroid gland	Fisher et al. (1967)
	Preston et al. (1966)		Lance (1967a)
	Taylor et al. (1966)		Shafey and Longmire (1967)
Kidney	Mitchell et al. (1967)	Ureter	Paccione et al. (1965)
	Murray et al. (1964)	Vessel	Robicsek et al. (1966)
	Sheil et al. (1968)		S. I. Schwartz et al. (1967)
	Simonsen (1953)		Znamensky and Odaryuk
Limb	Goldwyn et al. (1966)		(1965)
Liver	Starzl et al. (1967, 1968)		
	Stuart et al. (1967)		
Lung	Beattie (1966)		
	Blumenstock et al. (1967)		
	Flax and Barnes (1966)		
	Veith (1968)		
	Zajtchuk et al. (1967)		

thoroughly studied, so we selected it to illustrate some aspects of transplantation immunology in dogs.

a. Clinical Aspects

Primary renal allografts seldom survive more than 3 weeks in immunologically unmodified recipients and are usually rejected within 9 days (Zukoski, 1968). Rejection is associated with oliguria, terminating in anuria and uremia. A second kidney transplanted to a sensitized recipient is normally rejected in 1 to 2 days and may never function successfully at all. Thus, the detection of imminent rejection at the earliest possible moment is of critical importance if it is to be reversed. Indications of rejection include proteinuria, elevated blood urea nitrogen, lymphocyturia, and evidence of tissue destruction at biopsy (Koo et al., 1965; Veith et al., 1967). Recently, elevated urinary or serum values of renal lactic dehydrogenase, alkaline phosphatase, and lysozyme activity have been found to correlate well with impending rejection (Koo et al., 1965; Najarian et al., 1965; Van Breda Vriesman et al., 1967).

b. Pathologic Changes of Rejection

During acute rejection of a primary renal allograft, mononuclear cell infiltration of the renal cortex, accompanied or preceded by endothelial damage to small intertubular vessels may be seen within 72 hours after transplanation (Kountz et al., 1963; Shorter and Hallenbeck, 1968). Damage to renal vessels progresses, and the blood supply to the kidney is compromised during day 3 through day 6. (Horowitz et al., 1965). Thrombosis of peritubular capillaries or larger vessels results in tubular destruction, infarction, hemorrhage, and complete rejection over the next several days.

Immunologic modification of the recipient, i.e., by immunosuppressive therapy, usually prolongs the course of rejection, and chronic rejection is characterized by chronic inflammation. Histologically, recurring episodes of vascular damage accompanied by mild inflammation progress to generalized renal fibrosis and atrophy (K. A. Porter et al., 1964; Sheil et al., 1968).

c. Cell-Mediated versus Humoral Rejection

The relative importance of cell-mediated versus humoral immunity in canine transplanation is unclear. Cell-mediated sensitivity against graft antigens probably dominates first-set rejection (Govaerts, 1960), whereas second-set rejection, which is basically a vascular thrombotic phenomenon, may be mediated by circulating antibodies (Perez-Tamayo and Kretschmer, 1965). Cytotoxic antibodies have been found in the serum of dogs during or following the rejection of tissue and organ allografts (Altman and Simonsen, 1964; Milgrom, 1966; Hampers et al., 1967; Dempster, 1968; Almgard and Svehag, 1968; Yamada and Kay, 1968; Clark et al., 1968), and it has recently been demonstrated that sensitization to canine renal allografts may be transferred by immune serum (Altman, 1963; Dubernard et al., 1968). Some investigators believe that renal antigens form immune complexes with circulating anti-kidney antibodies to produce vascular damage during rejection (Horowitz et al., 1965; Lowenhaupt and Nathan, 1968). The role of serum factors is further amplified in xenograft rejection. Porcine renal xenografts transplanted to dogs are rejected peracutely, i.e., in 10 to 20 minutes, apparently due to endothelial damage from performed anti-porcine cytotoxic antibody present in dog serum with the participation of complement (Gewurz et al., 1966; Perper and Najarian, 1966; Nelson, 1966). In the end, both humoral and cell-mediated effector mechanisms may be found necessary for full manifestation of primary allograft rejection as suggested by Gewurz and associates (1966).

3. Modification of Rejection

Immunologic modification of graft recipients is essential for successful transplantation of organs between allogeneic animals such as dogs. Two basic procedures have become popular for this purpose: suppression of host effector mechanisms (lymphoreticular system) and establishment of immunologic tolerance by pretransplanation treatment of the host with donor antigens.

a. Immunosuppression

Immunosuppressive therapy induces a generalized hyporesponsive state in the lymphoreticular system, and thus represents the crudest and perhaps most dangerous of the modifying regimens. Nevertheless, judicious use of chemical and physical immunosuppressants can prolong graft survival without comprising the host.

Chemical immunosuppressants used in canine transplantation include azathioprine (Murray et al., 1964; Starzl et al., 1967; Stuart et al., 1967; Diethelm et al., 1968), 6-mercaptopurine (Zukoski and Ende, 1965), methotrexate (E. D. Thomas et al., 1963b; Storts et al., 1968), cyclophosphamide (Storb et al., 1969), azaserine (Haxhe et al., 1967; Diethelm et al., 1968), actinomycin (Stuart, et al., 1967), corticosteroids (Kountz and Cohn, 1967; Diethelm et al., 1968), and phytohemagglutinin (Calne et al., 1965; Gertner et al., 1969). Azathioprine (Imuran), a purine analog, is currently considered the chemical immunosuppressant of choice for dogs and may be used alone or in combination with other immunosuppressive agents (Murray et al., 1964; Diethelm et al., 1968). Azathioprine may be hepatoxic at pharmacologic levels, so dose ranges and schedules must be tailored for individual dogs to attain maximal immunosuppression without untoward side effects (Starzl et al., 1967). Dosages can usually be cut in half for maintenance, once a graft is well established (Murray et al., 1964). Additional discussion of the pharmacology and use of chemical immunosuppressants is provided by Gabrielsen and Good (1967).

Antilymphocytic serum (ALS) is a promising new immunosuppressive agent, which, unlike most chemical immunosuppressants, does not depend on generalized depletion of lymphoreticular cells to be effective. Anti-canine ALS has been produced in horses (Iwasaki et al., 1967), sheep (Fox et al., 1968), goats (Simons, 1968), and rabbits (Shorter et al., 1968) by immunization with lymph node cells (Russell and Monaco, 1967), thymocytes (Braf et al., 1967; Shorter et al., 1968), or thoracic duct lymphocytes (Herman and Schloerb, 1967). Unmodified ALS, which contains antibodies to many antigens, may cause undesirable side effects such as anemia, anaphylaxis, or serum sickness, so it is normally absorbed with canine erythrocytes and may be fractionated to antilymphocytic globulin before use (Iwasaki et al., 1967; Russell and Monaco, 1967).

The immunosuppressive potency of ALS *in vivo* does not correlate well with either its cytotoxic potency and leukoagglutinability *in vitro* (Russell and Monaco, 1967) or the degree of lymphopenia it produces *in vivo* (Jeejeebhoy, 1967). Thus, the effectiveness of ALS must be determined through clinical trials (Russell and Monaco, 1967). ALS is usually administered in combination with other chemical immunosuppressants, such as azathioprine, beginning several days before transplantation, for maximal effect (Murray et al., 1964; Starzl et al., 1967).

Long-term side effects, such as intercurrent bacterial infection, are rare during ALS therapy (Fateh-Moghadam et al., 1967). Conversely, the development of distemper and hepatitis in vaccinated dogs given ALS has been reported (Abaza et al., 1966). ALS is also known to potentiate viral infections in rodents (reviewed by Hirsch and Murphy, 1968). The current status of ALS has been reviewed by James (1969).

Physical methods for immunosuppression include irradiation, thoracic duct drainage, and thymectomy.

Whole body irradiation, at exposures required for effective prolongation of graft survival, is usually lethal for dogs unless supplemented by allogeneic bone marrow infusions (E. D. Thomas et al., 1963a). Local x-irradiation of grafts (Wolf et al., 1967) and intraarterial implantation of yttrium-90 pellets have been used in immunosuppressive therapy with equivocal results (Wolf and Hume, 1965). Extracorporeal irradiation of blood produces lymphoid cell depletion and may be capable of reversing early, but not late, stages of rejection (Donahoo et al., 1967; Maginn and Bullimore, 1968). Hume and Wolf (1967) have reviewed the immunosuppressive effects of irradiation.

Thoracic duct drainage of lymphocytes has been reported to enhance survival of canine skin and kidney allografts (Singh et al., 1965; Parker et al., 1966), and, when used in combination with chemical immunosuppressants such as azathioprine, it may reduce the time and dose of drugs required for therapy (Vega et al., 1968). Thoracic duct cannulas are, however, difficult to maintain for extended periods and are esthetically unappealing (Kozuszek, 1967).

Thymectomy, although without detectable effect on immune responsiveness of adults by itself, has been used successfully with immunosuppressive chemotherapy to maintain grafts longer than if drugs alone had been employed (Kiskin, 1966; Furuse et al., 1967).

b. Tolerance

Tolerance may be defined as specific immunologic unresponsiveness to antigenic stimulation. This definition assumes that an animal rendered tolerant to donor transplantation antigens, need not have its immunologic competence to all environmental antigens comprised in order to maintain allografted tissue. Thus, induction of specific immunologic tolerance to tissue allografts remains a central goal in transplantation immunology.

Attempts to induce tolerance in dogs have taken two general forms, exposure of neonatal or adult dogs to antigen, frequently in massive doses, and exposure of immunosuppressed dogs to antigen followed by withdrawal of imunosuppressive therapy.

Tolerance by Pregrafting Exposure to Antigen. Some species, notably rodents, are immunologically immature at birth and can be rendered tolerant to many antigens provided exposure to these antigens occurs during the first day or 2 of life (Hasek et al., 1961). Dogs are considered immunologically mature to most antigens at birth, so generally speaking, efforts to induce tolerance in canine neonates by injection of tissue extracts have failed (Fowler et al., 1961; Grosjean and Otte, 1966b). Puza and Gombos (1958) and Gombos and associates (1962) were able to induce tolerance to skin and kidney allografts by giving exchange transfusions of donor blood to 3- to 12-day-old puppies, but this technique seems rather heroic for general use. J. M. Anderson (1965) described a state of "immunologic inertia" existing between a bitch and her progeny during the week after parturition, whereby maternal skin grafts were accepted by pups for exceptionally long periods, occasionally more than a year. These results could also be explained by assuming that favorable histocompatibility relationships existed between the dam and her litter.

Predictably, preexposure of adult recipients to donor antigens in order to induce tolerance has also met with little success. Furthermore, prolonged graft survival in these instances may be due to immunologic enhancement rather than tolerance (Section VI,5) (Halasz et al., 1964, 1966; Kekis et al., 1964; Zimmerman et al., 1965; Linn, 1966; Grosjean and Otte, 1966a; Calne et al., 1966).

Tolerance through Immunosuppression. Murray et al. (1964), in reporting the results of 1000 canine renal allografts, observed that most dogs rejected kidneys after being withdrawn from immunosuppressive therapy, but some grafts were retained for more than a year. These results could not be wholly attributed to harmony between donor and recipient antigenic profiles, since a second kidney transplanted from the original donor could be rejected while the first one continued to function. Furthermore, persisting renal allografts were permanently accepted if retransplanted to original donors, indicating that expression of new antigens was not responsible for tolerance of the graft by the allogeneic host. Calne (1968) suggested that the results reported by Murray's group could be explained either by antigenic deletion occurring in the renal allograft or by masking of transplantation antigens on the donor kidney by anti-renal antibodies formed in the recipient. The latter phenomenon resembles enhancement as mentioned above. Nevertheless, tolerance to allogeneic tissues in adult dogs appears easier to produce if recipients are initially given immunosuppressive therapy. This principle was further supported by Epstein and associates (1967) who produced permanent tolerance to allogeneic bone marrow in 2 lethally irradiated adult male dogs.

Antigenic Specificity in Tolerance. Antigenically complex canine tissue extracts compound the difficulties of tolerance induction in dogs since unresponsiveness may ensue to some antigens in the mixture only to be negated by sensitization to others (Calne, 1968). Thus, injections of isolated and standardized major transplantation antigens could facilitate tolerance while reducing adverse responses to minor antigens. Solubilized transplantation antigens have been used to prolong survival of renal allografts in dogs (R. E. Wilson *et al.*, 1969), but the biologic and chemical characterization of these preparations has not been completed (Kahan and Reisfeld, 1969). This approach to tolerance in transplantation is additionally promising, since minute quantities of solubilized protein fractions can be used to produce immunologic tolerance in adult animals (Dresser and Mitchison, 1968). Some strains of bacteria also appear to contain antigens which can sensitize recipients against donor tissues, but whether they can substitute for canine transplantation antigens in the induction of tolerance remains to be investigated (Zabriskie, 1967).

4. Histocompatibility

a. General Considerations

If immunologic modification of a graft recipient is to be minimized, then donor and recipient must be reasonably histocompatible. In other words, methods must be developed to identify and match the major transplantation antigens of donor–recipient pairs. Erythrocytic typing before transfusion is an example of this approach to donor–recipient pairing. It looked for a time as if similar typing for solid tissue grafting would be a hopeless task in genetically heterogeneous species, but the discovery that leukocyte antigens can be used for histocompatibility testing has reduced the problem to manageable size (Bach, 1968). Thus, what appears to be the major histocompatibility locus of man has recently been identified (Dausset and Rapaport, 1968).

Similar advances in histocompatibility testing of dogs have been painfully slow despite the widespread use of dogs in transplantation studies. Nevertheless, numerous accounts exist of prolonged allograft survival in immunologically unaltered dogs. For example, Hurley and Kosek (1968) reported the 5-month survival of a cardiac allograft transplanted between littermates. Koo and associates (1966) studied a dog which had maintained a renal allograft without immunosuppressive therapy for 123 days when it died from unrelated causes. We have transplanted skin allografts between littermates in a closed inbred Beagle colony and recorded graft survivals of up to 125 days (Jacoby and Dennis, 1969). These results can be explained by assuming that donor–recipient pairs were more histocompatible than would be expected on the basis of random selection.

b. Canine Blood Groups

Swisher, Young, and associates have pioneered the study of canine blood groups, and their comprehensive reviews of the subject are only briefly summarized here (Swisher and Young, 1961; Swisher et al., 1962). The seven major canine blood groups, designated alphabetically A through G appear to be inherited as autosomal dominants. The A group consists of two subgroups, A_1 and A_2, and is expressed in about 63% of a random dog population. Most clinically significant transfusion reactions follow infusion of A-positive blood in isoimmunized A-negative donors. Reactions may include tremors, emesis, fever, urinary and fecal incontinence, hemoglobinemia, hemoglobinuria, thrombocytopenia, asthmatic breathing, convulsions, hives, and transient prostration. Nevertheless, animals usually recover within 24 hours without the renal injury often associated with transfusion reactions in man. Infusion of blood from isoimmunized A-negative donors in A-positive recipients may cause similar reactions.

Swisher et al. (1962) indicated that only a small risk is involved by primary transfusion of incompatible canine blood since less than 10% of the dog population possesses naturally occurring isoantibodies to major blood group antigens. Cross-matching for A antigen, however, reduces the risk involved with either single or multiple transfusions. Beyond this, use of unsensitized A-negative donors is encouraged.

Incompatibility reactions may also occur in A-positive neonatal pups that are suckling isoimmunized A-negative dams who were mated with A-positive sires (L. E. Young *et al.*, 1951). The syndrome is precipitated by absorption of colostral isoantibodies against A-factor and is characterized clinically by hemolytic anemia and a positive direct antiglobulin test. Transplacental passage of isoantibodies does not appear to be significant in this condition.

c. Canine Leukocytes in Histocompatibility Testing

It was hoped originally that canine blood group antigens could be used in histocompatibility testing for transplantation of other tissues. Enthusiasm for this prospect was dampened by reports indicating that little correlation existed between blood group matching and graft survival (Kasakura *et al.*, 1964; E. D. Thomas *et al.*, 1964). Rubinstein and associates (1968) have described a new class of erythrocytic antigens which appear to act as histocompatibility markers, but their findings are presently unconfirmed by other workers. Still, erythrocyte cross-matching of donor–recipient pairs is practiced by some investigators in order to reduce side reactions accompanying transplantation (Kasakura *et al.*, 1964; Serre and Clot, 1968). Evidence indicates that canine leukocyte antigens will be useful histocompatibility markers.

Histocompatibility testing, as a general technique, can be divided generally into two categories: matching procedures and typing procedures. Matching tests give a rough estimation of the extent of antigenic similarity between two individuals, whereas leukocyte typing implies precise identification of specific antigens (Russell *et al.*, 1966; Bach, 1968). Among the matching tests applied to dogs are (1) the normal lymphocyte transfer test, (2) the irradiated hamster test, and (3) the mixed lymphocyte culture test.

In the normal lymphocyte transfer test, recipient lymphocytes are injected in the dermis of donor skin. If the transformed cells recognize donor tissue as foreign, a delayed skin reaction occurs whose intensity and size may correlate with the duration of graft survival (Gray and Russell, 1965). Hornick and Sensenig (1968) found an inverse relation between reaction intensity and skin allograft survival among adult mixed breed dogs. Streilein and Barker (1967) and Hinchey and Bliss (1965) also observed delayed skin reactions in dogs, but they did not correlate their findings with graft survival.

The irradiated hamster test is based on the fact that leukocytes of antigenically dissimilar individuals provoke a delayed inflammatory reaction if they are mixed and injected in the skin of an irradiated, immunologically unreactive, hamster (Ramseier and Streilein, 1965). This procedure has been used sparingly in dogs and with conflicting results.

Cabasson and associates (1967) reported good correlation between results of the irradiated hamster test and survival of canine cardiac allografts in several animals, whereas Streilein and Barker (1967) found that mixed canine leukocytes produced only weak reactions in hamster skin and test results were not useful in selecting animals for renal transplants.

The mixed leukocyte culture test depends on the finding that lymphocytes from antigenically dissimilar individuals have a reciprocal mitogenic effect on one another when mixed *in vitro* (Bain and Lowenstein, 1964). After several days of incubation, the intensity of reaction may be gauged histologically by counting blast forms in the culture or quantitated by determining the uptake by cells of radiolabeled amino acids from the culture medium. This test appears to correlate well with the results of other matching procedures in dogs (Serre and Clot, 1968), but it has not been evaluated in clinical transplantation trials.

At least three major drawbacks are associated with leukocyte matching procedures. First, they are only semiquantitative, since multiple incompatibilities at weak loci may elicit the same results as a single incompatibility across a strong histocompatibility barrier. Second, they may not indicate the polarity of incompatibility reactions, since donor leukocytes may provoke reactions if they recognize recipient leukocyte antigens as foreign. Third, leukocytes from azotemic patients, such as those patients presented for kidney transplantation, do not respond well to antigenic stimulation (Mannick *et al.*, 1960). Main and co-workers (1967) simplified interpretation of the mixed canine leukocyte test by converting it from a "two-way" to a "one-way" reaction. They first inactivated donor cells by x-irradiation or freeze-thawing, so that only recipient leukocytes in the mixture could undergo blastogenesis.

Leukocyte typing with specific anitsera appears to hold great promise as a histocompatibility test (van Rood and Eernisse, 1969), and several attempts have been made to design typing tests for dogs. Briefly, donor and recipient cells are exposed to immune sera. If agglutination or cytotoxicity is detected for both or neither groups of cells, they are assumed to be antigenically similar. If one group is affected and the other is not, they are assumed to be antigenically dissimilar. Epstein and associates (1968) prepared cytotoxic antileukocytic antibodies of limited specificity by immunizing dogs with leukocytes from their littermates. Bone marrow donor–recipient pairs were purposefully matched or "mismatched" according to the results of leukocyte "typing" tests using 4 antisera and then the recipients were x-irradiated. Bone marrow allografts survived significantly longer in "histocompatible" than "histoincompatible" recipients (Epstein *et al.*, 1968; Storb *et al.*, 1968). Mollen and associates (1968) prepared 12 cytotoxic antisera largely by reciprocal exchange of skin grafts and peripheral blood leukocytes between litter-mates. These antisera detected leukocytic antigens which seemed to be inherited as Mendelian autosomal dominants in a colony of closely inbred Beagles. Subsequent skin grafting experiments indicated that animals detected as being antigenically dissimilar from their donors rejected grafts nearly twice as fast as animals which were antigenically similar to donors. Furthermore, typing of 3 donor–recipient pairs who had main-tained either lung, kidney, or bone marrow allografts for long periods revealed their detectable leukocyte antigens to be identical.

The number of major canine tissue antigens that would require match-ing is unknown, but E. D. Thomas and associates (1936b) suggest, on the basis of survival rates of dogs after bone marrow allografting, that it may be small. Further encouragement is derived from knowing that only a single major histocompatibility barrier, albeit with multiple alleles, has been identified in each of the other species studied thus far (Kahan and Reisfeld, 1969). Moreover, parents have restricted gene pools, so natural segregation of genes should result in a sibling being histocompat-ible with 1 of 4 littermates (Amos, 1968).

VII. Tumor Immunity

1. General Considerations

Cells undergoing neoplastic transformation acquire tumor-specific neoantigens which may provoke an immune response by the host. When these antigens occur on cell surfaces, they can act as weak transplanta-tion antigens called tumor-specific transplantation antigens (TSTA). Thus, responses to neoplastic cells may closely resemble responses to normal tissue allografts. In fact, Burnet (1968) hypothesized that the evolutionary significance of cell-mediated immunity may be primarily related to surveillance and elimination of aberrant cells, since allograft rejection responses are artificially elicited by human interference.

In virus-induced tumors, all cells transformed by a given virus have a common TSTA regardless of the morphology of the tumor or its host of origin, but the TSTAs of tumors induced by different viruses are im-munologically distinct. Conversely, tumors induced by chemical or physical carcinogens are usually antigenically heterogeneous so that, on a given animal, 2 tumors induced by a single carcinogen may be anti-genically unrelated. Other tumor-specific antigens associated with virus-induced tumors include T-antigens, i.e., complement-fixing nuclear anti-gens, and virion-specific antigens. Although they may elicit immune responses by the host, they probably have little influence on acceptance or rejection of neoplastic cells (Klein, 1968; Smith, 1968).

2. Transplantation of Canine Neoplasms

Tumor allografting in dogs presents formidable problems. First, dog populations are genetically heterogeneous, so canine tumors must be transplanted across normal histocompatibility barriers as well as across tumor-specific antigenic barriers. Second, dogs are able to reject tissue allografts from the time of birth. As a result, most attempts to establish transplantable tumors in dogs without the aid of devastating immunosuppressive regimens have failed (Allam *et al.*, 1956; Nielsen and Cole, 1961; Spencer and Leader, 1962). Successful transmission has been restricted to tumors of proved or suspected viral causation such as the oral papilloma (DeMonbreun and Goodpasture, 1932; LeBouvier *et al.*, 1966), venereal sarcoma (Stubbs and Furth, 1934; Karlson and Mann, 1952), lymphosarcoma (Moldovanu *et al.*, 1966; Kakuk *et al.*, 1968), and mastocytoma (Lombard and Moloney, 1959; Lombard *et al.*, 1963; Rickard and Post, 1968). Presumably, tumor transplantation between histocompatible dogs with the help of selective immunosuppressive agents such as ALS (Phillips and Gazet, 1967) would prove more feasible than current "shotgun" methods to establish experimental tumor lines.

3. Tumor-Specific Antigens

Tumor-specific antigens are most easily identified by transplanting tumor cells between syngeneic animals, since only neoantigens will be recognized as foreign by the host. In dogs, tumor-specific neoantigens must be separated from normal antigenic constituents present on tumor cells, a task of considerable dimensions. Nevertheless, demonstration of antigenic identity among groups of canine tumors would implicate viral participation in the neoplastic process. Recently, several investigators have tried to identify neoantigens in canine tumors. McKenna and Prier (1966) detected a soluble antigen associated with 10 of 51 spontaneous canine neoplasms of different types. They also demonstrated antibodies against canine venereal sarcoma antigens by conglutinating complement absorption tests in nearly all dogs carrying this tumor. Powers (1968) claimed to have demonstrated specific antibody against venereal sarcoma in dogs by immunoprecipitation and passive cutaneous anaphylaxis. He did not, however, absorb sera with normal tissues so his results, while interesting, are not conclusive. Yurko and collaborators (1969) found that dogs may produce tumor-specific antibodies against autochthonous tumors. The antibodies did not react with either normal autologous tissues or embryonic tissues. Southam (1967) and Klein (1968) have reviewed the status of tumor-specific transplantation antigens in man, and their approaches to the problem apply as well to dogs.

4. Host Responses

Several types of naturally occurring canine neoplasms including oral papillomas, venereal sarcomas, and histiocytomas normally regress spontaneously, and affected animals are then immunologically resistant to further induction of tumor growth (Stubbs and Furth, 1934; Karlson and Mann, 1952; Chambers and Evans, 1959; Mulligan, 1963). Little correlation appears to exist between regression and the presence of circulating cytotoxic antitumor antibodies, at least in the case of solid tumors (Karlson and Mann, 1952; Chambers et al., 1960; Prier and Brodey, 1963). Powers (1968), however, was able to effect a decrease in maximal size and accelerate rejection of venereal sarcomas by passively immunizing dogs with serum from immune donors. Furthermore, if immune serum and tumor cells were transferred to a susceptible animal simultaneously, tumors failed to grow.

The role of cell-mediated immunity in spontaneous regression of canine tumors has received only cursory attention (Chambers et al., 1960) despite the fact that tumors are frequently circumscribed or infiltrated by mononuclear cells. In vitro correlates of cell-mediated immunity could be used to clarify this issue. Thus, it may be possible to demonstrate cytotoxic reactions of autologous lymphoid cells against monolayers of autochthonous tumor cells (Rosenau, 1968). Alternatively, autochthonous tumor extracts may specifically inhibit migration of autologous macrophages on glass (Kronman et al., 1969). These methods could also prove helpful in identifying tumor-specific antigens.

The question arises as to why all tumors are not rejected, if they contain antigens foreign to the host. There are many factors bearing on this aspect of the host–tumor relationship such as antigenic concentration on tumor cell surfaces, rate of cell proliferation versus rate of host response, vertical transmission (tolerance) of oncogenic viruses from mother to progeny and enhancement (Smith, 1968). Howard (1967) found that dogs with recurrent mastocytomas had defective immune responses to Brucella abortus strain 19 vaccine. Other workers have shown that leukemogenic viruses and chemical carcinogens are capable of immunosuppressive activity in mice (Ceglowski and Friedman, 1967; Stjernwärd, 1967). It has even been suggested that an oncogen can enhance its own pathogenicity by suppressing a host's lymphoreticular system while initiating neoplastic transformation (R. S. Schwartz and Andre-Schwartz, 1968). The implications of these findings for canine neoplasia remain to be studied. Similarly, R. E. Wilson and co-workers (1968) warn that neoplastic cells, inadvertently transferred to immunosuppressed patients during allografting procedures, may continue to proliferate.

Genetic predisposition to neoplasia may occur in dogs. The Boxer breed, for example, has a significantly higher incidence of tumors, particularly of the lymphoreticular system, than the random dog population and Boxers are more liable to develop multiple, morphologically distinct tumors (Howard and Nielsen, 1965; Priester, 1967). It would be interesting to determine whether the multiple tumors occurring in Boxer dogs shared common tumor-specific antigens, since this might suggest the existence of a multipotential oncogenic virus in this breed.

5. Immunization against Neoplasia

Immunization against virus-induced canine tumors appears feasible, since the antigenicity of tumor and virus would remain relatively constant from animal to animal. In contrast, nonvirus-induced tumors represent a problem, because each may be antigenically distinct and therefore unresponsive to mass-produced vaccine (Smith, 1968). Minton and associates (1967) tried to circumvent this obstacle by immunizing dogs with autogenous tumor cells coupled to rabbit γ-globulin and emulsified in Freund's adjuvant. They succeeded in preventing recurrence of a partially excised hemangiopericytoma and thyroid adenocarcinoma in 2 dogs, 10 and 8 months after "vaccination," respectively. There is risk associated with immunization particularly against solid tumors, since tumor growth may be accelerated rather than abrogated. This enhancement phenomenon probably results from masking of tumor cells by antibody which is produced during injections of tumor material. The masked cells go undetected by the host's immune mechanisms and continue to proliferate (Kaliss, 1965).

VIII. Conclusions

Immunologic injury deserves increased attention from veterinarians as an effector of canine disease. Hypersensitivity, autosensitivity, tissue allograft rejection, and tumor regression in dogs are now well recognized phenomena and offer useful models for study in both canine medicine and comparative medicine.

Although many types of immunologic injury are mediated by humoral antibody, an equal, if not greater, variety of such lesions are probably evoked by sensitized immunocompetent cells. Hence, many experimentally induced hypersensitivity states can be transferred from affected to normal animals only with cells and not with serum. Furthermore, passive transfer of sensitivity with cells frequently constitutes the critical demonstration of the existence of hypersensitivity.

Unfortunately, dogs, being genetically and therefore antigenically heterogeneous, are not amenable to cell transfer experiments. This point is dramatically demonstrated by the failure of canine tissue allografts to survive for prolonged periods without substantial immunosuppressive chemotherapy. Consequently, a single problem hampers research of hypersensitivity states and allotransplantation in dogs, namely, lack of knowledge about canine histocompatibility antigens. It is now time for a cooperative effort by veterinarians to characterize the histocompatibility antigens of dogs and develop reliable tissue typing procedures for donor–recipient pairing in clinical and investigative canine medicine. To this end, workshops could be organized by veterinary immunologists, as has been done by physicians, to facilitate comparison and standardization of typing tests. Moreover, selective inbreeding of closed dog colonies should increase the chances of attaining monovalent typing sera in a relatively short time.

REFERENCES

Abaza, H. M., Nolan, D., Watt, J. G., and Woodruff, M. F. A. (1966). Effect of anti-lymphocytic serum on the survival of renal homotransplants in dogs. *Transplantation* **4**, 618–632.

Akcasu, A., and West, G. B. (1960). Anaphylaxis in the dog. *International Archives of Allergy and Applied Immunology* **16**, 326–335.

Alarcon-Segovia, D., Wakim, K. G., and Worthington, J. W. (1967). Clinical and experimental studies on the hydralazine syndrome and its relationship to systemic lupus erythematosus. *Medicine* **46**, 1–33.

Allam, M. W., Lombard, L. S., Stubbs, F. L., and Shirer, J. F. (1956). Transplantability of a canine thyroid carcinoma through thirty generations in mixed-breed puppies. *Journal of the National Cancer Institute* **17**, 123–129.

Almgard, L. E., and Svehag, S. E. (1968). Humoral antibodies in canine renal transplantation. *Acta Pathologica et Microbiologica Scandinavica* **73**, 605–618.

Alper, C. A., Rosen, F. S., and Janeway, C. A. (1966). The gamma globulins. II. Hypergammaglobulinemia. *New England Journal of Medicine* **275**, 591–596 and 652–658.

Altman, B. (1963). Tissue transplantation: Circulating antibody in the homotransplantation of kidney and skin. *Annals of the Royal College of Surgeons of England* **33**, 79–104.

Altman, B., and Simonsen, M. (1964). Cytotoxic antibody and hemagglutinin in canine homotransplantation. *Annals of the New York Academy of Sciences* **120**, 28–35.

Alvord, E. C., Sudduth, W. H., Hruby, S., and Hughes, K. (1968). A search for brain antigens in canine distemper. *Neurology* **18**, 112–116.

Amos, B. (1968). Immunologic factors in organ transplantation. *American Journal of Medicine* **44**, 767–775.

Anderson, J. M. (1965). Immunological inertia in pregnancy. *Nature* **206**, 786–787.

Anderson, L. J. (1967). Experimental reproduction of canine interstitial nephritis. *Journal of Comparative Pathology* **77**, 413–418.

Anderson, L. J. (1968). The glomeruli in canine interstitial nephritis. *Journal of Pathology and Bacteriology* **95**, 59–65.

Angell, M. E., Relman, A. S., and Robbins, S. L. (1968). "Active" chronic pyelonephritis without evidence of bacterial infection. *New England Journal of Medicine* **278**, 1303–1308.

Appel, M. J. G. (1969). Pathogenesis of canine distemper. *American Journal of Veterinary Research* **30**, 1167–1182.

Arey, L. B. (1941). Throttling veins in the livers of certain animals. *Anatomical Record* **8**, 21–35.

Arkins, J. A., Bukosky, R. J., and Fink, J. N. (1967). The characterization of skin-sensitizing antibody induced in nonsensitive dogs. *Journal of Allergy* **40**, 50–56.

Arrocha, R., Wittwer, J. W., and Gargiulo, A. W. (1968). Tissue response to heterogenous bone implantation in dogs. *Journal of Periodontology* **39**, 162–166.

Attaran, S. E., Hodges, C. V., and Crary, L. S., Jr. (1966). Homotransplants of the testis. *Journal of Urology* **95**, 387–389.

Austen, K. F. (1965). Anaphylaxis: Systemic, local cutaneous, and *in virto*. In "The Inflammatory Process" (B. W. Zweifach, L. Grant, and R. T. McCluskey, eds.), pp. 587–612. Academic Press, New York.

Bach, F. H. (1968). Transplantation: Problems of histocompatability testing. *Science* **159**, 1196–1198.

Baer, R. L., and Harber, L. C. (1965). Allergic eczematous contact dermatitis. *In* "Immunological Diseases" (M. Samter and H. L. Alexander, eds.), pp. 646–653. Little, Brown, Boston, Massachusetts.

Bain, B., and Lowenstein, L. (1964). Genetic studies on the mixed leukocyte reaction. *Science* **145**, 1315–1316.

Baker, E. (1966). Allergy skin testing in the dog. *Journal of the American Veterinary Medical Association* **148**, 1160–1162.

Baker, E. (1969). Management of allergic disease by hyposensitization. *Journal of the American Veterinary Medical Association* **154**, 491–494.

Baker, J. A., Robson, D. S., Gillespie, J. H., Burgher, J. A., and Doughty, M. F. (1959). A nomograph that predicts the age to vaccinate puppies against distemper. *Cornell Veterinarian* **49**, 158–167.

Baldini, M. (1965). Acute ITP in isoimmunized dogs. *Annals of the New York Academy of Sciences* **124**, 543–549.

Baltch, A. L., Osborne, W., Canarile, L., Hassirdjian, A., and Bunn, P. A. (1962). Serum properdin, complement and agglutinin changes in dogs with staphylococcal bacteremia. *Journal of Immunology* **88**, 361–368.

Baltch, A. L., Lepper, M. H., and Lolans, V. T. (1966). Influence of corticosteroid therapy on serum complement, agglutinins, free-boundary electrophoresis, total protein and blood counts in dogs with S staphylococcal bacteremia. *Journal of Immunology* **96**, 149–158.

Barac, G. (1967). Expériences sur les surrénales homotransplantées au cou chez le chien et chez le chat. *Comptes rendus des séances de la société de biologie* **161**, 1138–1142.

Beattie, E. J., Jr. (1966). Some observations on lung transplantation. *American Surgeon* **32**, 818–820.

Beckett, S. D., Burns, M. J., and Clark, C. H. (1964). A study of blood glucose, serum transaminase and electrophoretic patterns of dogs with infectious canine hepatitis. *American Journal of Veterinary Research* **25**, 1186–1190.

Beierwaltes, W. H., and Nishiyama, R. H. (1968). Dog thyroiditis—occurrence and similarity to Hashimoto's struma. *Endocrinology* **83**, 501–508.

Benacerraf, B., and Green, I. (1969). Cellular hypersensitivity. *Annual Review of Medicine* **20**, 141–154.

Ben-Efraim, S., and Torten, M. (1968). Experimental induction of delayed ocular reactions resembling post-leptospirosis ophthalmia. *Journal of General Microbiology* **50**, Suppl. 7–8.

Benjamini, E., Feingold, B. F., and Kartman, L. (1960). Allergy to flea bites. III. The experimental induction of flea bite sensitivity in guinea pigs by exposure to flea bites and by antigen prepared from whole flea extracts of *Ctenocephalides felis felis*. *Experimental Parisitology* **10**, 214–222.

Benjamini, E., Feingold, B. F., and Kartman, L. (1961). Skin reactivity in guinea pigs sensitized to flea bites: The sequence of reactions. *Proceedings of the Society for Experimental Biology and Medicine* **108**, 700–702.

Benjamini, E., Feingold, B. F., Young, J. D., Kartman, L., and Shimizu, M. (1963). Allergy to flea bites. IV. *In vitro* collection and antigenic properties of the oral secretion of the cat flea, *Ctenocephalides felis felis* (Bouche). *Experimental Parisitology* **13**, 1143–1154.

Benninghoff, D. L., Korostoff, A. J., and Herman, P. G. (1968). The microcirculation of the lymph node. Its role in the fourth circulation. *American Journal of Roentgenology, Radium Therapy and Nuclear Medicine* **102**, 891–889.

Bicks, R. O., and Walker, R. H. (1962). Immunologic "colitis" in dogs. *American Journal of Digestive Diseases* **7**, 574–584.

Bliss, J. Q., Johns, D. G., and Burger, A. S. V. (1959). Transfusion reactions due to plasma incompatibility in dogs. *Circulation Research* **7**, 79–85.

Bloch, K. J. (1967). The anaphylactic antibodies of mammals including man. *Progress in Allergy* **10**, 84–150.

Blumenstock, D. A., Grosjean, O. V., Otte, H. P., and Mulder, M. A. (1967). Experimental allotransplantation of the lung. *Journal of Thoracic & Cardiovascular Surgery* **54**, 807–814.

Boguth, W. (1953). Papierelektrophoretische Serumuntersuchungen bei Haussaugetieren (1 Mitteilung). *Zentralblatt für Veterinärmedizin* **1**, 168–187.

Bossak, E. T., Wang, C., and Aldersberg, D. (1955). Effect of cortisone on plasma globulins in the dog. Studies by paper electrophoresis. *Proceedings of the Society for Experimental Biology and Medicine* **88**, 634–636.

Böttger, G. (1966). Ersatz von Femurschaftanteilen durch homologe Knochentransplantate. Tier-experimentelle Untersuchungen. *Langenbecks Archiv für klinische Chirurgie* **316**, 531–537.

Braf, Z. F., Smellie, W. A., and Williams, G. M. (1967). Preparation of specific, potent antilymphocyte serum in the horse using dog thymocytes. *Surgical Forum* **18**, 227–229.

Brambell, F. W. R. (1958). The passive immunity of the young animal. *Biological Reviews of the Cambridge Philosophical Society* **33**, 488–531.

Brambell, F. W. R. (1966). The transmission of immunity from mother to young and the catabolism of immunoglobulins. *Lancet* **II**, 1087–1093.

Brunner, M., Altman, I., and Bowman, K. (1944). Canine sensitivity to ascaris antigen. *Journal of Allergy* **15**, 2–7.

Bukosky, R. J., Hogan, M. R., and Arkins, J. A. (1968). Characterization of ragweed antibodies induced in nonatopic dogs. *Journal of Laboratory and Clinical Medicine* **72**, 383–391.

Burnet, F. M. (1959). "The Clonal Selection Theory of Acquired Immunity." Cambridge Univ. Press, London and New York.

Burnet, F. M. (1968). Evolution of the immune process in vertebrates. *Nature* **218**, 426–430.

Cabasson, J., Joos, H. A., and Dureau, G. (1967). Histocompatibilité et transplantation cardiaque. *Presse médicale* **75**, 2825-2828.

Calne, R. Y. (1968). The present position and future prospects of organ transplantation. *Annals of the Royal College of Surgeons of England* **42**, 283-306.

Calne, R. Y., Wheeler, J. R., and Hurn, B. A. L. (1965). Combined immunosuppressive action of phytohemagglutinin and azothiopurine (imuran) on dogs with renal homotransplants. *British Medical Journal* **II**, 154-155.

Calne, R. Y., Davis, D. R., Medawar, P., and Wheeler, J. R. (1966). Effect of donor antigen on dogs with renal homotransplants. *Transplantation* **4**, 742-746.

Carmichael, L. E. (1964). The pathogenesis of ocular lesions of infectious canine hepatitis. I. Pathology and virological observations. *Pathologia Veterinaria (Basel)* **1**, 73-95.

Carmichael, L. E. (1965). The pathogenesis of ocular lesions of infectious canine hepatitis. II. Experimental ocular hypersensitivity produced by the virus. *Pathologia Veterinaria (Basel)* **2**, 344-359.

Carmichael, L. E., Robson, D. S., and Barnes, F. D. (1962). Transfers and decline of maternal infectious hepatitis antibody in puppies. *Proceedings of the Society for Experimental Biology and Medicine* **109**, 677-681.

Ceglowski, W., and Friedman, H. (1967). Suppression of the primary antibody plaque response of mice following infection with Friend disease virus. *Proceedings of the Society for Experimental Biology and Medicine* **126**, 662-666.

Chambers, V. C., and Evans, C. A. (1959). Canine oral papillomatosis. I. Virus assay and observations on the various stages of the experimental infection. *Cancer Research* **19**, 1188-1195.

Chambers, V. C., Evans, C. A., and Weiser, R. S. (1960). Canine oral papillomatosis. II. Immunologic aspects of the disease. *Cancer Research* **20**, 1083-1093.

Chertkov, I. L., Maximenko, A. S., and Novikova, M. N. (1965). Bone marrow allografts in thymectomized x-irradiated dogs. *Nature* **208**, 399-400.

Chiba, C., Kondo, M., and Rosenblatt, M. (1966). Serum electrophoretic changes following heart allotransplantation. *Proceedings of the Society for Experimental Biology and Medicine* **123**, 746-751.

Chou, C. C. (1965). Mechanism of anaphylactic shock. *Journal of the Oklahoma Medical Association* **58**, 419-420.

Chretien, P. B., Behar, R. J., and Kohn, Z. (1967). The canine lymphoid system—a study of the effect of surgical excision. *Anatomical Record* **159**, 5-15.

Cirstea, M., Suhaciu, G., and Butculescu, I. (1966). Evaluation du role de la bradykinine dans le choc anaphylactique. *Archives internationales de physiologie et de therapie* **159**, 18-33.

Clark, D. S., Foker, J. E., Good, R. A., and Varco, R. L. (1968). Humoral factors in canine renal allograft rejection. *Lancet* **I**, 8-10.

Cleveland, R. J., Madge, C. E., and Lower, R. R. (1967). Homovital graft replacement of the aortic valve. *Surgical Forum* **18**, 124-125.

Cluff, L. E., and Johnson, J. E. (1965). Poststreptococcal disease. *In* "Immunological Diseases" (M. Samter and H. L. Alexander, eds.), pp. 418-429. Little, Brown. Boston, Massachusetts.

Cochrane, C. G. (1968). The role of immune complexes and complement in tissue injury. *Journal of Allergy* **42**, 113-129.

Cohen, A. S. (1967). Amyloidosis. *New England Journal of Medicine* **277**, 522-530, 574-583, and 628-638.

Comens, P. (1956). Experimental hydralazine disease and its similarity to disseminated lupus erythromatosus. *Journal of Laboratory and Clinical Medicine* **47**, 444–454.

Connell, J. T. (1969). Role of antibodies in allergic disease. *New York State Journal of Medicine* **69**, 551–560.

Cooper, D. K. (1968). Experimental development of cardiac transplantation. *British Medical Journal* **IV**, 174–181.

Cooper, M. D., Gabrielsen, A. E., and Good, R. A. (1967). Role of the thymus and other central lymphoid tissues in immunological disease. *Annual Review of Medicine* **18**, 113–138.

Cortez, J., Brunner, M., and Altman, I. (1947). Skin tests in dogs with common allergens. *Journal of Allergy* **18**, 305–310.

Csaba, B., Szilágyi, T., Damjanovich, S., and Kövér, A. (1963). Anaphylactic shock and peptone shock in the dog. I. The role of histamine in anaphylactic shock. *Acta Physiologica Academiae Scientiarum Hungaricae* **23**, 363–369.

Csaba, B., Miltenyi, L., and Foldes, I. (1966). Antigen distribution in the tissues of dogs in anaphylactic shock. *Acta Physiologica Academiae Scientiarum Hungaricae* **30**, 99–105.

Cummings, J. F., and Haas, D. C. (1967). Coonhound paralysis. An acute idiopathic polyradiculoneuritis in dogs resembling the Landry-Guillain-Barre syndrome. *Journal of the Neurological Sciences* **4**, 51–81.

Dammin, G. J., Wheeler, H. B., Montague, A. C. W., Dealy, J. B., Greenberg, J. B., and Moore, F. D. (1962). The splenic homograft: Its course in the unmodified and modified canine recipient. *Annals of the New York Academy of Sciences* **99**, 861–869.

Daniels, J. C., Ritzmann, S. E., and Levin, W. C. (1968). Lymphocytes: Morphological, developmental and functional characteristics in health, disease and experimental study—an analytical review. *Texas Reports on Biology and Medicine* **26**, 5–92.

Dausset, J., and Rapaport, F. T. (1968). The Hu-1 system of human histocompatability. *In* "Human Transplantation" (F. T. Rapaport and J. Dausset, eds.), pp. 369–382. Grune & Stratton, New York.

David, J. R. (1967). Interactions between immunocompetent cells and target cells or antigens. *Bulletin of the New York Academy of Medicine* [2] **43**, 949–958.

DeMonbreun, W. A., and Goodpasture, E. W. (1932). Infectious oral papillomatosis of dogs. *American Journal of Pathology* **8**, 43–55.

Dempster, W. J. (1968). Renal allograft rejection. *Lancet* **I**, 145–146.

Dennis, R. A., Jacoby, R. O., and Griesemer, R. A. (1969a). Development of immunity in fetal dogs. Skin allograft rejection. *American Journal of Veterinary Research* **30**, 1511–1516.

Dennis, R. A., Jacoby, R. O., and Griesemer, R. A. (1969b). Development of immunity in fetal dogs. Effects of thymectomy. *American Journal of Veterinary Research* **30**, 1517–1522.

de Wael, J. (1956). Application of paper electrophoresis to the differential diagnosis of canine diseases. *Ciba Found. Symp., Paper Electrophoresis* pp. 22–29.

Diethelm, A. G., Dubernard, J. M., Busch, G. J., and Murray, J. E. (1968). Critical re-evaluation of immunosuppressive therapy in canine renal allografts. *Surgery, Gynecology and Obstetrics* **126**, 723–736.

Dillman, R. C., and Coles, E. H. (1966). A canine serum fraction analogous to human C-reactive protein. *American Journal of Veterinary Research* **27**, 1769–1775.

Ditchfield, W. J. B. (1968). Systemic mycoses. *In* "Canine Medicine" (E. J. Catcott, ed.), pp. 170–181. Am. Vet. Publ., Santa Barbara, California.

Dixon, F. J. (1968). The pathogenesis of glomerulonephritis. *American Journal of Medicine* 44, 493–498.

Dixon, F. J., Talmage, D. W., Maurer, P. H., and Deichmiller, M. P. (1952). The half-life of homologous gammaglobulin (antibody) in several species. *Journal of Experimental Medicine* 96, 313–318.

Donahoo, J. S., Wilkinson, C. P., and Weldon, C. S. (1967). The production of lymphocytopenia by selective irradiation in dogs. A comparison of two techniques. *Journal of Surgical Research* 7, 475–480.

Dresser, D. W., and Mitchison, N. A. (1968). The mechanism of immunological paralysis. *Advances in Immunology* 8, 129–181.

Dubernard, J. M., Carpenter, C. B., and Busch, G. J. (1968). Rejection of canine renal allografts by passive transfer of sensitized serum. *Surgery* 64, 752–760.

Dubois, E. L., Katz, Y. J., Freeman, V., and Garbak, F. (1957). Chronic toxicity studies of hydralazine (Apresoline) in dogs with particular reference to the production of the "hydralazine syndrome." *Journal of Laboratory and Clinical Medicine* 50, 119–126.

Edgington, T. S., Glassock, R. J., and Dixon, F. J. (1967). Autologous immune-complex pathogenesis of experimental allergic glomerulonephritis. *Science* 155, 1432–1434.

Engle, R. L., Jr., and Woods, K. R. (1960). Comparative biochemistry and embryology of the plasma proteins. *In* "The Plasma Proteins" (F. W. Putnam, ed.), Vol. 2, pp. 183–265. Academic Press, New York.

Epstein, R. B., Bryant, J., and Thomas, E. D. (1967). Cytogenic demonstration of permanent tolerance in adult outbred dogs. *Transplantation* 5, 267–272.

Epstein, R. B., Storb, R., Ragde, H., and Thomas, E. D. (1968). Cytotoxic typing antisera for marrow grafting in littermate dogs. *Transplantation* 6, 45–58.

Fateh-Moghadam, A., Pichlmayr, R., and Morell, C. (1967). Verhalten der Immunoglobulinie und der Antikörperbildung während der Behandlung mit heterologen Antilymphocytenserum. *Klinische Wochenschrift* 45, 665–670.

Filkins, M. E., and Gillette, D. D. (1966). Initial dietary influences on antibody absorption in newborn puppies. *Proceedings of the Society for Experimental Biology and Medicine* 122, 686–688.

Fisher, B., Fisher, E. R., Feduska, N., and Sakai, A. (1967). Thyroid and parathyroid implantation—an experimental re-evaluation. *Surgery* 62, 1025–1038.

Flax, M. H., and Barnes, B. A. (1966). The role of vascular injury in pulmonary allograft rejection. *Transplantation* 4, 66–78.

Fowler, R., Nathan, P., and West, C. D. (1961). The fate of skin homografts following inoculation of homologous donor leucocytes into newborn puppies. *Transplantation Bulletin* 28, 81–85.

Fox, M., Diethelm, A. G., Orr, W. M., Dammin, G. J., Glassock, R. J., and Murray, J. E. (1968). The effect of sheep antilymphocyte plasma on the survival of dog renal allografts. *Proceedings of the Royal Society of Medicine* 61, 877–879.

Fukuda, M., Greene, J. A., Jr., and Vander, A. J. (1968). Plasma renin activity during development of experimental antiserum glomerular nephritis. *Journal of Laboratory and Clinical Medicine* 71, 148–152.

Furuse, A., Uei, I., and Nakamura, K. (1967). Heterotopic allotransplantation of heart in adult dog treated with thymectomy and intralymphatic administration of 6-mercaptopurine. *Japanese Heart Journal* 8, 58–66.

Gabrielsen, A. E., and Good, R. A. (1967). Chemical suppression of adaptive immunity. *Advances in Immunology* **6**, 91–229.

Gertner, H. R., Harrah, J. D., Sample, W. F., and Chretien, P. B. (1969). Synergistic effect of phytohemagglutinin (PHA) and immunosuppressive regimens on skin allograft survival in adult dogs. *Federation Proceedings* **28**, 582.

Gewurz, H., Clark, D. S., Finstadt, J., Kelley, R. L., Varco, R. L., Good, R. A., and Gabrielsen, A. E. (1966). Role of the complement system in graft rejections in experimental animals and man. *Annals of the New York Academy of Sciences* **129**, 673–713.

Gibson, J. P., Griesemer, R. A., and Koestner, A. (1965). Experimental distemper in the gnotobiotic dog. *Pathologia Veterinaria (Basel)* **2**, 1–19.

Gillespie, J. H., Baker, J. A., Burgher, J., Robson, D. S., and Gilman, G. (1958). The immune response of dogs to distemper virus. *Cornell Veterinarian* **48**, 103–126.

Gillette, D. O., and Filkins, M. (1966). Factors affecting antibody transfer in the newborn puppy. *American Journal of Physiology* **210**, 419–422.

Gocke, D. J., Preisig, R., Morris, T. Q., McKay, D. G., and Bradley, S. E. (1967). Experimental viral hepatitis in the dog—production of persistent disease in partially immune animals. *Journal of Clinical Investigation* **46**, 1506–1517.

Godfrey, W. D., Neely, W. A., and Elliott, R. L. (1966). Canine heartworms in experimental cardiac and pulmonary surgery. *Journal of Surgical Research* **6**, 331–336.

Goldwyn, R. M., Beach, P. M., and Feldman, D. (1966). Canine limb homotransplantation. *Plastic and Reconstructive Surgery* **37**, 184–195.

Gombos, A., Tischler, V., Jacina, J., and Skokan, J. (1962). Successful homotransplanted kidneys in dogs. *Annals of the New York Academy of Sciences* **99**, 787–794.

Good, R. A., and Papermaster, B. W. (1964). Ontogeny and phylogeny of adaptive immunity. *Advances in Immunology* **4**, 1–115.

Govaerts, A. (1960). Cellular antibodies in kidney homotransplantation. *Journal of Immunology* **85**, 516–522.

Gray, J. G., and Russell, P. S. (1956). The lymphocyte transfer test in man. *National Academy of Sciences—National Research Council, Publication* **1229**, 105–116.

Greenfield, J. G., and Norman, R. M. (1963). Demyelinating diseases. *In* "Greenfield's Neuropathology" (W. Blackwood *et al.*, eds.), pp. 475–519. Williams & Wilkins, Baltimore, Maryland.

Grosjean, O., and Otte, H. (1966a). Tentative de production de paralysis et de facilitation immunologique chez le chien adulte. *Comptes rendus des séances de la société de biologie* **160**, 442–446.

Grosjean, O., and Otte, H. (1966b). Tolérance immunologique induite chez le chien par des injections néonatales uniques ou répétées de moelle osseuse de donneurs adultes non apparentés. *Comptes rendus des séances de la société de biologie* **160**, 216–220.

Guttman, P. H., and Andersen, A. D. (1968). Progressive intercapillary glomerulosclerosis in aging and irradiated Beagles. *Radiation Research* **35**, 45–60.

Halasz, N. A., Orloff, M. J., and Hirose, F. (1964). Increased survival in renal homografts in dogs after injection of graft donor blood. *Transplantation* **2**, 453–458.

Halasz, N. A., Seifert, L. N., and Rosenfield, H. A. (1966). The effects of antigen overloading on survival of renal allografts. *Proceedings of the Society for Experimental Biology and Medicine* **123**, 924–929.

Hampers, C. L., Kolker, P., and Hager, E. B. (1967). Isolation and characterization of antibodies and other immunologically reactive substances from rejecting renal allografts. *Journal of Immunology* **99**, 514–525.

Hanna, M. G., Nettesheim, P., Ogden, L., and Makinodan, T. (1967). Reduced immune potential of aged mice: Significance of morphologic changes in lymphatic tissue. *Proceedings of the Society for Experimental Biology and Medicine* **125**, 882–886.

Hašek, M., Lengerová, A., and Hraba, T. (1961). Transplantation immunity and tolerance. *Advances in Immunology* **1**, 1–66.

Haxhe, J. J., Alexandre, G. P., and Kestens, P. J. (1967). The effect of imuran and azaserine on liver function tests in the dog. Its relation to the detection of graft rejection following liver transplantation. *Archives internationales de pharmacodynamie* **168**, 366–372.

Hayes, T. G. (1968). Development of ellipsoids in the spleen of the dog. *American Journal of Veterinary Research* **29**, 1245–1250.

Hennes, A. R., Sevelius, H., Lewellyn, T., Joel, W., Woods, A. H., and Wolf, S. (1962). Atrophic gastritis in dogs. *Archives of Pathology* **73**, 281–287.

Herman, A. H., and Schloerb, P. R. (1967). The effect of thoracic duct lymphocyte antiserum on canine renal allografts. *Transplantation* **5**, 732–733.

Heymann, W., Hunter, J. L. P., and Hackel, D. B. (1962). Experimental autoimmune nephrosis in rats. III. *Journal of Immunology* **88**, 135–141.

Highman, B., Roshe, J., and Altland, P. D. (1958). Endocarditis and glomerulonephritis in dogs with aortic insufficiency. *A.M.A. Archives of Pathology* **65**, 388–394.

Hinchey, E. J., and Bliss, J. Q. (1965). The lymphocyte transfer test in the dog. *Canadian Journal of Physiology and Pharmacology* **43**, 1025–1027.

Hirasawa, Y., Marmor, L., and Liebes, D. (1968). Irradiated experimental nerve heterografts pretreated with specific antiserum. *Journal of Neurosurgery* **28**, 233–240.

Hirsch, M. S., and Murphy, F. A. (1968). Effects of anti-lymphoid sera on viral infections. *Lancet* **II**, 27–40.

Hobson, H. P., and Ellett, E. W. (1968). Bacterial diseases. *In* "Canine Medicine" (E. J. Catcott, ed.), pp. 150–158. Am. Vet. Publ., Santa Barbara, California.

Hornick, D. N., and Sensenig, D. M. (1968). Applicability of the normal lymphocyte transfer test to the dog. *American Surgeon* **34**, 457–460.

Horowitz, R. E., Burrows, L., Paronetto, F., Dreiling, D., and Kark, A. (1965). Immunologic observations on homografts. II. The canine kidney. *Transplantation* **3**, 318–325.

Hottendorf, G. H., and Nielsen, S. W. (1966). Collagen necrosis in canine mastocytomas. *American Journal of Pathology* **49**, 501–513.

Hottendorf, G. H., and Nielsen, S. W. (1968). Pathologic report of 29 necropsies on dogs with mastocytoma. *Pathologia Veterinaria (Basel)* **5**, 102–121.

Howard, E. B. (1967). Immunologic defect in mastocytoma-bearing dogs. *Journal of the American Veterinary Medical Association* **151**, 1308–1310.

Howard, E. B., and Kenyon, A. J. (1965). Canine mastocytoma-altered alphaglobulin distribution. *American Journal of Veterinary Research* **26**, 1132–1137.

Howard, E. B., and Nielsen, S. W. (1965). Neoplasia of the Boxer dog. *American Journal of Veterinary Research* **26**, 1121–1131.

Hudson, B. W., Feingold, B. F., and Kartman, L. (1960). Allergy to flea bites. I. Experimental induction of flea-bite sensitivity in guinea pigs. *Experimental Parasitology* **9**, 18–24.

Hughes, F. W., Richards, A. B., and Solow, E. B. (1966). Similar factors occurring in the *ordinary* and the hyperacute form of experimental allergic encephalomyelitis in the rat and the dog. *Life Sciences* **5**, 137–148.

Hume, D. M., and Wolf, J. S. (1967). Modification of renal homograft rejection by irradiation. *Transplantation* **5**, Suppl., 1174–1191.

Hurley, E. J., and Kosek, J. C. (1968). Atypical rejection of the canine heart. *Transplantation* **6**, 895–903.

Idezuki, Y., Feemster, J. A., Dietzman, R. H., and Lillehei, R. C. (1968a). Experimental pancreaticoduodenal preservation and transplantation. *Surgery, Gynecology and Obstetrics* **126**, 1002–1014.

Idezuki, Y., Lillehei, R. C., and Feemster, J. A. (1968b). Pancreaticoduodenal allotransplantation in dogs. *Vascular Diseases* **5**, 78–89.

Ikeda, K. (1966). Successful peripheral nerve homotransplantation by use of high-voltage electron irradiation. *Archiv für japanische Chirurgie* **35**, 679–705.

Ikeda, S., Sealy, W. C., and Cline, R. E. (1967). Aortic valve homograft to subcoronary and pulmonic positions. *Annals of Thoracic Surgery* **4**, 412–419.

Innes, J. R. M., and Saunders, L. Z. (1962). "Comparative Neuropathology," pp. 373–384. Academic Press, New York.

Inou, T., Ota, K., and Mori, S. (1968). Manifestations of rejection of pancreaticoduodenal allografts. *Transplantation* **6**, 503–513.

Irfan, M. (1967). The electrophoretic pattern of serum proteins in normal animals. *Research in Veterinary Science* **8**, 137–142.

Isacson, P. (1967). Myxoviruses and autoimmunity. *Progress in Allergy* **10**, 256–292.

Iwasaki, Y., Porter, K. A., Amend, J. R., Jr., Marchioro, T. L., Zühlke, V., and Starzl, T. E. (1967). The preparation and testing of horse antidog and antihuman antilymphoid plasma or serum and its protein fractions. *Surgery, Gynecology and Obstetrics* **124**, 1–24.

Jackson, B. T. (1967). Immunologic aspects of the fetus and fetal-maternal relationships. *Surgery* **62**, 232–237.

Jacoby, R. O., and Dennis, R. A. (1969). Unpublished data.

Jacoby, R. O., Dennis, R. A., and Griesemer, R. A. (1969). Development of immunity in fetal dogs. Humoral responses. *American Journal of Veterinary Research* **30**, 1503–1510.

James, K. (1969). The preparation and properties of antilymphocytic sera. *Progress in Surgery* **7**, 140–216.

Jeejeebhoy, H. F. (1967). The relationship of lymphopenia production and lymphocyte agglutinating and cytotoxic antibody titers to the immunosuppressive potency of heterologous antilymphocyte plasma. *Transplantation* **4**, Suppl., 1121–1126.

Johnson, J. S., and Vaughan, J. H. (1967). Canine immunoglobulins. I. Evidence for six immunoglobulin classes. *Journal of Immunology* **98**, 923–934.

Johnson, J. S., Vaughan, J. H., and Swisher, S. N. (1967). Canine immunoglobulins. II. Antibody activities in six immunoglobulin classes. *Journal of Immunology* **98**, 935–940.

Jones, T. C., and Zook, B. C. (1965). Aging changes in the vascular system of animals. *Annals of the New York Academy of Sciences* **127**, 671–684.

Joshua, J. O. (1956). Some allergic conditions in the dog and cat. *Veterinary Record* **68**, 682–685.

Kahan, B. D., and Reisfeld, R. A. (1969). Transplantation antigens. *Science* **164**, 514–521.

Kakuk, T. J., Hinz, R. W., Langham, R. F., and Conner, G. H. (1968). Experimental transmission of canine malignant lymphoma to the Beagle neonate. *Cancer Research* **28**, 716–723.

Kaliss, N. (1965). Immunological enhancement—the immunologically induced prolongation of tumor homograft survival. *Proceedings of the 10th Congress of the International Society of Blood Transfusion, Stockholm, 1964* pp. 91–103. Karger, Basel.

Karlson, A. G., and Mann, F. C. (1952). The transmissable venereal tumor of dogs: Observations on forty generations of experimental transfers. *Annals of the New York Academy of Sciences* **54**, 1197–1213.

Kasakura, S., Thomas, E. D., and Ferrebee, J. W. (1964). Leukocytotoxic isoantibodies in the dog. *Transplantation* **2**, 274–280.

Kekis, B. P., Nabseth, D. C., Rowe, M. I., Apostolou, K., Gottlieb, L. S., and Deterling, R. A. (1964). Parabiosis with cross circulation in adult mongrel dogs. *Annals of the New York Academy of Sciences* **120**, 367–378.

Kelly, W. D. (1963). The thymus and lymphoid morphogenesis in the dog. *Federation Proceedings* **22**, 600.

Kiskin, W. A. (1966). Skin allograft survival in the thymectomized, azathioprine-treated adult mongrel. *Archives of Surgery* **92**, 386–387.

Kissileff, A. (1938). The dog flea as a causative agent in summer eczema. *Journal of the American Veterinary Medical Association* **93**, 21–27.

Kissileff, A. (1962). Relationship of dog fleas to dermatitis. *Veterinary Medicine/Small Animal Clinician* **2**, 1132–1135.

Klein, G. (1968). Tumor-specific transplantation antigens. *Cancer Research* **28**, 625–635.

Koffler, D., and Kunkel, H. G. (1968). Mechanisms of renal injury in systemic lupus erythematosus. *American Journal of Medicine* **45**, 165–169.

Kondo, Y., Chaptal, P. A., Gradel, F. O., Cottle, H. R., and Kantrowitz, A. (1967). Fate of orthotopic canine heart transplants. *Journal of Cardiovascular Surgery* **8**, 155–161.

Koo, G. C., Monaghan, E. D., Gault, M. H., and MacLean, L. D. (1965). Comparative value of lymphocyturia, serum, and urinary enzymes in the diagnosis of renal homograft rejection. *Surgical Forum* **16**, 256–258.

Koo, G. C., Monaghan, E. D., Gault, M. H., Pirozynski, W. J., and MacLean, L. D. (1966). A unique instance of canine renal homotransplantation with remission of rejection crisis and prolonged survival. *Transplantation* **4**, 500–505.

Kosek, J. C., Hurley, E. J., and Lower, R. R. (1968). Histopathology of orthotopic canine cardiac homografts. *Laboratory Investigation* **19**, 97–112.

Kountz, S. L., and Cohn, R. B. (1967). Successful intrarenal treatment of the allograft reaction. *Surgical Forum* **18**, 251–252.

Kountz, S. L., Williams, M. A., Williams, P. L., Kapros, C., and Dempster, W. J. (1963). Mechanism of rejection of homotransplanted kidneys. *Nature* **199**, 257–260.

Kozma, C. K., Pelas, A., and Salvador, R. A. (1967). Electrophoretic determination of serum proteins of laboratory animals. *Journal of the American Veterinary Medical Association* **151**, 865–869.

Kozuszek, W. (1967). Die Beeinflussung der Immuntoleranz bei experimentellen homologen Nierentransplantationen durch mechanische Lymphableitung. *Ärztliche Forschung* **21**, 280–286.

Krakower, C. A., and Greenspon, S. A. (1954). Factors leading to variation in concentration of "nephrotoxic" antigen(s) of glomerular basement membrane. *A.M.A. Archives of Pathology* **58**, 401–432.

Krohn, K. (1968a). Experimental gastritis in the dog. I. Production of atrophic gastritis and antibodies to parietal cells. *Annales Medicinae Experimentalis et Biologiae Fenniae (Helsinki)* **46**, 249–258.

Krohn, K. (1968b). Experimental gastritis in the dog. II. Production of antibodies to a gastric B_{12}-binding auto-antigen. *Annales Medicinae Experimentalis et Biologiae Fenniae (Helsinki)* **46**, 259–272.

Kronman, B. S., Wepsic, H. T., Churchill, W. H., Zbar, B., Borsus, T., and Rapp, H. J. (1969). Tumor-specific antigens detected by inhibition of macrophage migration. *Science* **165**, 296–297.

Kruvskii, I. L. (1967). Vograstne osobennosti construkchii regionarnich Lymfaticheshich uzlov sobaki. *Arkhiv Anatomii, Gistologii i Embriologii* **53**, 25–34.

Kwong, K. H., Paton, B. C., and Hill, R. B., Jr. (1967). Experimental use of immuno-suppression in aortic valve homografts and heterografts. *Journal of Thoracic & Cardiovascular Surgery* **54**, 199–212.

Lance, E. M. (1967a). A functional and morphologic study of intracranial thyroid allografts in the dog. *Surgery, Gynecology and Obstetrics* **125**, 529–539.

Lance, E. M. (1967b). A functional and morphological study of intracranial parathyroid allografts in the dog. *Transplantation* **5**, 1471–1483.

Langr, F., Fixa, B., and Komarkova, O. (1967). Morphology of the gastric mucosa of the dog after immunization with autologous gastric juice. I. Histological study. *Pathologia et Microbiologia* **30**, 419–424.

Larin, N. M., Gaddum, R., and Orbell, W. G. (1957). The complement activity of canine serum. *Journal of Hygiene* **55**, 402–413.

Larrivee, D. H., Benjamini, E., Feingold, B. F., and Shimizu, M. (1964). Histologic studies of guinea pig skin: Different stages of allergic reactivity to flea bites. *Experimental Parasitology* **15**, 491–502.

Lázár, L., Maros, T., and Kovács, I. (1966). Uber Gewisse Eigentumlichkeiten des Physikalischen Abbaus der Markscheide bei der experimentellen allergischen Ensephalomyelitis der Hunde. *Acta Morphologica Academiae Scientiarum Hungaricae* **14**, 87–98.

LeBouvier, G. L., Sussman, M., and Crawford, L. V. (1966). Antigenic diversity of mammalian papillomaviruses. *Journal of General Microbiology* **45**, 497–501.

LeVeen, H. H., Falk, G., and Schatman, B. (1961). Experimental ulcerative colitis produced by anticolon sera. *Annals of Surgery* **154**, 275–280.

Lewis, R. M. (1965). Clinical evaluation of the lupus erythematosus cell phenomenon in dogs. *Journal of the American Veterinary Medical Association* **147**, 939–943.

Lewis, R. M. (1968). Models of auto-immunity. Spontaneous diseases of lower animals. *Postgraduate Medicine* **43**, 143–149.

Lewis, R. M., and Hathaway, J. E. (1967). Canine systemic lupus erythematosus—presenting with symmetrical polyarthritis. *Journal of Small Animal Practice* **8**, 273–284.

Lewis, R. M., Henry, W. B., Thorton, G. W., and Gilmore, C. E. (1963). A syndrome of auto-immune hemolytic anemia and thrombocytopenia in dogs. *Scientific Proceedings of the 100th Meeting of the American Veterinary Medical Association, New York* pp. 140–163.

Lewis, R. M., Schwartz, R. S., and Henry, W. B. (1965a). Canine systemic lupus erythematosus. *Blood* **25**, 143–160.

Lewis, R. M., Schwartz, R. S., and Gilmore, C. E. (1965b). Autoimmune diseases in domestic animals. *Annals of the New York Academy of Sciences* **124**, 178–200.

Lillehei, R. C., Idezuki, Y., Feemster, J. A., Dietzman, R. H., Kelley, W. D., Merkel. F. K., Goetz, F. C., Lyons, G. W., and Manax, W. G. (1967). Transplantation of stomach, intestine, and pancreas-experimental and clinical observations. *Surgery* **62**, 721–741.

Linn, B. S. (1966). Renal allografts and donor spleen cells-survival according to schedule of infusion. *Annals of Surgery* **164**, 223–226.

Lombard, L. S., and Moloney, J. B. (1959). Experimental transmission of mast cell sarcoma in dogs. *Federation Proceedings* **18**, 490.

Lombard, L. S., Moloney, J. B., and Rickard, C. G. (1963). Transmissable canine mastocytoma. *Annals of the New York Academy of Sciences* **108**, 1086–1105.

Long, J. F., and Koestner, A. (1969). Unpublished data.

Lowenhaupt, R., and Nathan, P. (1968). Platelet accumulation observed by electron microscopy in the early phase of renal allo-transplant rejection. *Nature* **220**, 822–825.

Lupulescu, A., Potorac, E., and Pop, A. (1968). Experimental investigations on immunology of the parathyroid gland. *Immunology* **14**, 475–482.

McCluskey, R. T., Vassalli, P., Gallo, G., and Baldwin, D. S. (1966). An immunofluorescent study of pathogenic mechanisms in glomerular diseases. *New England Journal of Medicine* **274**, 695–701.

McDonald, J. C. (1966). Serum antibodies in transplantation. *New York State Journal of Medicine* **66**, 1631–1635.

McIntyre, W. I. M., and Montgomery, G. L. (1952). Renal lesions in *Leptospiro canicola* infection in dogs. *Journal of Pathology and Bacteriology* **64**, 145–160.

Mackay, I. R., and Burnet, F. M. (1963). "Autoimmune Diseases." Thomas, Springfield, Illinois.

McKelvie, D. H., Powers, S., and McKim, F. (1966). Microanalytical procedures for blood chemistry long-term study on Beagles. *American Journal of Veterinary Research* **27**, 1405–1412.

McKenna, J. M., and Prier, J. E. (1966). Some immunologic aspects of canine neoplasms. *Cancer Research* **26**, 137–142.

Maginn, R. R., and Bullimore, J. A. (1968). Extracorporeal irradiation of the blood in renal homograft rejection. *British Journal of Radiology* **41**, 127–133.

Magrane, H. J., Magrane, W. G., and Ross, J. R. (1959). Idiopathic thrombocytopenic purpura in a dog—a case report. *Journal of the American Veterinary Medical Association* **135**, 520–522.

Main, R. K., Cole, L. J., and Jones, M. J. (1967). DNA synthesis in mixed cultures of dog leukocytes—differential effect of x-radiation and freeze-thawing on cellular isoantigenicity. *Journal of Immunology* **98**, 417–424.

Mannick, J. A., Powers, J. H., Mithoefer, J., and Ferrebee, J. W. (1960). Renal transplantation in azotemic dogs. *Surgery* **47**, 340–345.

Mantovani, A., and Kagan, I. G. (1967). Fractionated *Dirofilaria immitis* antigens for the differential diagnosis of canine filariasis. *American Journal of Veterinary Research* **28**, 213–217.

Marchioro, T. L., Rowlands, D. T., Rifkind, D., Waddell, W. R., and Starzl, T. E. (1964). Splenic homotransplantation. *Annals of the New York Academy of Sciences* **120**, 626–651.

Maros, T., Kovács, V. V., Lázár, L., and Marinica, D. (1967). Contributions au probleme de l'influence des facteurs météorologiques sur l'evolution de l'encéphalomyélite allergique expérimentale. *Journal of the Neurological Sciences* **4**, 217–225.

Mason, J. H., Dalling, T., and Gordon, W. S. (1930). Transmission of maternal immunity. *Journal of Pathology and Bacteriology* **33**, 783–797.

Mellors, R. C. (1968). Autoimmune disease and neoplasia of NZB mice. Implication of murine leukemia-like virus. *Perspectives in Virology* **6**, 239–258.

Merler, E., and Rosen, F. S. (1966). The gammaglobulins. I. Structure and synthesis of the immunoglobulins. *New England Journal of Medicine* **275**, 480–486.

Michaeli, D., and Goldfarb, S. (1968). Clinical studies on the hyposensitization of dogs and cats to flea bites. *Australian Veterinary Journal* **44**, 161–165.

Michaeli, D., Benjamini, E., de Buren, F. P., Larrivee, D. H., and Feingold, B. F. (1965). The role of collagen in the induction of flea bite hypersensitivity. *Journal of Immunology* **95**, 162–167.

Michaeli, D., Benjamini, E., Miner, R. C., and Feingold, B. F. (1966). *In vitro* studies on the role of collagen in the induction of hypersensitivity to flea bites. *Journal of Immunology* **97**, 402–406.

Michaelson, S. M., Shively, J. N., and Haydock, I. C. (1966). Radiation-induced changes in the properdin system of the dog and a critical analysis of the general problem. *Radiation Research* **28**, 60–70.

Milgrom, F. (1966). Tissue-specific antigens and isoantigens. *Annals of the New York Academy of Sciences* **129**, 767–775.

Miller, G., Firth, G. F., Swisher, S. N., and Young, L. E. (1957). Studies on the destruction of red blood cells by canine autoantibodies in normal dogs and in a dog with naturally occurring autoimmune hemolytic disease. *American Journal of Diseases of Children* **93**, 35–36.

Miller, M. E., Christensen, G. C., and Evans, H. E. (1964). "Anatomy of the Dog," pp. 433–434. Saunders, Philadelphia, Pennsylvania.

Minton, J. P., Wilson, G. P., Geyer, V. B., Bigley, N. J., and Dodd, M. C. (1967). Nucleic acid antibody and tumor growth following autogenous tumor vaccination in dogs. *Surgical Forum* **18**, 96–98.

Mitchell, G. F., and Miller, J. F. A. P. (1968). Cell to cell interaction in the immune response. II. The source of hemolysin-forming cells in irradiated mice given bone marrow and thymus or thoracic duct lymphocytes. *Journal of Experimental Medicine* **128**, 821–837.

Mitchell, R. M., Stevens, B. G., and Kelly, M. M. (1967). Progress in experimental kidney transplantation. *Medical Journal of Australia* **2**, 303–308.

Moegle, H., Boguth, W., and Bierbaum, A. (1956). Serum-Eiweissuntersuchungen bei nierenkranken Hunden unter besonderer Berücksichtigung des nephrotischen Syndroms. *Zentralblatt für Veterinärmedizin* **3**, 662–696.

Mohri, H., Reichenbach, D. D., and Barnes, R. W. (1967). A biologic study of the homologous aortic valve in dogs. *Journal of Thoracic & Cardiovascular Surgery* **54**, 622–628.

Moldovanu, G., Moore, A. E., Friedman, M., and Miller, D. G. (1966). Cellular transmission of lymphosarcoma in dogs. *Nature* **210**, 1342–1343.

Mollen, N., Cannon, F. D., and Ferrebee, J. W. (1968). Lymphocyte typing in allografted Beagles. *Transplantation* **6**, 939–940.

Moog, F. (1953). The functional differentiation of the small intestine. III. The influence of the pituitary-adrenal system on the differentiation of phosphatase in the duodenum of the suckling mouse. *Journal of Experimental Zoology* **124**, 329–346.

Moulton, J. E. (1956). Fluorescent antibody studies of demyelination in canine distemper. *Proceedings of the Society for Experimental Biology and Medicine* **91**, 460–464.

Movat, H. Z., McGregor, D. D., and Steiner, J. W. (1961). Studies of nephrotoxic nephritis. II. The fine structure of the glomerulus in acute nephrotoxic nephritis of dogs. *American Journal of Clinical Pathology* **36**, 306–321.

Muller, G. H. (1961). Flea allergy dermatitis. *Veterinary Medicine/Small Animal Clinician* **1**, 185–192.

Muller, G. H. (1967). Contact dermatitis in animals. *Archives of Dermatology* **96**, 423–426.

Müller-Eberhard, H. J. (1968). Chemistry and reaction mechanisms of complement. *Advances in Immunology* **8**, 1–80.

Mulligan, R. M. (1963). Comparative pathology of human and canine cancer. *Annals of the New York Academy of Sciences* **108**, 642–690.

Murray, J. E., Sheil, A. G., Moseley, R., Knight, P., McGavic, J. D., and Dammin, G. J. (1964). Analysis of mechanism of immunosuppressive drugs in renal homotransplantation. *Annals of Surgery* **160**, 449–473.

Musser, E. A., and Graham, W. R. (1968). Familial occurrence of thyroiditis in purebread Beagles. *Laboratory Animal Care* **18**, 58–68.

Najarian, J. S., Noble, R. E., Braby, P., and Brainerd, H. D. (1965). Lysozyme determination as a measure of rejection of kidney homotransplants. *Surgical Forum* **16**, 258–260.

Nelson, R. A., Jr. (1966). A new concept of immunosuppression in hypersensitivity reactions and in transplantation immunity. *Survey of Ophthalmology* **11**, 498–505.

Nielsen, S. W., and Cole, C. R. (1961). Homologous transplantation of canine neoplasms. *American Journal of Veterinary Research* **22**, 663–672.

Norman, J. C., Covelli, W. H., and Sise, H. S. (1968). Transplantation of the spleen. *Annals of Internal Medicine* [N.S.] **68**, 700–704.

Okoshi, S., Tomoda, I., and Makimura, S. (1967). Analysis of normal dog serum by immunoelectrophoresis. *Japanese Journal of Veterinary Science* **29**, 233–244.

Oldstone, M. B. A., and Dixon, F. J. (1969). Pathogenesis of chronic disease associated with persistent lymphocytic choriomeningitis viral infection. I. Relationship of antibody production to disease in neonatally infected mice. *Journal of Experimental Medicine* **129**, 483–505.

Oliveras, F. E., Kelley, W. D., Merchant, C., and Good, R. A. (1963). Effect of thymectomy on immune reactions in adult dogs. *Surgical Forum* **14**, 184–186.

Osborne, C. A., Johnson, K. H., Perman, V., and Schall, W. D. (1968a). Renal amyloidosis in the dog. *Journal of the American Veterinary Medical Association* **153**, 669–688.

Osborne, C. A., Perman, V., Sautter, J. H., Stevens, J. B., and Hanlon, G. F. (1968b). Multiple myeloma in the dog. *Journal of the American Veterinary Medical Association* **153**, 1300–1319.

Ota, Y., Camishion, R. C., and Gibbon, J. H. (1962). *Dirofilaria immitis* (heartworms) and *Dipetalonema* species as causes of "transfusion reaction" in dogs. *Surgery* **51**, 518–526.

Ovary, Z., Bloch, K. J., and Benacerraf, B. (1964). Identification of rabbit, monkey and dog antibodies with PCA activity for guinea pigs. *Proceedings of the Society for Experimental Biology and Medicine* **116**, 840–845.

Paccione, F., Enein, A. A., and Shikata, T. (1965). Changes in the transplanted ureter. *British Journal of Experimental Pathology* **46**, 519–529.

Parker, R. L., Fish, J. C., and Sarles, H. E. (1966). Skin allograft survival in lympho-cyte-depleted dogs. *Texas Reports on Biology and Medicine* **24**, 647–654.

Paterson, P. Y. (1966). Experimental allergic encephalomyelitis and autoimmune disease. *Advances in Immunology* **5**, 131–208.

Paterson, P. Y. (1968). Infectious and immune synergistic factors in tissue injury. Parallels between chronic obstructive respiratory disease and chronic pyelo-nephritis. *Yale Journal of Biology and Medicine* **40**, 550–556.

Paterson, P. Y. (1969). Immune processes and infectious factors in central nervous system disease. *Annual Review of Medicine* **20**, 75–100.

Patterson, R. (1960). Investigations of spontaneous hypersensitivity of the dog. *Journal of Allergy* **31**, 351–363.

Patterson, R. (1968). Animal models demonstrating respiratory responses to inhalant antigens. *Yale Journal of Biology and Medicine* **40**, 495–500.

Patterson, R., and Sparks, D. B. (1962). The passive transfer to normal dogs of skin reactivity, asthma and anaphylaxis from a dog with spontaneous ragweed pollen hypersensitivity. *Journal of Immunology* **88**, 262–268.

Patterson, R., Pruzansky, J. J., and Chang, W. W. Y. (1963a). Spontaneous canine hypersensitivity to ragweed. Characterization of the serum factor transferring skin, bronchial and anaphylactic sensitivity. *Journal of Immunology* **90**, 35–42.

Patterson, R., Chang, W. W. Y., Pruzansky, J. J., and Portney, G. L. (1963b). The immunologic response of dogs to soluble protein antigens. *Journal of Immunology* **91**, 129–135.

Patterson, R., Chang, W. W. Y., and Pruzansky, J. J. (1963c). The Northwestern colony of atopic dogs. *Journal of Allergy* **34**, 455–459.

Patterson, R., Pruzansky, J. J., and Janis, B. (1964). Biologic activity of canine nonprecipitating and precipitating antibody. *Journal of Immunology* **93**, 51–58.

Patterson, R., Tennenbaum, J. I., Pruzansky, J. J., and Nelson, V. L. (1965). Canine antiragweed serum. Demonstration of "blocking" activity by *in vivo* and *in vitro* techniques. *Journal of Allergy* **38**, 138–146.

Patterson, R., Roberts, M., and Pruzansky, J. J. (1968). Types of canine serum immunoglobulins. *Journal of Immunology* **101**, 687–694.

Patterson, R., Roberts, M., and Pruzansky, J. J. (1969). Comparisons of reaginic antibodies from three species. *Journal of Immunology* **102**, 466–475.

Peng, M. T., and Pi, W. P. (1967). Emesis in horse serum anaphylactic shock in dogs. *American Journal of Physiology* **212**, 131–134.

Perey, D. Y. E., and Good, R. A. (1968). Experimental arrest and induction of lymphoid development in intestinal lymphoepithelial tissues of rabbits. *Laboratory Investigation* **18**, 15–26.

Perez-Tamayo, R., and Kretschmer, R. R. (1965). Inflammation in homograft rejection. *In* "The Inflammatory Process" (B. W. Zweifach, L. Grant, and R. T. McCluskey, eds.), pp. 685–730. Academic Press, New York.

Perper, R. J., and Najarian, J. S. (1966). Experimental renal heterotransplantation. I. In widely divergent species. *Transplantation* **4**, 377–388.

Pette, E. (1968). Measles virus: A causative agent in multiple sclerosis? *Neurology* **18**, 168–169.

Pette, E., Mannweiler, K., Polacios, O., and Mütze, B. (1965). Phenomena of the cell membrane and their possible significance for the pathogenesis of so-called autoimmune diseases of the nervous system. *Annals of the New York Academy of Sciences* **122**, 417–428.

Phillips, B., and Gazet, J. C. (1967). Growth of two human tumor cell lines in mice treated with antilymphocyte serum. *Nature* **215**, 548–549.

Porter, D. D., and Larsen, A. E. (1968). Virus-host interactions in Aleutian disease of mink. *Perspectives in Virology* **6**, 173–187.

Porter, K. A., Calne, R. Y., and Zukoski, C. F. (1964). Vascular and other changes in two hundred canine renal homotransplants treated with immunosuppressive drugs. *Laboratory Investigation* **13**, 809–824.

Portier, P., and Richet, C. (1902). De l'action anaphylactique de certains venins. *Comptes rendus des séances de la société de biologie* **54**, 170–172.

Powers, R. D. (1968). Immunologic properties of canine transmissible venereal sarcoma. *American Journal of Veterinary Research* **29**, 1637–1645.

Preston, F. W., Macalalad, F., Wachowski, T. J., Randolph, D. A., and Apostol, J. V. (1966). Survival of homografts of the intestine with and without immunosuppression. *Surgery* **60**, 1203–1210.

Prier, J. E., and Brodey, R. S. (1963). Canine neoplasia. A prototype for human cancer study. *Bulletin of the World Health Organization* **29**, 331–344.

Priester, W. A. (1967). Canine lymphoma—relative risk in the Boxer breed. *Journal of the National Cancer Institute* **39**, 833–845.

Puza, A., and Gombos, A. (1958). Acquired tolerance to skin homografts in dogs. *Transplantation Bulletin* **5**, 30–32.

Ramseier, H., and Streilein, J. W. (1965). Homograft sensitivity reactions in irradiated hamsters. *Lancet* **I**, 622–624.

Rickard, C. G., and Post, J. E. (1968). Cellular and cell-free transmission of a canine mast cell leukemia. *Bibliotheca Haematologica* **30**, 279–281.

Robertshaw, G. E., Madge, G. E., and Willams, G. M. (1967). Nephrotoxic activity of hyperimmune homologous dog immune serum. *Surgical Forum* **18**, 276–278.

Robicsek, R., Sanger, P. W., and Gallucci, V. (1966). Transplantation of coronary arteries. An experimental study. *Annals of Thoracic Surgery* **2**, 243–249.

Rockey, J. H., and Schwartzman, R. M. (1967). Skin sensitizing antibodies—a comparative study of canine and human PK and PCA antibodies and a canine myeloma protein. *Journal of Immunology* **98**, 1143–1151.

Rosen, F. S., and Janeway, C. A. (1966). The gamma globulins. III. The antibody deficiency syndromes. *New England Journal of Medicine* **275**, 709–715 and 769–775.

Rosenau, W. (1968). Target cell destruction. *Federation Proceedings* **27**, 34–38.

Rowlands, D. T., Jr., Vanderbeek, R. B., and Seigler, H. F. (1968). Rejection of canine cardiac allografts. *American Journal of Pathology* **53**, 617–629.

Rubinstein, P., Morgado, F., Blumenstock, D. A., and Ferrebee, J. W. (1968). Isohemagglutinins and histocompatibility in the dog. *Transplantation* **6**, 961–969.

Russell, P. S., and Monaco, A. P. (1965). "The Biology of Tissue Transplantation." Little, Brown, Boston, Massachusetts.

Russell, P. S., and Monaco, A. P. (1967). Heterologous antilymphocyte sera and some of their effects. *Transplantation* **5**, Suppl., 1086–1099.

Russell, P. S., Nelson, S. D., and Johnson, G. J. (1966). Matching tests for histocompatibility in man. *Annals of the New York Academy of Sciences* **129**, 368–385.

Samoylina, N. L., and Chertkov, I. L. (1966). Graft-versus-host specificity of lymphoid cells transformed from bone marrow allograft in supralethally x-irradiated dogs. *Nature* **210**, 108.

Schnappauf, H., and Schnappauf, U. (1968). Drainage des Ductus Thoracicus und Grösse der "leicht mobilisierbaren" Lymphozyten bei Kälbern, Schafen und Hunden. *Blut* **16**, 209–220.

Schwartz, R. S., and Andre-Schwartz, J. (1968). Malignant lympho-proliferative diseases: Interactions between immunological abnormalities and oncogenic viruses. *Annual Review of Medicine* 19, 269–282.

Schwartz, S. I., Kutner, F. R., Neistadt, A., Barner, H., Resnicoff, S., and Vaughan, J. (1967). Antigenicity of homografted veins. *Surgery* 61, 471–477.

Schwartzman, R. M. (1965). Atopy in the dog. *In* "Comparative Physiology and Pathology of the Skin" (A. J. Rook and G. S. Walton, eds.), pp. 317–331. Davis, Philadelphia, Pennsylvania.

Schwartzman, R. M., and Rockey, J. H. (1967). Atopy in the dog. *Archives of Dermatology* 96, 418–422.

Seddon, J. A., and Howard, J. M. (1966a). The exocrine behavior of the homotransplanted pancreas. *Surgery* 59, 226–234.

Seddon, J. A., and Howard, J. M. (1966b). The endocrine function of the homotransplanted pancreas. *Surgery* 59, 235–242.

Serre, A., and Clot, J. (1968). Les tests d'histocompatibilité chez le chien en vue de l'éxperimentation des greffes d'organes. *Revue francaise d'études cliniques et biologiques* 13, 109–1022.

Shafey, O. A., and Longmire, W. P., Jr. (1967). Experience in autologous and allogenetic thyroid grafts. *Journal of Surgical Research* 7, 247–249.

Shean, F. C., Barker, W. F., and Fonkalsrud, E. W. (1964). Studies on active and passive antibody induced colitis in the dog. *American Journal of Surgery* 107, 337–339.

Sheil, A. G., Dammin, G. J., Mitchell, R. M., Moseley, R. V., and Murray, J. E. (1968). The management, function and histology of long functioning renal allografts in dogs on immunosuppressive drug therapy. *Annals of Surgery* 167, 467–485.

Shibata, S., Nagasawa, T., and Takuma, T. (1966a). Isolation and properties of the soluble antigen specific for the production of nephrotoxic glomerulonephritis. I. Immunopathological demonstration of the complete antigenicity of the soluble antigen. *Japanese Journal of Experimental Medicine* 36, 127–142.

Shibata, S., Nagasawa, T., and Takuma, T. (1966b). Isolation and properties of the soluble antigen specific for the production of nephrotoxic glomerulonephritis. II. Purification of the active principle from the soluble antigen. *Japanese Journal of Experimental Medicine* 36, 143–159.

Shorter, R. G., and Hallenbeck, G. A. (1968). The histopathologic features of rejection in the allogeneically transplanted kidney in dog and man—a review. *Journal-Lancet* 88, 162–167.

Shorter, R. G., Hallenbeck, G. A., Nava, C., O'Kane, H. O., DeWeerd, J. H., and Johnson, W. J. (1968). Antilymphoid sera in renal allotransplantation. *Archives of Surgery* 97, 323–329.

Simons, M. J. (1968). Antilymphocyte serum. *Lancet* I, 866–867.

Simonsen, M. (1953). Biological incompatability in kidney transplantation in dogs. *Acta Pathologica et Microbiologica Scandinavica* 32, 36–84.

Singh, L. N., Vega, R. E., Makin, G. S., and Howard, J. M. (1965). External thoracic duct fistula and canine renal homograft. *Journal of the American Medical Association* 191, 1009–1011.

Smith, R. T. (1968). Tumor-specific immune mechanisms. *New England Journal of Medicine* 278, 1207–1214, 1268–1275, and 1326–1331.

Snow, L. M., Burns, M. J., and Clark, C. H. (1966). Serum protein electrophoresis and serum transaminase activity of dogs with canine distemper. *American Journal of Veterinary Research* **27**, 70–73.

Southam, C. M. (1967). Evidence for cancer-specific antigens in man. *Progress in Experimental Tumor Research* **9**, 1–39.

Spector, W. S. (1956). "Handbook of Biological Data," pp. 55–56. Saunders, Philadelphia, Pennsylvania.

Spencer, G. R., and Leader, R. W. (1962). Effect of cell-free tumor materials on irradiated and newborn animals. *American Journal of Veterinary Research* **23**, 587–591.

Spink, W. W., Davis, R. B., Potter, R., and Chartrand, S. (1964). The initial stage of canine endotoxin shock as an expression of anaphylactic shock: Studies on complement titers and plasma histamine concentration. *Journal of Clinical Investigation* **43**, 696–704.

Starzl, T. E., Marchioro, T. L., Porter, K. A., and Brettschneider, L. (1967). Homotransplantation of the liver. *Transplantation* **5**, Suppl., 790–803.

Starzl, T. E., Brettschneider, L., and Martin, A. J., Jr. (1968). Organ transplantation, past and present. *Surgical Clinics of North America* **48**, 817–838.

Steblay, R. W. (1963). Some immunologic properties of human and dog glomerular basement membranes. III. Production of glomerulonephritis in juxtamedullary glomeruli of neonatal pups with rabbit anti-human glomerular basement membrane sera. *Laboratory Investigation* **12**, 432–442.

Sterzl, J., and Silverstein, A. M. (1967). Developmental aspects of immunity. *Advances in Immunology* **6**, 337–459.

Stickler, G. B., Khalil, G. W., and McKenzie, B. F. (1956). Canine experimental nephrosis. *Journal of Laboratory and Clinical Medicine* **48**, 866–878.

Stjernswärd, J. (1967). "Studies on Host Immune Status and Tumor-host Relationships in Hydrocarbon Carcinogenesis." Tryckeri Balder, Stockholm.

Storb, R., Epstein, R. B., Bryant, J., Ragde, H., and Thomas, E. (1968). Marrow grafts by combined marrow and leukocyte infusions in unrelated dogs selected by histocompatibility typing. *Transplantation* **6**, 587–594.

Storb, R., Epstein, R. B., Rudolph, R. H., and Thomas, E. D. (1969). Allogeneic canine bone marrow transplantation following cyclophosphamide. *Transplantation* **7**, 378–386.

Storts, R. W., Koestner, A., and Dennis, R. A. (1968). The effects of canine distemper virus on explant tissue cultures of canine cerebellum. *Acta Neuropathologica* **11**, 1–14.

Streilein, J. W., and Barker, C. F. (1967). Transplantation immunity and delayed cutaneous hypersensitivity reactions in dogs. *Journal of Immunology* **98**, 601–608.

Stuart, F. P., Torres, E., and Hester, W. J. (1967). Orthotopic autotransplantation and allotransplantation of the liver—functional and structural patterns in the dog. *Annals of Surgery* **165**, 325–340.

Stubbs, E. L., and Furth, J. (1934). Experimental studies on venereal sarcoma of the dog. *American Journal of Pathology* **10**, 275–286.

Sudduth, W. H. (1955). Allergy: The possible etiological basis of distemper encephalitis. *North American Veterinarian* **36**, 292–294.

Swisher, S. N., and Young, L. E. (1961). The blood grouping systems of dogs. *Physiological Reviews* **41**, 495–520.

Swisher, S. N., Young, L. E., and Trabold, N. (1962). *In vitro* and *in vivo* studies of the behavior of canine erythrocyte-isoantibody systems. *Annals of the New York Academy of Sciences* **97**, 15–25.

Taylor, R. M., Watson, J. W., and Walker, F. C. (1966). Prolongation of survival of jejunal homografts in dogs treated with azathioprine (Imuran). *British Journal of Surgery* **53**, 134–138.

Tennenbaum, J. I., Patterson, R., and Pruzansky, J. J. (1963). Canine antiserums analogous to human allergic and "blocking" antiserums. *Science* **142**, 589–590.

Terplan, K. L., Witebsky, E., Rose, N. R., Paine, J. R., and Egan, R. W. (1960). Experimental thyroiditis in rabbits, guinea pigs and dogs, following immunization with thyroid extracts of their own and heterologous species. *American Journal of Pathology* **36**, 213–231.

Than, M. M., Bina, P. R. C., Martinez, C., and Absolon, K. B. (1962). The age factor and tolerance of full thickness skin homografts in normal and thymecto-mized canine littermates. *Surgical Forum* **13**, 53–55.

Thomas, E. D., Collins, J. A., Kasakura, S., and Ferrebee, J. W. (1963a). Lethally irradiated dogs given infusions of fetal and adult hematopoietic tissue. *Transplantation* **1**, 514–520.

Thomas, E. D., Kasakura, S., Cavins, J. A., and Ferrebee, J. W. (1963b). Marrow transplants in lethally irradiated dogs: The effect of methotrexate on survival of the host and the homograft. *Transplantation* **1**, 571–574.

Thomas, E. D., Kasakura, S., Cavins, J. A., Swisher, S. N., and Ferrebee, J. W. (1964). Significance of blood groups in homotransplantation of marrow in the dog. *Annals of the New York Academy of Sciences* **120**, 362–366.

Thomas, L., Paterson, P. Y., and Smithwick, B. (1950). Acute disseminated en-cephalomyelitis following immunization with homologous brain extracts. I. Studies on the role of a circulating antibody in the production of the condition in dogs. *Journal of Experimental Medicine* **92**, 133–152.

Thomas, L., Murray, J. E., and Couch, N. P. (1957). Consecutive skin homografts in the dog. *Transplantation Bulletin* **4**, 156–157.

Thompson, J. C., Daves, I. A., and Nemhauser, G. M. (1966). Survival and function of canine gastric allografts. *Transplantation* **4**, 452–464.

Tocantins, L. M., and Stewart, H. L. (1939). Pathological anatomy of experimental thrombocytopenic purpura in the dog. *American Journal of Pathology* **15**, 1–23.

Torten, M., Ben-Efraim, S., and Shenberg, E. (1967). Experimental induction of ocular reaction resembling post leptospiral ophthalmia and its relation to skin reactions and circulating antibodies. *Clinical and Experimental Immunology* **2**, 573–580.

Trautwein, G. (1965). Vergleichende Untersuchungen über das Amyloid und Para-myloid verschiedener Tierarten. I. Histomorphologie und färberische Eigen-schaften des Amyloids und Paramyloids. *Pathologica Veterinaria (Basel)* **2**, 297–327.

Uhr, J. W. (1966). Delayed hypersensitivity. *Physiological Reviews* **46**, 359–419.

Vaerman, J-P., and Heremans, J. F. (1968). The immunoglobulins of the dog. I. Identification of canine immunoglobulins homologous to human IgA and IgM. *Immunochemistry* **5**, 425–432.

Van Breda Vriesman, P. J., Vink, M., and Willighagen, R. G. (1967). Histochemical studies of canine renal homotransplants with special reference to alkaline phos-phatase and its isoenzymes. *Transplantation* **5**, 420–434.

Van de Water, J. M., and Katzman, H. (1964). Studies of the immune mechanism in thymectomized pups. *Journal of Surgical Research* **4**, 387–389.

van Rood, J. J., and Eernisse, J. G. (1969). The detection of transplantation antigens in leukocytes. *Progress in Surgery* **7**, 217–252.

Vega, R. E., Daniele, R. P., and Chaya, A. (1968). Treatment of renal allograft rejection in dogs. Combined thoracic duct fistula and immunosuppressive chemotherapy. *Archives of Surgery* **96**, 344–348.

Veith, F. J. (1968). Lung transplantation 1968. *American Review of Respiratory Diseases* **98**, 769–775.

Veith, F. J., Stenzel, K. H., and Thompson, D. D. (1967). Urinary proteins from dog kidney transplants. *Transplantation* **5**, 1459–1470.

Vesselinovitch, S. D. (1959). The analysis of serum proteins of domestic animals by filter-paper electrophoresis. A review. *Cornell Veterinarian* **49**, 82–96.

Waksman, B. H., and Adams R. D. (1955). Allergic neuritis: An experimental disease of rabbits induced by the injection of peripheral nervous tissue and adjuvants. *Journal of Experimental Medicine* **102**, 213–236.

Waksman, B. H., and Adams, R. D. (1962). Infectious leukoencephalitis. A critical comparison of certain experimental and naturally-occurring leukoencephalitides with experimental allergic encephalomyelitis. *Journal of Neuropathology and Experimental Neurology* **21**, 491–518.

Walton, G. S. (1965). Contact dermatitis in domestic animals. *In* "Comparative Physiology and Pathology of the Skin" (A. J. Rook and G. S. Walton, eds.), pp. 515–519. Davis, Philadelphia, Pennsylvania.

Walton, G. S. (1966). Allergic dermatoses of the dog and cat. *Journal of Small Animal Practice* **7**, 749–754.

Walton, G. S. (1967). Skin responses in the dog and cat to ingested allergens. Observations on one hundred confirmed cases. *Veterinary Record* **81**, 709–713.

Waye, J. W. (1960). ITP in a dog. *Canadian Veterinary Journal* **1**, 569–571.

Webb, H. E., and Smith, C. E. G. (1966). Relation of immune response to development of central nervous system lesions in virus infections of man. *British Medical Journal* **II**, 1179–1181.

West, C. D., Fowler, R., and Nathan, P. (1960). The relationship of serum globulins to transplant rejection in the dog studied by paper and immunoelectrophoretic techniques. *Annals of the New York Academy of Sciences* **87**, 522–537.

Whipple, G. H., Hill, R. B., Terry, R., Lucas, F. V., and Yuile, C. L. (1955). The placenta and protein metabolism. Transfer studies using carbon [14]-labeled proteins in dogs. *Journal of Experimental Medicine* **101**, 617–626.

Wilson, D. B., and Billingham, R. E. (1967). Lymphocytes and transplantation immunity. *Advances in Immunology* **7**, 189–273.

Wilson, R. E., Hager, E. B., Hampers, C. L., Carson, J. M., Merrill, J. P., and Murray, J. E. (1968). Immunologic rejection of human cancer transplanted with a renal allograft. *New England Journal of Medicine* **278**, 479–483.

Wilson, R. E., Rippin, A., Dagher, R. K., Kinneart, P., and Busch, G. J. (1969). Prolonged canine renal allograft survival after pretreatment with solubilized antigen. *Transplantation* **7**, 360–371.

Witebsky, E. (1959). Historical roots of present concepts of immunopathology. *Immunopathology, 1st International Symposium, Basal/Seelisburg, 1958* pp. 1–13. Benno Schwabe, Basel.

Wittich, F. W. (1941). Spontaneous allergy (atopy) in the lower animal. Seasonal hay fever (Fall type) in a dog. *Journal of Allergy* **12**, 247–251.

Wolf, J. S., and Hume, D. M. (1965). Transplant immunity in animals with lymphocytopenia induced by indwelling beta irradiation. *Surgical Forum* **16**, 202–204.

Wolf, J. S., McGavic, J. D., and Hume, D. M. (1967). Inhibition of the effector mechanism in transplant immunity by local graft irradiation. *Surgical Forum* **18**, 249–250.

Wright, N. G. (1967a). The relationship between the virus of infectious canine hepatitis and interstitial nephritis. *Journal of Small Animal Practice* **8**, 67–70.

Wright, N. G. (1967b). Experimental infectious canine hepatitis. IV. Histological and immunofluorescence studies of the kidney. *Journal of Comparative Pathology* **77**, 153–158.

Yamada, T., and Kay, J. H. (1968). Kidney homotransplantation with special reference to cytotoxic antibody response. *Surgery* **63**, 637–645.

Young, J. D., Benjamini, E., Feingold, B. F., and Moller, H. (1963). Allergy to flea bites. V. Preliminary results of fractionation, characterization and assay for allergenic activity of material derived from the oral secretion of the cat flea. Ctenocephalides *felis felis*. *Experimental Parasitology* **13**, 155–166.

Young, L. E., Christian, R. M., Ervin, D. M., Davis, R. W., O'Brien, W. A., Swisher, S. N., and Yuile, C. L. (1951). Hemolytic disease in newborn dogs. *Blood* **6**, 291–313.

Yurko, L. E., Bigley, N. J., and Wilson, G. P. (1969). Tumor-group specificity of autoantibodies produced in neoplastic canines. *Federation Proceedings* **28**, 632.

Zabriskie, J. B. (1967). Mimetic relationships between group A streptococci and mammalian tissues. *Advances in Immunology* **7**, 147–188.

Zajtchuk, R., Gago, O., and Adams, W. E. (1967). Homotransplantation of the lung. Influence of quantity of antigen on survival of the graft. *Journal of Thoracic Cardiovascular Surgery* **53**, 109–115.

Zimmerman, C. E., Stuart, F. P., and Wilson, R. E. (1965). Dog renal homografts prolonged by antigenic pretreatment. *Surgical Forum* **16**, 267–269.

Znamensky, M. S., and Odaryuk, T. S. (1965). Homotransplantation of arteries based on total blood exchange to overcome tissue incompatibility (experimental study). *Acta Chirurgiae Plasticae* **7**, 228–235.

Zukoski, C. F. (1968). Experimental suppression of allograft rejection—background and application. *Journal-Lancet* **88**, 159–161.

Zukoski, C. F., and Ende, N. (1965). Membranous glomerular nephritis complicating prolonged survival of a homografted kidney. *Transplantation* **3**, 118–122.

Glucose Synthesis in Ruminants

R. A. LENG*

*Department of Biochemistry and Nutrition, School of Rural Science,
University of New England, Armidale, N.S.W., Australia*

I. Introduction

The animal benefits from the microbial population of the rumen in the following ways: (1) fermentation of cellulose and other structural components of plants occurs to yield readily metabolizable substrates; (2) synthesis by the bacteria of all essential amino acids takes place and in some instances synthesis occurs from nonprotein nitrogen, which allows the animal to be independent of protein quality of the feed; and (3) synthetic activity of the microorganisms provides all vitamins of the B complex required by the animal. Against this, the animal loses an appreciable proportion of the energy of the feed as the heat of fermentation (Walker and Forrest, 1964; Houpt, 1968). Because of the anaerobic conditions of

* The author is Associate Professor of Nutritional Biochemistry at the University of New England, Armidale, N.S.W. 2351, Australia.

the rumen, oxidative phosphorylation is absent, and hydrogen gas is liberated to be converted to methane by methanogenic bacteria present in the rumen. The anaerobic conditions of the rumen also impose other restrictions on the animal. The storage of polysaccharides in bacteria in the rumen appears to be low (Gunsalus and Shuster, 1961), and the amount of these reaching the lower digestive tract is extremely small (Heald, 1951). There also appears to be a loss of storage polysaccharide from microorganisms in the omasum before passage to the lower digestive tract (Weller and Pilgrim, 1953). Because of the rapid fermentation of glucose and starches in the rumen, little if any glucose of dietary origin reaches the small intestines for absorption in animals on roughage diets. However, the quantities of glucose reaching the small intestines in sheep and cattle may be affected by a number of factors as discussed in detail elsewhere in this review.

The majority of the world's ruminants are dependent on grazing for their food intake and as such ingest carbohydrates that are resistant to digestion in the small intestine. However, where ruminants are held under intensive conditions they may be given a high proportion of grain in their diet. That ruminants absorb little glucose on diets of grass or similar products has resulted in suggestions that glucose was quantitatively less important in ruminants than in other animals. However, the recognition that there is a substantial requirement for glucose by the central nervous system and also for the nutrient supply of the fetus and for sustenance of lactation and synthesis of lactose has resulted in suggestions that the carbohydrate economy of ruminants is precarious (Lindsay, 1959). Recent publications have shown that relatively large quantities of glucose are synthesized by the ruminant. These quantities are similar to those in postabsorptive monogastric animals when they are compared on a metabolic body weight basis (i.e., $Wt^{3/4}$) (Ballard et al., 1969). In this review the discussions will show that glucose synthesis in ruminants varies with diet and with physiologic condition of the animal.

It is now well established that the supply of glucose or, more specifically, the supply of glucose precursors is of great importance in ruminant metabolism. When the supply of glucogenic precursors is limited by reduced food intake, metabolic disturbances occur, particularly when glucose demands are high as during pregnancy and lactation (Reid, 1968).

The significance of carbohydrate in ruminant metabolism was last reviewed by Lindsay (1959) and Armstrong (1965); there have been considerable advances in this field since then.

II. Glucose Metabolism by the Whole Animal

The advent of isotopic tracer techniques for monogastric animals brought forward new techniques for studying carbohydrate metabolism, and these techniques were soon applied to ruminants. The work of Steele *et al.* (1956) on dogs has had considerable influence on the approach to isotopic tracer techniques to study glucose entry rate and metabolism of ruminants. There are basically three variations of the isotope dilution technique that can be applied to study pool size and rate of entry of glucose to the body glucose pool, but surprisingly few studies have been done to compare and critically evaluate the various techniques.

An attempt will be made in this review to compare the techniques used in ruminants for measuring entry rate and pool size of glucose.

1. Nomenclature and Definitions

Many terms have been employed for the description of parameters estimated by using isotopic tracers, and, in order to clarify the situation, some discussion of terms is made here.

Single injection of isotope refers to a small quantity of material of high specific radioactivity injected over a short finite time, i.e., one minute or less, and is the same as pulse labeling. The repeated single injection used by Hetenyi *et al.* (1961) to study glucose entry rate in dogs is not basically different from the single injection technique.

Continuous infusion of isotope refers to the infusion of a small quantity of isotopically labeled material at a precisely controlled rate.

Primed infusion of isotope is a continuous infusion which is primed at the commencement of infusion by a single injection. Usually there is a balance between the injected amount and the rate of infusion such that the specific radioactivity in plasma glucose reaches a "plateau" in a short time as compared with a continuous infusion.

Entry rate of glucose. The rate parameters of turnover estimated from primed or continuous infusions or single injections have been termed turnover rate, transfer rate, utilization rate, entry rate, inflow-outflow rate, flux, renewal rate, or irreversible disposal. These measurements are probably all synonymous with irreversible loss or disposal (Baker *et al.*, 1959; R. G. White *et al.*, 1969) which more correctly describes the parameter. In this review, the words entry rate are often loosely used to describe all of these parameters, and the total entry rate is reserved for describing the rate of appearance of glucose in the body pool. Entry rates are the total entry rate minus the recycling of carbon i.e., the return of ^{14}C to plasma glucose which has previously left the glucose pool, and recycling causes an underestimation of total glucose entry rate. Recycling is discussed in more detail elsewhere.

Total glucose entry rate is the rate at which glucose enters the sampled pool of glucose.

Irreversible loss is the rate at which glucose carbon, which does not return to the glucose pool during the course of the experiment, leaves the glucose pool.

Turnover rate. The concept of turnover rate is one that is confused by many workers in this field. Kleiber (1967) has defined it as the rate at which a pool of substrate turns over, i.e., it is the total entry rate divided by the pool size. Turnover time is the reciprocal of turnover rate (Kleiber, 1967), i.e.,

$$\text{turnover time} = \frac{1}{\text{turnover rate}} = \frac{\text{pool content}}{\text{total entry rate}}$$

Kleiber argues the points in this way, "Isometrically built animals have metabolic pools proportional to their body weights. Isokinetically behaving animals have rates of intermediary transfer proportional to the metabolic body size or the three fourths power of body weight." Therefore,

$$\text{entry rate} = K_1 W^{\frac{3}{4}} \quad \text{and} \quad \text{pool size} = K_2 W$$
$$\text{turnover rate} = K_3 W^{-\frac{1}{4}} \quad \text{or} \quad \text{turnover time} = K_4 W^{\frac{1}{4}}$$

Thus, the "metabolic time" for isokinetic animals is proportional to the fourth root of body weight (Kleiber, 1965). If results of experiments between animals of different weights and with different time base are to be compared then a basis for this would be the concept of the sheep hour, or the rat hour, or the cow hour. For instance, comparisons of time bases in a 500 g. rat, a 40 kg. sheep, and a 400 kg. cow can be done as follows:

$$\frac{W^{\frac{1}{4}} \text{ sheep}}{W^{\frac{1}{4}} \text{ rat}} = \frac{1}{x}$$

where x is the time in a rat equivalent to 1 hour in a sheep; 1 hour for a sheep then becomes equivalent to 0.32 hour in a rat or 1.72 hour in a cow of the above weights.

Glucose pool is the quantity of body glucose with which injected isotopically labeled glucose mixes.

Glucose space is the volume of fluid through which the glucose pool is distributed.

Half time is the time for half the glucose pool to turn over.

2. General Considerations

In monogastric animals, glucose entry rate and pool size have been studied by all techniques mentioned above, but the two techniques that appear to be most widely used are the primed infusion and the single injection. The single injection method in which the isotope disappearance was assumed to be a first-order single exponential function was discarded by many investigators because significantly higher glucose entry rates were obtained by this method than by infusion (Searle *et al.*, 1954, 1956). The use of primed infusion for studying glucose metabolism was first advocated by Searle and his colleagues. However, Steele *et al.* (1956) extended the technique and developed a more sophisticated analysis of the data, apparently allowing more accurate estimation of some of the parameters of glucose metabolism in dogs. For a review of this method, the reader is referred to the publication by Steele (1964).

In research with ruminants, two groups of investigators can be distinguished, those using the single injection and those depending largely on the primed infusion. Continuous infusions of (^{14}C)glucose apparently have also been successfully used for the measurement of gluose entry rate in sheep (Leng *et al.*, 1967). Surprisingly few comparisons have been made of the various techniques and, until recently, where they have been made, large differences have been found in glucose entry rate measured by a single injection, using a single exponential function, and by primed infusion (Annison and White, 1961). Partly the large differences have been due to the fact that analysis of data from a single injection was oversimplified and lacked a multicompartmental approach (Baker, 1969). In a direct comparison of techniques, Annison and White (1961) determined the specific radioactivity of plasma glucose between 20 and 60 minutes (R. R. White, 1963) following a single injection of (U-^{14}C)glucose in sheep and estimated glucose entry rate, turnover time, and pool size by assuming this portion of the curve to be linear on a semilogarithmic plot, and obey first-order kinetics. In addition, it was assumed that recycling was negligible. Kronfeld and Simesen (1961a) arbitrarily showed that the time interval from 40 to 160 minutes in sheep after the single injection of (U-^{14}C)glucose could be used and that recycling of carbon back to glucose was apparently insignificant over this time period. However, R. G. White *et al.* (1969) have published multicompartmental analyses of single injection data of sheep in which the specific radioactivity of plasma glucose was followed up to 24 hours after the initial injection.

3. Mathematical Treatment of Isotope Dilution Data

a. Single Injection

The isotope dilution curve obtained after an intravenous injection of (^{14}C)glucose in sheep is described as a sum of exponential terms as follows (R. G. White *et al.*, 1969):

$$SR_t = \sum_{i=1}^{n} A_i e^{-m_i t} \quad \text{(see Fig. 1)} \tag{1}$$

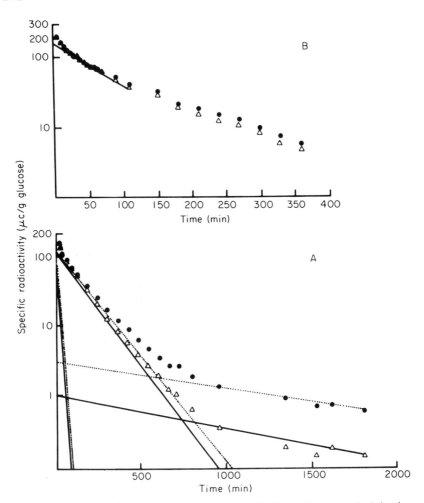

Fig. 1. (A) Glucose specific radioactivities with time after a single injection of 1 mc. of each of (U-¹⁴C)- and (3-T)glucose in goats.   (B) Expanded part of the early portion of the isotope dilution curve. ●, (¹⁴C)glucose; △, tritiated glucose. In (B) the early part of the isotope dilution curve is shown with a single exponential function fitted to the data. In (A) the whole curve is shown with the three exponential functions for each isotope. The exponents for ¹⁴C are shown as dotted lines whereas those for tritium are shown as solid lines. (From Leng and Black, 1970.)

where

SR_t = specific radioactivity of plasma glucose at time t (mμc/mg. C)

A = zero-time intercept of each component (mμc/mg. C)

m = rate constant of each component (min.⁻¹)

n = number of exponential components
i = exponential-component number
t = time (min.)

The number of exponential terms is determined by the shape of the observed specific radioactivity time curve (Steele *et al.*, 1956) and on the basis of a postulated model (see Baker *et al.*, 1959). The term *model* is used in both a physical and mathematical sense (Berman, 1963) to represent any set of equations or functions that describes the behavior of a tracer in a system. The parameters of a model are the arbitrary constants of the functions or equations. The formulation and testing of models has been discussed by Berman (1963), and it is not the purpose of this review to set this problem out in detail.

Berman (1963) has pointed out that it is not possible to derive the number of independent functions of a model on the basis of the data alone, because any model that is compatible with the data can always be interpreted as a degenerate case for one of higher order. However, the minimal components can be chosen from biologic considerations so that the model chosen is probably the one with the smallest number of compartments compatible with the data. When the model has been defined, a set of values that best predict the data must be derived and the goodness of fit must be tested. No data for the rates of flow between pools are available on this, for the model describing glucose metabolism in sheep (Fig. 2).

In studies of glucose metabolism of animals, a number of models are available for describing the movement of glucose carbon in the body. Generally, it is fairly well established that a 2 or 3 compartmental model is the simplest one to fit (^{14}C)glucose isotope dilution data in rats (Baker *et al.*, 1959; Steele, 1964; Skinner *et al.*, 1959) and in sheep (R. G. White *et al.*, 1969). The injected (^{14}C)glucose appears to mix quite rapidly with the body pool of glucose, and this is discernible up to 5 minutes in rats and up to 15 minutes in sheep. A second and third process also appears to be acting continuously, which is compatible with recycling of ^{14}C back to glucose from several substrate pools. Glucose is metabolized in a number of ways and the carbon of glucose enters a large number of substrate pools, many or all of which are capable of returning the ^{14}C back to glucose. Recycling of ^{14}C will alter the shape of the dilution curve from a straight line log. specific radioactive time relationship. As time progresses, the proportion of ^{14}C in the glucose pool that is recycled becomes greater until it is virtually 100%.

The model that appears to most likely describe the isotope dilution curve is shown in Fig. 2. The rate parameters between the various pools

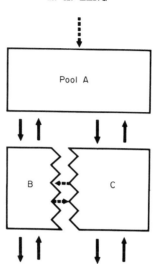

Fig. 2. Model for glucose metabolism in sheep. The model is based on the exponential analysis of the isotope dilution curves after a single injection of (U-^{14}C)-glucose and also on other biologic considerations. Compartment A represents the body pool of glucose which is reversibly interconnected with precursor pools B and C. The precursor pools may sometimes be indistinguishable from one another and are therefore assumed to be reversibly interconnected. Entry of exogenous glucose to pool A is shown as a broken line since in these sheep only a small quantity of glucose is absorbed from the digestive tract. The glucose carbon entering compartment A arises from the precursor pools B and C, and all irreversible loss occurs through these pools. Pools B and C are probably made up of all glucogenic precursors, i.e., glucogenic amino acids, lactate, propionate, and glycerol, and CO_2 and glycogen. (From R. G. White *et al.*, 1969.)

in the model have not been estimated, but this is possible with further experimentation and with the use of computer programs such as SAAM22 (Baker, 1969). There are considerable difficulties associated with fitting data to models, and the general solution of a model can only be used if all the slopes and intercepts that describe the model can be ascertained from the data. These difficulties, i.e., defining all components, suggest the use of curve-fitting computer techniques where the individual component slopes within a complex curve need not be clearly defined (Berman, 1963). In the simple situation, as may be applied to glucose kinetics in sheep, solutions of the three compartmental model are readily available in published form (Skinner *et al.*, 1959; Rescigno and Segre, 1966).

The irreversible loss of glucose can be calculated from the following

$$\text{irreversible loss (mg. C/min.)} = \frac{Q}{\sum\limits_{i=1}^{n} \dfrac{A'_i}{m_i}} \tag{2}$$

$$\text{pool size, } Q \text{ (mg. C)} = \frac{P}{\sum_{i=1}^{n} (A_i)} \qquad (3)$$

where P is injected dose of radioactivity and A'_i is fractional zero-time intercepts; therefore,

$$A'_2 = \frac{A_2}{\sum_{i=1}^{n} A_i} \qquad \text{and} \qquad \sum_{i=1}^{n} A'_i = 1$$

(see Baker *et al.*, 1959; Segal *et al.*, 1961; Steele, 1964; Baker and Rostami, 1969). The equations hold for any model regardless of the number of compartments or how they are interconnected provided the tracer is injected in circulating blood and steady state conditions exist (Baker and Rostami, 1969; Shipley *et al.*, 1967).

Calculation of total entry rate of glucose from single injection isotope dilution data is dependent to some extent on the model chosen (Baker *et al.*, 1959; Baker and Schotz, 1967). However, for most three compartmental models and for the model proposed in this review the total entry rate (T.E.R.) of glucose may be calculated from the equation

$$\text{T.E.R. (mg. C/min.)} = Q\Sigma A'_i m_i \qquad (4)$$

Where total entry rates have been studied, the results have been variable (R. G. White *et al.*, 1969; Leng and Black, 1970).

Insufficient samples have been taken over too short a time period in many experiments for accurate analysis of single injection data.

b. *Continuous Infusion*

The continuous infusion techniques used in sheep (Leng *et al.*, 1967; R. G. White *et al.*, 1969) have relied on a simple mathematical treatment. In these studies the specific radioactivity of glucose was found to come to a "plateau" after 180–240 minutes. The infusion rate of radioactivity divided by this mean specific radioactivity gave an estimate of irreversible loss. This is a simplification of the actual isotope dilution curve since the curve is described by the following equation (Steele *et al.*, 1956; Steele, 1964),

$$SR_t = \frac{F}{Q} \sum_{i=1}^{n} \frac{A'_i}{m_i} (1 - e^{-m_i t}) \qquad (5)$$

where F is infusion rate (mμc./min.) and Q is pool size (mg. C). As time approaches infinity during a continuous infusion of isotopically labeled

materials a plateau specific radioactivity is obtained which is described
as

$$SR_\infty = \frac{F}{Q} \sum_{i=1}^{n} \frac{A'_i}{m_i} \tag{6}$$

If the SR_∞ is used to calculate irreversible loss of glucose, then

$$\text{irreversible loss} = \frac{\text{infusion rate (m}\mu\text{c./min.)}}{SR_\infty \text{ (m}\mu\text{c./mg. C)}}$$

$$= \frac{F}{\dfrac{F}{Q} \displaystyle\sum_{i=1}^{n} \dfrac{A'_i}{m_i}} = \frac{Q}{\displaystyle\sum_{i=1}^{n} \dfrac{A'_i}{m_i}} \tag{7}$$

An objection to the use of the plateau specific radioactivity of plasma
glucose after 180 to 240 minutes of a continuous infusion of (U-^{14}C)-
glucose is that the attainment of plateau specific radioactivity may take
considerable time. The error involved, however, has been estimated to
be an overestimation of 1.5–6% (Steel, 1969) which is probably not a
major problem sufficiently high to be a serious error in most experimental
data (R. G. White et al., 1969).

c. Primed Infusion

The analysis of primed infusion data has been largely influenced by
the method of Steele et al. (1956) which is based on evidence that the
glucose pool of the dog is distributed in two compartments of the extracellular fluid. Steele (1964) showed that when the priming injection (P)
and the infusion rate (F) of (^{14}C)glucose were balanced so that $P/F = 1/m_2$ (where m_2 is the rate constant of the second (terminal) exponential
term in Eq. 1) extrapolation of a straight line relationship of specific
radioactivity with time between 60 and 180 minutes of the infusion to the
zero time intercept gave a value for specific radioactivity (SR_{tp}) from
which "pool size" was calculated as follows:

$$\text{pool size} = \frac{\text{priming injection (P)}}{SR_{tp}}$$

The priming injection to infusion rate was usually balanced so that
the line drawn between the points from 60 to 180 minutes had a slight
negative or positive slope. The curve was then extrapolated to an asymptote value by using a computer program to solve the equation

$$SR_t = X - Y^{-bt}$$

Here X is the asymptote value for specific radioactivity of plasma glucose (mμc./mg. C), and

$$X - Y = \text{intercept specific radioactivity (m}\mu\text{c./mg. C)}$$
$$b = \text{rate constant}$$

R. G. White *et al.* (1969) demonstrated that this procedure estimates the irreversible loss, as might be expected, from the equation describing primed infusion data which is the sum of the equation of the curves describing the specific radioactivity time relations when continuous infusion and single injections of (^{14}C) glucose are given (Steele, 1964). Therefore

$$SR_t = \frac{1}{Q} \sum_{i=1}^{n} \left[\left(P - \frac{F}{m_i} \right) A'_i e^{-m_i t} \right] + \left[\frac{F}{Q} \sum_{i=1}^{n} \frac{A'_i}{m_i} \right] \tag{8}$$

If the prediction of the asymptote, which has assumed a more simplified form, is close to the asymptote predicted by Eq. 8, then the equation for irreversible loss of glucose is the same as that for a continuous infusion or for single injection (R. G. White *et al.*, 1969). Hence, it becomes obvious that the three techniques for measuring "entry rate" actually estimate the same parameter, irreversible loss, which has been proved experimentally by R. G. White *et al.* (1969) (see Table I).

The data for isotope dilution curves obtained by single injection have indicated that in sheep, glucose in plasma and interstitial fluid constitutes a single well-mixed pool and that recycling of glucose carbon from peripheral pools results in a multiexponential curve. Consequently, the use of primed infusion to calculate pool size appears to be unsound on theoretic grounds.

It has been experimentally shown, and is theoretically feasible, that the irreversible loss of glucose can be estimated from isotope dilution

TABLE I

COMPARISON OF DATA FROM THREE TECHNIQUES OF ISOTOPE DILUTION FOR
ESTIMATING PARAMETERS OF GLUCOSE METABOLISM IN FEEDING SHEEP[a]

Technique	Number of experiments	Irreversible loss (mg./min.)	Pool size (g.)	Space (% B. Wt.)
Single injection	9	58 ± 4.1^b	4.5 ± 0.21^c	18 ± 0.8^c
Primed infusion	12	55 ± 1.5^b	5.4 ± 0.26^c	24 ± 0.9^c
Continuous infusion	6	63 ± 4.7^b		

[a] From R. G. White *et al.* (1969).
[b] Not significant at $P = 0.05$; Students "t" test.
[c] $p < 0.01$; Students "t" test.

curves obtained after single injections, continuous infusions, or primed infusions of (U-^{14}C) glucose, provided the data can be fitted to the appropriate equation, which usually requires the services of a digital computer.

4. Use of Tritium and Carbon-14 Labeled Glucose

Glucose labeled with ^{14}C has been used almost universally for measuring entry rates of glucose in conscious animals. However, the difficulties of interpretation of results because of the recycling of ^{14}C led to investigations of the use of tritium labeled glucose. Katz and Dunn (1967) and Dunn et al. (1967) used 6T and 2T labeled glucose to study glucose metabolism of rats and have shown that tritiated and ^{14}C labeled glucose had different half times and that recycling of ^{14}C back to glucose occurred soon after injection of the tracer. Leng and Black (1970) studied glucose entry rates in goats fasted for 18 hours using mixtures of (U-^{14}C)- and (3-T) glucose or (U-^{14}C)- and (6-T) glucose as single injections, primed or continuous infusions. There was apparently little difference in the results obtained with either 6-T or 3-T labeled glucose. The ratio of ^{14}C/T in circulating glucose was taken to indicate the relative recycling of ^{14}C to T. The ratio of ^{14}C/T with time after single injection of (U-^{14}C)- and (3-T) glucose is shown in Fig. 3. Typical isotope dilution curves for the two tracers are shown in Fig. 1.

The data from single injection of the mixed isotope were analyzed as indicated in the above section. Generally, the irreversible loss of glucose estimated by using (^{14}C) glucose was approximately 15% less than that estimated by using (3-T)- or (6-T) glucose. This difference is represented by the rate of recycling of carbon through a three carbon pool other than glycerol since the tritium from (3-T) glucose is lost on conversion of glucose to triose phosphates and lactate in the Embden–Meyerhoff pathway of glycolysis. (6-T) Glucose apparently behaved isotopically in a similar way to (3-T) glucose. The apparently successful use of (6-T)-glucose and its similarity to (3-T) glucose is in contrast to the results of Dunn and Strahs (1965) and Hetenyi et al. (1966) where an apparent isotope effect was believed to be the cause of differences observed in isotope dilution between 6-T and ^{14}C labeled glucose in the rat and dog, respectively.

(3-T) Glucose and (U-^{14}C) glucose infusions or primed infusions in fasted goats showed that although the specific radioactivity of tritiated glucose in plasma came to a plateau, the (^{14}C) glucose specific radioactivity continued to increase up to 9 hours, which is contrary to the results observed in feeding sheep (Leng et al., 1967), indicating that recycling is a major process in the fasting animal where precursors from the digestive tract are reduced in quantity (Annison et al., 1967).

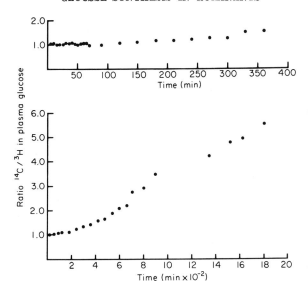

Fig. 3. The relationship of the ratio of $^{14}C/T$ in plasma glucose with time following a single injection of $(U-^{14}C)$- and $(3-T)$glucose (1 mc. of each). (From Leng and Black, 1970.)

It appears that tritium labeled glucose is a useful tool for investigating glucose metabolism in ruminants and that the use of mixed isotopes will enable more information to be gained on recycling through lactate.

The ratio of ^{14}C to tritium in plasma glucose did not change for up to 60 minutes following a single injection of (^{14}C)- and $(3-T)$glucose (Fig. 3). The loss of tritium from the glucose molecule on cleavage to three carbon units indicates that recycling through such compounds is not appreciable over this period of time (Leng and Black, 1970). It is suggested that this part of the isotope dilution curve may be considered as being due solely to dilution of radioactivity by glucose synthesis, i.e., the total entry rate of glucose (Leng and Black, 1970). This part of the curve appeared to obey first-order kinetics and pool size, and the total entry rate was calculated from the zero time intercept and slope as follows:

$$SR_t \text{ (m\mu c./mg. glucose)} = A_s e^{-m_s t} \qquad (9)$$

$$\text{pool size } (Q) = \frac{\text{injected dose}}{A_s} \qquad (10)$$

$$\text{total entry rate of glucose (mg. glucose/min.)} = Q \times m_s \qquad (11)$$

There was good agreement between estimates using the different isotopes (Leng and Black, 1970).

Although there is need for more work it appears that the early part of an isotope dilution curve may give meaningful results for these parameters of glucose metabolism. More work is required also before this analysis can be recommended as a routine tool. Hetenyi *et al.* (1961) advocated a similar part of the isotope dilution curve for studies with the dog based on measured glucose entry rates in eviscerated dogs loaded with glucose. Similar parts of the isotope dilution curve have been used by Annison and White (1961), R. R. White (1963), and Jarrett *et al.* (1964) in studies with sheep and by Head *et al.* (1965) and Kronfeld and Raggi (1964) with cows.

It should be possible to measure both the irreversible loss and total entry rate of glucose from data after a single injection of (U-¹⁴C) glucose provided sufficient samples of blood are taken over the time period from 10 to 60 minutes and through to 24 hours.

III. Glucose Entry Rates in Nonpregnant Sheep and Cattle

Glucose entry rates and pool size in ruminants have been studied by numerous workers who used isotope dilution techniques (Tables II and III). Usually sheep and cattle were either fed once or twice daily or not fed on the day of the trial. However, Bergman *et al.* (1966), Leng *et al.* (1967), Judson *et al.* (1968), and R. G. White *et al.* (1969) fed sheep at hourly intervals during the experimental periods. It is difficult to compare results among laboratories since most investigators have used different feeding or nutritional regimes; thus quoted glucose entry rates vary considerably (Tables II and III). Also, it has been shown that entry rates of glucose are increased during pregnancy (Bergman, 1963; Steel and Leng, 1968) and during lactation (Bergman and Hogue, 1967). Furthermore, Ford (1965) and Judson and Leng (1968) showed that glucose entry rates of sheep are dependent to some extent on the quantity of food eaten. Comparisons of glucose entry rates are usually made on a metabolic body weight basis ($Wt^{3/4}$) (Ballard *et al.*, 1969). This appears to be justified for comparisons between species of animals that are postabsorptive; however, the ruminant is not truly postabsorptive 24 hours after the latest ingestion of feed, since the rumen is a large store for feed materials. A 2- to 4-day postfeeding ruminant has been subjected to an ever decreasing supply of glucose precursors from the digestive tract and is mobilizing body reserves at an increasing rate, whereas a monogastric animal is completely dependent on its body reserves after 24 hours. Also, to compare animals such as the rat with a large dog or large ruminant, the period without food should be in proportion to their weights raised to one fourth power as has been discussed previously (Kleiber, 1965). Changes in irreversible loss of glucose with starvation are shown in Fig. 4.

Table II shows the collated results of most reported results for glucose

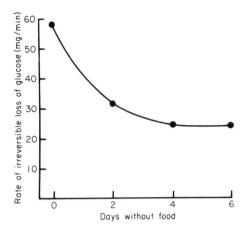

Fɪɢ. 4. Irreversible loss of glucose in feeding sheep and in the same sheep after 2, 4 and 6 days starvation (Steel, 1970).

entry rates in nonpregnant sheep. There is considerable variation and it may be due to (1) the techniques used, (2) the experimental treatment of the animal, and (3) the nutritional regime to which the animal was subjected. The headings of the tables are critical for evaluation of an investigator's results, and omissions are indicated within the table.

Diet and physiologic condition of the animal have a considerable effect on glucose entry rates. The effect of nutritional regimen on glucose entry rate is one that appears to have been neglected by most workers, and much of the variation in Tables II and III can be attributed to the nutritional and feeding regimens of the animals involved. Only a few attempts have been made to compare glucose entry rates in ruminants on different nutritional regimens (Ford, 1965; Judson et al., 1968; Judson and Leng, 1968; Steel and Leng, 1968). However, it appears that glucose entry rates increase with increasing digestible energy intake (Fig. 5). This is probably a factor related mainly to the supply of precursors since the higher the digestible energy intake the higher the absorption of glucogenic precursors. Also, it has been shown that infusions of propionate (Bergman et al., 1966; Judson and Leng, 1970) or lactate (Chapman and Black, 1969) increases gluconeogenesis even in well-fed animals, whereas, glucose infusions were found to inhibit gluconeogenesis (Annison and White, 1961; Bartley and Black, 1966; West and Passey, 1967). This raises an important consideration when comparing results between laboratories. Much of the work done on glucose metabolism in sheep and cattle in the United States used high concentrate diets, whereas in British and Australian laboratories workers have largely used animals given roughage

TABLE II

Glucose Entry Rates in Nonpregnant, Nonlactating Sheep[a]

Reference[b] and technique	Ration or diet, and feeding regimen	Time after last feed (hr.)	No. of expt.	Animal Wt (kg.)	Plasma glucose conc. (mg./100 ml.)	Glucose pool size (g.)	(mg./kg.)	Glucose space (% B. Wt)	Glucose entry rate (mg./min.)	(mg./kg./min.)	(mg./kg.$^{3/4}$/min.)	Glucose oxidized (%)	CO_2 output from glucose (%)
1. (PI)	400 g. alfalfa, once daily	24–27	5	33.5^c	59	4.7^d	140^d	22	44^d	1.3	3.2^d		11–
1. (PI)	400 g. alfalfa + 500 g. maize, once daily	24–27	7	33.5^c	59	4.5^d	134^d	23	54^d	1.6	3.9^d		19
1. (PI)	400 g. alfalfa, once daily	2–5	1	36.6^c	85	6.8^d	186^d	22	95^d	2.6	6.4^d		
1. (PI)	400 g. alfalfa + 500 g. maize, once daily	2–5	6	36.6^c	88	9.0^d	246^d	28	99^d	2.7	6.6^d		22–
1. (SI)	400 g. alfalfa, once daily	24–27	3	33.5^c	71	4.0^d	119^d	17	94^d	2.8	6.8^d		23
1. (SI)	400 g. alfalfa + 500 g. maize, once daily	24–27	3	33.5^c	82	5.2^d	155^d	19	87^d	2.5	6.2^d		
2. (SI)	Hay and grain, ad lib.	16	6	54	50	7.5	139^d	27	123	2.3^d	6.1		
2. (SI)	Alfalfa pellets, ad lib.	16	2	44	48	6.7	152^d	31	81	1.8^d	4.7		
2. (SI)	Alfalfa pellets, ad lib.	1	2	44	52	6.3	143^d	27	79	1.8^d	4.7		
2. (SI)	Alfalfa pellets, ad lib.	96	2	44	53	6.7	152^d	31	56	1.3^d	3.1		
2. (PI)	Alfalfa pellets, ad lib.	16	2	44	49	6.0	136^d	26	87	2.0^d	5.0		
3. (PI)	Hay plus ¼–⅓ lb. maize, once daily	4	2	48	57	7.4	157	27	67	1.4^d	3.7	31	10
3. (PI)	Hay plus ¼–⅓ lb. maize once daily	120	2	49	56	5.3	110	20	45	0.9^d	2.5	32	8
4. (PI)	Pasture + hay + concentrate, ad lib.	4	2	65	82				118	1.8	5.2	4	3
5. (PI)	1000 g. hay and 200 g. oats, once daily		3							1.8		6	4
5. (PI)	1500 g. alfalfa + 300 g. maize, once daily		3							2.8		7	7
5. (PI)	10,000 g. fresh grass, once daily		3							4.3		7	9
6. (SI)	660 g. wheaten chaff, once daily	24	3	30	53	5.6	185	35	54	2.0	4.2^d		
6. (PI)	334 g. alfalfa, once daily	24	2	31	51	4.4	143	28	37	1.2	2.8^d		
7. (PI)	800 g. pelleted alfalfa, cont. over 24 hr.		4	54	58	8.5^d	157^d	27	63	1.2	3.2^d	32	8
8. (PI)	480 g. alfalfa + 320 g. grain, once daily	0–4	4	59	62	9.5	158	25	80	1.4^d	3.8	34	9
9. (CI)	800 g. alfalfa, cont. over 12 hr.		4	37	68				59	1.6^d	3.9^d		

Diet description											
9. (PI) 800 g. alfalfa, cont. over 12 hr.	3–7	4	35	72			58	1.7[d]	4.0[d]		
10. (PI) 800 g. alfalfa + 100 g. maize, once daily	24–30	2	32	81			67	2.1	5.0	33	9
10. (PI) 800 g. alfalfa + 100 g. maize, once daily		4	35	69			54	1.6	3.8	33	11
11. (CI) 400 g. maize, cont. over 12 hr.		3	33	82			53	1.6	3.8[d]		
11. (CI) 250 g. alfalfa + 260 g. maize, cont. over 12 hr.		4	35	76			65	1.9	4.5[d]		
11. (CI) 400 g. alfalfa + 200 g. maize, cont. over 12 hr.		3	33	68			59	1.8	4.3[d]		
12. (SI) 800 g. alfalfa, cont. over 12 hr.		9	37	68	18	122	58	1.6	3.9		
12. (PI) 800 g. alfalfa, cont. over 12 hr.		12	35	66	24	154	55	1.6	3.8		
12. (CI) 800 g. alfalfa, cont. over 12 hr.		6	37	68			93	1.7	4.2		
12. (SI) 800 g. alfalfa, once daily	2–24	4	34	79	16	121	64	1.9	4.5		

[a] The data shown were collated from different studies on the basis that the work had used a different ration, diet, or technique for measurements. Only a few results were excluded because the measurements had been repeats of previous work.

[b] Reference

[c] Mean weight of all starved or fed sheep.

[d] Calculated from the mean values in the table, and therefore these results are not necessarily identical when calculations are made for each individual animal and then averaged since the expected value of the ratio x/y is given by

$$E\left(\frac{x}{y}\right) = \frac{E(x)}{E(y)} - \frac{\text{covariance }(x, y)}{E(y)^2} + \frac{E(x)}{E(y)^3}\text{ variance } y.$$

1. Annison and White (1961)
2. Kronfeld and Simesen (1961a)
3. Bergman (1963)
4. Ford (1963)
5. Ford (1965)
6. Jarrett et al. (1964)
7. Bergman et al. (1966)
8. Bergman and Hogue (1967)
9. Leng et al. (1967)
10. Annison et al. (1967)
11. Judson et al. (1968)
12. R. G. White et al. (1969)

However, authors have tended to select their animals to be of a like weight and therefore the error may be expected to be small.

TABLE III

Glucose Metabolism in Lactating and Nonlactating Cows

Reference[a] and technique	Ration or diet	Milk production (gal./day)	Feeding regimen	Time after last feed (hr.)	No. of expt.	Animal Wt (kg.)	Plasma glucose conc. (mg./100 ml.)	Glucose pool size (g.)	Glucose pool size (mg./kg.)	Glucose space (% B. Wt)	Glucose entry rate (mg./min.)	Glucose entry rate (mg./kg./min.)	Glucose entry rate (mg./kg.$^{3/4}$/min.)	Glucose oxidized to CO$_2$ (%)	Respired CO$_2$ from glucose oxidation (%)
1. (SI)[b]	Not stated	—	Fed	48–120	8	493	58	76	154[f]	27	1030	2.1[f]	9.8[f]		
1. (SI)		—	Fasted		4	465	48	56	120[f]	25	500	1.1[f]	5.0[f]		
2. (SI)[c]	Not stated	—	Fed		4	514	62	75	146[f]	25	1025	2.0[f]	9.5[f]		
3. (SI)[d]	Not stated	10	Not stated		1	457		62	136[f]	14	1173	2.6[f]	10.2	40	9–12
4. (SI)[e]	Ad lib. hay	—	Twice daily	2–4	4	561	83	84	151	18	814	1.5	7.0		
4. (PI)	Restricted grain	—	Twice daily	2–4	4	584	74	77	132	18	658	1.1	6.5		
5. (PI)[e]	Not stated	—	Not stated	24	3	166	81	28	169	21	289	1.7	6.3[f]		

[a] Reference

1. Kronfeld and Raggi (1964)   4. Head et al. (1965)
2. Kronfeld et al. (1959)   5. Davis and Brown (1962)
3. Baxter et al. (1955)

[b] Single injection of (U-^{14}C)glucose was used and the log specific radioactivity time relationship was assumed to be a straight line from 45–150 minutes.

[c] As above but log specific radioactivity was assumed to be a straight line from 30–180 minutes.

[d] The final component left after "peeling" a single injection curve was assumed to represent the entry rate of glucose into the body glucose pool.

[e] Nonlactating, nonpregnant cows.

[f] Estimated.

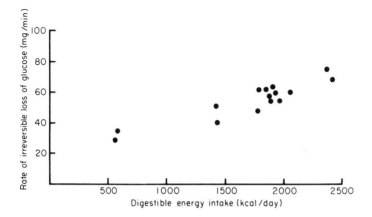

Fig. 5. Relationship between digestible energy intake and the measured irreversible loss of glucose in sheep. (Judson and Leng, 1970; see also Judson and Leng, 1968.)

diets. Most studies have been done with animals given a ration once a day. If glucose is being absorbed in animals on grain rations, once a day feeding may result in glucose absorption at particular times and presumably when this occurs gluconeogenesis will be reduced as will recycling of glucose carbon. Also, the availability of peak quantities of propionate and bacterial protein may effect the rate of gluconeogenesis. This may explain some of the variation in results, particularly when the single injection technique was applied. Judson *et al.* (1968) have demonstrated that the irreversible losses of glucose in sheep were apparently constant on diets of different starch content but having approximately the same digestible energy value and have suggested that glucose absorption was responsible for the observed decrease in gluconeogenesis from propionate.

It is obvious from Table II that despite considerable criticism of the isotope dilution technique which employs a simple analysis of data from a single injection experiment, the results of Kronfeld and Simesen (1961a) for glucose entry rates are within the range of estimates obtained using a primed infusion. Kronfeld and Simesen (1961a) used a single exponential function through the specific radioactivity values of the plasma glucose between 40 and 160 minutes, which should have involved some recycling. However, these same authors demonstrated that glucose entry rates determined from single exponential functions fitted to the data from 20 to 40 minutes 40 to 80 minutes, 80 to 160 minutes, and 40 to 160 minutes of an isotope dilution curve, after a single injection of (U-^{14}C)glucose, gave identical results. In these studies recycling apparently caused decrease in the slope of the line through the log. specific radioactivity values such that extrapolated specific radioactivity (SR_{to}) decreased as the time interval increased and this increased estimates of pool size. The rate constant of the function decreased such that, in the estimation of entry rate, the errors associated with these two parameters were cancelled resulting in a "quasi" constant glucose entry rate. Thus, although entry rate data may be reliable for these studies, the estimates of pool size and space are probably erroneous.

Jarrett et al. (1964) used a single exponential function from 10 to 60 minutes and Annison and White (1961) used the data from 20 to 60 minutes after a single injection of $(U-{}^{14}C)$ glucose to calculate the parameters of glucose metabolism in sheep. Since the time intervals chosen coincide with the time interval in which no recycling was found in goats (Leng and Black, 1970), these estimates are probably closer to total entry rate values of glucose and, therefore, may be expected to be higher than the irreversible loss estimated by the primed infusion technique.

Similarly, the time interval chosen in studies with cows (Table III) may be more correct for analysis of total entry rate for these animals since the time interval from 30 to 180 minutes may have been little affected by recycling (Kronfeld and Raggi, 1964; Head et al., 1965).

Since it has been demonstrated that the primed infusion technique measures irreversible loss, and that the estimate of the plateau specific radioactivity includes recycled $({}^{14}C)$ glucose, the estimates of pool size and space from this technique are probably unreliable, especially since a wide range of priming dose to infusion rates have been used, i.e., from 50:1 to 120:1 and in all, or most, studies a plateau specific radioactivity was apparently obtained between 60 and 180 minutes.

In conclusion, it appears that the variation in glucose entry rate observed by numerous workers in this field is attributable to technique, food intake, diet, and feeding regimen of the animal.

IV. Glucose Entry Rates in Pregnant and Lactating Animals

Estimates of the parameters of glucose metabolism in pregnant ruminants are shown in Table IV. Again there is considerable variation between studies, and it may be due to duration of pregnancy, to nutrition, and to the techniques that have been applied.

Investigations which have systematically studied the interaction between stage of pregnancy and nutrition on glucose metabolism in sheep illustrated that these factors had considerable effect, and a summary of these results are shown in Fig. 6 (Steel and Leng, 1968). The effects of starvation on glucose entry rate in pregnant animals is of considerable interest since they presumably represent the ability of the animal to mobilize body reserves of glucose precursors. In animals given alfalfa

TABLE IV
GLUCOSE METABOLISM IN PREGNANT SHEEP

Reference[a] and technique	Ration or diet, and feeding regimen	Days before lambing	Time after last feed (hr.)	No. of expt.	Sheep Wt (kg.)	Plasma glucose conc. (mg./100 ml.)	Glucose pool size (g.)	Glucose pool size (g./kg.)	Glucose space (% B. Wt)	Glucose entry rate (mg./min.)	Glucose entry rate (mg./kg./min.)	Glucose entry rate (mg./kg.$^{3/4}$/min.)	Glucose oxidized to CO_2 (%)	CO_2 output from glucose (%)
1. (PI)	Hay + ¼ to ½ lb maize, once daily	1–10[b]	0–4	5	69	47	8.6	127	28	112	1.6[f]	4.7	37	11
		1–10[b]	72–144	5	69	31[c]	5.6	85	27	73	1.1[f]	3.2	31	8
2. (PI)	Pasture + concentrate, once daily	5–15[d]	4	4	78	45				105	1.4	4.0	6	2
		5–15[d]	up to 96	4	68	35[e]				83	1.2	3.5	8	2
3. (SI)[d]	?	2–4	0	4	60–70	57	14.2			200				
		18–56	0	3	60–70	44	8.4			103				
		14–17	fasted	2	60–70	42	3.9			60				
4. (SI)[e]	Alfalfa chaff *ad lib.*, cont. over 12 hr.	67	0	4	37	69	5.6	153	22	80	2.2	5.3		
		46	0	4	38	72	5.6	147	20	85	2.2	5.6		
		8	0	4	41	66	5.4	132	20	108	2.7	6.7		
	Alfalfa chaff *ad lib.*, cont. over 12 hr.	63	96	4	33	47	3.9	105	23	41	1.1	3.0		
		42	96	4	33	45	3.6	94	21	46	1.2	3.3		
		5	96	3	36	31	2.5	60	20	44	1.1	3.0		
	800 g. alfalfa chaff, cont. over 12 hr.	71	0	4	33	65	4.1	126	19	59	1.8	4.3		
		52	0	4	33	67	4.5	137	21	64	2.0	4.6		
		11	0	4	36	61	4.3	121	21	77	2.2	5.2		
	250 g. alfalfa chaff + 250 g. wheaten chaff, over 12 hr.	68	0	4	32	61	4.8	149	24	47	1.5	3.5		
		47	0	4	32	51	3.6	120	25	49	1.6	3.6		
		5	0	4	32	46	4.2	137	28	58	1.9	4.3		

[a] Reference

1. Bergman (1963)   3. Kronfeld and Simesen (1961b)
2. Ford (1963)   4. Steel and Leng (1968)

[b] Only ewes carrying twins were used.
[c] Animals showed signs of pregnancy toxemia.
[d] Kronfeld and Simesen (1961b) used the single injection technique using a single exponential analysis of the results between 15–160 minutes. Steel and Leng (1968) adopted a compartmental analysis approach and these measurements were of irreversible loss.
[e] Irreversible loss of glucose estimates were based on a compartmental analysis of the data.
[f] Estimated from the mean data presented.

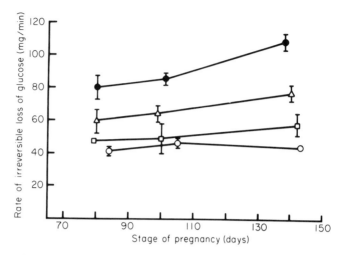

FIG. 6. The effects of stage of pregnancy on the irreversible loss of glucose in sheep. Sheep were given rations of ●, alfalfa chaff *ad libitum;* △, 800 g. alfalfa chaff; □, 250 g. alfalfa chaff + 250 g. wheaten chaff; ○, alfalfa chaff *ad libitum* and starved for 4 days. (Steel and Leng, 1968.)

chaff *ad libitum,* then starved for 4 days, glucose entry rates were fairly constant around 45 mg./minute at 63, 42, and 5 days before lambing (Table IV) probably indicating the upper limit of mobilization of body reserves for gluconeogenesis (Steel and Leng, 1968). In similar experiments and with larger pregnant and nonpregnant sheep, Nolan and Leng (1968) estimated from measured urea entry rates (Cocimano and Leng, 1967) that the upper limit of glucose synthesis from deaminated amino acids of the underfed sheep was 40 mg./minute. This calculation was based on the assumptions that the protein catabolized contained 6.25% nitrogen and that 100 g. of a protein degraded, the nitrogen gives rise to 35 g. urea and the carbonaceous residues to 50–60 g. of glucose (Krebs, 1964a). Thus, starved, pregnant animals appear to have quite a low ability to synthesize glucose from mobilized body reserves. In contrast, the fetus appears to have a high requirement for glucose on which it is dependent for the majority of its energy requirements, and it has been suggested that the fetus drains about 32 g. of glucose per day during late pregnancy (Kronfeld, 1958). The entry rates of glucose in pregnant ruminants are therefore probably dependent to a large extent on food intake, and the requirements of the animal for glucose depends to some extent on the size and number of fetuses (Reid, 1968).

Garber and Ballard (cited by Ballard *et al.,* 1969) suggested that the fetus of the ruminant may be less dependent on maternal glucose than the fetuses of nonruminants because of the ability of the liver of the fetus to convert pyruvate to glucose at approximately the same rate as the adult liver can. The liver of the fetus is fairly small and weighs approximately 80 g. as against 750 g. for the liver of the adult sheep (Filsell *et al.*, 1963). Calculations of potential glucose synthesis from pyruvate in adult sheep liver and fetal liver by extrapolating from the results of Garber and Ballard (cited in Ballard *et al.*, 1969) indicates a net production of 13 g. and 1 g. of glucose per day in the isolated preparations, respectively. If this is indicative of the relative rates of glucose synthesis by the two livers *in vivo*, in a pregnant sheep synthesizing 80 g. of glucose per day, the fetus could only synthesize 6.5 g per day, which is considerably less than the estimated requirements of the fetus (Kronfeld, 1958) or the increase in irreversible loss of glucose over the last 60 days of pregnancy in sheep (Steel and Leng, 1968).

The effects of lactation on glucose entry rates in sheep and goats have been investigated by Annison and Linzell (1964) and Bergman and Hogue (1967). No nutritional studies have been made, but it has been demonstrated that the lactose drain is a large proportion of the glucose entry, approximately 60% of the glucose entry rate being drained by the mammary gland for lactose synthesis (Annison and Linzell, 1964; Bergman and Hogue, 1967). It is well established that plasma glucose is the major source of milk lactose (Kleiber *et al.*, 1955).

The results of Bergman and Hogue (1967) and Annison and Linzell (1964) are shown in Table V. Bergman and Hogue (1967) concluded that lactation is a much greater stimulus to gluconeogenesis than pregnancy. However, a comparison of glucose entry rates in animals with the same energy intake in pregnancy and lactation has not been made. It is notable that glucose entry rates were three times greater in lactating sheep than in nonlactating sheep, but the lactating animals were eating approximately three times the quantity of food. Annison and Linzell (1964) found no differences between lactating and nonlactating goats, though only one dry animal was examined, and its food intake was not reported.

In the reviewer's opinion, the glucose entry rates reported for feeding animals are largely a product of the food intake, and it is the supply of glucose precursors and, indirectly, the control of appetite that affects the glucose entry rate. A recent publication by Baile *et al.* (1969) showed that goats that were hyperphagic due to hypothalmic lesions had twice the glucose entry rate of intact goats which tends to support the above conclusions. It would be interesting to compare glucose entry rates of sheep given a high plane of nutrition and force fed in addition.

V. Gluconeogenesis in Ruminants

There are a number of reported investigations in which it is suggested that in ruminants given high grain rations significant quantities of glu-

TABLE V

GLUCOSE ENTRY RATES IN LACTATING GOATS AND SHEEP

Reference[a] and animal	Ration or diet	Lactation period (weeks)	No. of expt.	Animal Wt (kg.)	Plasma glucose conc. (mg./100 ml.)	Glucose pool size (g.)	Glucose pool size (mg./kg.)	Glucose space (% B. Wt)	Lactose production (mg./min.)	Glucose entry rate[b] (mg./min.)	Glucose entry rate[b] (mg./kg./min.)	Glucose entry rate[b] (mg./kg.$^{3/4}$/min.)	Glucose oxidized to CO_2 (%)	CO_2 output from glucose (%)
1. Sheep	3000 g./day alfalfa hay plus concentrate	2.5	4	61	56	8.6	142	25	127	197	3.2[c]	9.0	23	8
		4	4	61	60	10.1	165	27	135	243	4.0[c]	11.1	25	9
		10	4	60	61	9.8	160	26	62	175	2.9[c]	8.1	29	9
	800 g. of above ration	0	5	59	62	9.5	158	25	0	80	1.4[c]	3.8		9
2. Goats	Ad lib. hay plus concentrate twice daily	6	1	68					145[c]	428[c]	5.3	18.1[c]	34	10
		17	1	69					92[c]	248[c]	3.6	10.4[c]		9
	according to milk yield	12–15	1	74					77[c]	222[c]	3.0	8.8[c]		11
		35	1	60					63[c]	186[c]	3.1	8.6[c]		8
		6–12	1	63					38[c]	202[c]	3.2	9.0[c]		7
		0	1	66					0[c]	238[c]	3.6	10.3[c]		14

[a] Reference

1. Bergman and Hogue (1967)
2. Annison and Linzell (1964)

[b] Since primed infusions were used the entry rate is the irreversible loss of glucose.

[c] Calculated from the reported studies.

cose may be absorbed from the digestive tract. Studies with animals given grain rations may be important; however, the majority of the world's domestic ruminants depend on roughage and in countries such as Australia, Africa, and South America, ruminants are largely maintained at pasture. In other countries, more intensive systems of management are usually applied. Ruminants are dependent largely on cellulose under one system, whereas in the other, they depend on grain starches for their energy supply.

1. Quantitative Aspects of Glucose Absorption from the Gastrointestinal Tract of Ruminants

Early studies of glucose absorption in ruminants generally showed that little glucose was absorbed from the digestive tract of sheep and cattle (McClymont, 1949; Heald, 1951; Schambye 1951a,b; and reviews of Lindsay, 1959 and Armstrong, 1965). Recently, considerable controversy has arisen concerning the quantity of glucose that may be absorbed. Some investigations have demonstrated that considerable quantities of glucose may be absorbed from the digestive tract of both sheep and cattle (Wright et al., 1966; Karr et al., 1966; Little et al., 1968; Tucker et al., 1968) whereas other studies (MacRae and Armstrong, 1966; Topps et al., 1968a,b; Sutton and Nicholson, 1968; Orskov and Fraser, 1968) appear to have demonstrated quite contrary results. However, the diets given to the animals may explain the large differences between these results. Tucker et al. (1968) used finely ground maize as the starch in the diet, whereas Topps et al. (1968a) used pelleted concentrates of which the starch was in the form of barley grain; MacRae and Armstrong (1966) used rolled barley and Sutton and Nicholson (1968) used flaked maize. If the fine grinding of grain resulted in a faster rate of passage of food through the rumen, even though the immediate effect of grinding may be more rapid fermentation, a greater proportion of starch may leave the rumen intact, particularly if the initial rapid fermentation was followed by a period of slow fermentation because of a reduction in ruminal pH. However, Orskov and Fraser (1968) found that with ground barley there was a decrease in starch appearing in the lower digestive tract. It appears logical that all these findings are correct, and that the type of food is the main factor controlling the quantities of starch that may escape fermentation. More investigations are required to clarify these effects, i.e., of feeding cracked, rolled, or finely ground grains (barley, wheat, or maize) in varying proportions to sheep and cattle and at different frequencies of feeding. The variety of grain used may be important particularly with wheat grains where hard and soft varieties are well recognized. A further consideration may be the degree of accustoming of the animal to the diet, which is not always clear in the publications. In many cases, the actual description of diets is omitted which hinders interpretations of the results of such experiments.

Since it may be assumed that a variable but small quantity of glucose is absorbed from the digestive tract of ruminants on concentrate rations and since the provision of a glucose load reduces gluconeogenesis (Annison and White, 1961; Bartley and Black, 1966; West and Passey, 1967), the need for gluconeogenesis may depend on the amount of, and the preparation and type of grain in the diet. However, on the majority of diets, absorption of glucose from the intestine must be low and irreversible loss of glucose is a good indication of net gluconeogenesis in the animal.

2. Gluconeogenesis from Propionate

It is now established that carbohydrates of the ration of sheep and cattle are fermented in the rumen to give rise mainly to the volatile fatty acids (VFA) acetic, propionic, and butyric acids. VFA production and absorption have been reviewed by Warner (1964), Hungate (1966), and Annison (1965), and isotope dilution techniques have been applied to the measurements of VFA production in the rumen (Gray et al., 1960, 1967; Bergman et al., 1965; Leng and Leonard, 1965; Leng and Brett, 1966; Esdale et al., 1968; Leng et al., 1968; Weston and Hogan, 1968). Continuous infusion of ^{14}C labeled acids has shown that VFA production is higher than previously estimated (Warner, 1964) and constitutes up to 60% of the digestible energy of a ration. These studies have been facilitated by continuously feeding the experimental animals; where animals have been fed frequently over 24 hours, VFA production can be estimated on a daily basis. However, Leng and Brett (1966) showed that there is a linear relationship between the production of VFA and their concentrations in the rumen of sheep.

Before the later studies on VFA production, it was believed that the rate of propionate production in the rumen was insufficient to meet the demands for gluconeogenesis and this led to suggestions that glucose may be synthesized from fatty acids with an even number of carbon atoms (butyrate and acetate). McCarthy et al. (1958) appeared to demonstrate that (^{14}C)butyrate was converted to (^{14}C)lactate by the rumen epithelium, but later work clearly illustrated that this was due to contamination of isolated lactate with (^{14}C)-β-hydroxybutyrate produced from (^{14}C)-butyrate (Holter et al., 1963). In subsequent work, Leng and Annison (1963) working with liver slices from sheep and Annison et al. (1963a) using sheep and Ramsey and Davis (1965) working with cows showed that the pattern of radioactivity that appeared in glucose from (^{14}C)-acetate or (^{14}C)butyrate was consistent with equilibration of that carbon in the tricarboxylic acid cycle, in order that there was no net conversion of these compounds to glucose (Weinman et al., 1957). Black et al. (1961) also showed that the labeling patterns of amino acids in milk caesin after specifically labeled (^{14}C) butyrate was injected into cows again was consistent with metabolism of these compounds in the tricarboxylic acid cycle. Indication of a separate pathway of conversion of acetone to lactate (propanediol pathway) to glucose in ruminants was suggested by the work of Luick et al. (1967), Leng and White (1964), and Lindsay and Brown (1966). However, this pathway is probably quantitatively insignificant and could not account for much of the glucose synthesis rate. The "propanediol pathway" (Miller and Bazzano, 1965) has not been investigated quantitatively in ketotic or ketonemic animals.

The recent studies on VFA production revealed that if all the propionate produced in the rumen of sheep was converted to glucose almost all the glucose entry rates in the sheep could be met (Table VI).

Bergman et al. (1966) infused (2-^{14}C) propionate in a ruminal vein and measured the specific radioactivity in the propionate of the portal vein and the amount of ^{14}C appearing in plasma glucose. They demonstrated that 27% of the glucose was being synthesized from absorbed propionate. In similar experiments with animals given similar quantities of feed, Leng et al. (1967) infused (U-^{14}C)-, (1-^{14}C)-, (2-^{14}C)-, and (3-^{14}C) propionate in the rumen of sheep in separate experiments and were able to estimate that 54% of the glucose was being synthesized from propionate. The apparent discrepancies between the two studies can be explained if appreciable propionate is converted to lactate in the rumen wall (Pennington and Sutherland, 1956). From the specific radioactivity of plasma glucose after (1-^{14}C)-, (2-^{14}C)-, or (U-^{14}C) propionate was infused in the rumen, it was suggested that 70% of the propionate that was converted to glucose was first converted to lactate (Leng et al., 1967). The sheep of these studies were fed their total ration (800 g. alfalfa) in 12 equal amounts over 12 hours, whereas in the studies of Bergman et al. (1966) the animals were fed at a constant rate throughout the 24 hours. In subsequent studies (Judson and Leng, 1968), the feeding regimen of Bergman et al. (1966) was used and in these studies a mean of 50–60% of the glucose was synthesized from propionate. In all studies from these laboratories, between 50 and 60% of the propionate was converted to glucose. It is thus obvious that there is considerably more substrate available in the animal than is required for gluconeogenesis. Glycerol (Bergman, 1968), and free fatty acid (West and Annison, 1964) entry rates are low in feeding animals. Thus, it appears that propionate and amino acids are the main source of glucose carbon in feeding sheep. The majority of the amino acids enter the tricarboxylic acid cycle before they are

TABLE VI

PRODUCTION RATES OF PROPIONATE IN THE RUMEN OF SHEEP AND COWS MEASURED BY ISOTOPE DILUTION AND THE POTENTIAL, AND MEASURED CONTRIBUTIONS OF PROPIONATE TO GLUCOSE SYNTHESIS[a]

Ref.[b]	Ration and feeding regimen	No. of expt.	Propionate prod. rate (mmole/min.)	(mole/day)	Potential glucose synthesis from propionate (mg./min.)	(g./day)	Glucose entry rate (mg./min.)	Glucose entry rate from propionate (%)	Propionate prod. rate converted to glucose (%)
1.	900 g. dried grass cubes, cont. over 24 hr.	4	0.70	1.0	63	90	60	—	—
2.	800 g. alfalfa, cont. over 12 hr.	3	1.17	—	105	—	60[c]	—	—
3.	800 g. alfalfa, cont. over 24 hr.	2	0.66	0.95	59	85	60[c]	—	—
4.	800 g. alfalfa, cont. over 12 hr.	4	0.98	—	88	—	—	—	—
	400 g. maize + 200 g. alfalfa, cont. over 12 hr.	4	0.74	—	67	—	—	—	—
	300 g. maize + 300 g. alfalfa, cont. over 12 hr.	3	0.58	—	52	—	—	—	—
	450 g. wheaten straw + 50 g. alfalfa, cont. over 12 hr.	4	0.34	—	31	—	—	—	—

5.	400 g. maize, cont. over 12 hr.	4	0.80	—	—	72	53	36	27
	250 g. alfalfa + 260 g. maize, cont. over 12 hr.	4	0.75	—	—	68	65	39	38
	400 g. alfalfa + 200 g. maize, cont. over 12 hr.	4	0.85	—	—	77	59	56	46
6.	1000 g. wheaten hay *ad lib.*	1	0.73[d]	—	—	66	—	—	—
7.	800 g. pelleted alfalfa, cont. over 24 hr.	4	0.4[e]	—	52	36	63	27	50
	400 g. pelleted alfalfa, cont. over 24 hr.	1	0.21[e]	—	27	19	—	—	—
8.	800 g. alfalfa, cont. over 12 hr.	8	1.24	—	—	112	59	54	32
9.	Silage hay, cont. over 24 hr.	2	4.65	—	603	419	738[f]	—	—
		2	3.61	—	468	325	738[f]	—	—

[a] Only results have been reported where the production of propionate has been made directly using an infusion of (^{14}C)propionate.

[b] Reference

1. Bergman *et al.* (1965)
2. Leng and Leonard (1965)
3. Leng (1970)
4. Leng and Brett (1966)
5. Judson *et al.* (1968)

6. Gray *et al.* (1960)
7. Bergman *et al.* (1966)
8. Leng *et al.* (1967)
9. Esdale *et al.* (1968)

[c] See Tables I and II.

[d] A single injection was used.

[e] Only absorbed propionate was measured.

[f] From Head *et al.* (1965).

oxidized or converted into glucose (see Fig. 7), and it may be assumed that the propionate entering the tricarboxylic acid cycle is diluted with amino acid carbon which is also entering the cycle. The extent of this dilution may be indicated by the specific radioactivity of plasma glucose since, if little glucose is synthesized from compounds entering the glycolytic scheme above phosphoenolpyruvate, the specific radioactivity of oxaloacetate in the liver cells should be similar to that of plasma glucose (see Fig. 7). During a continuous infusion of (2-^{14}C)propionate into the rumen, the plasma glucose attained a specific radioactivity approximately 50% of that of ruminal propionate; according to the cited arguments the specific radioactivity of oxaloacetate in the liver cells should be similar, which would indicate that the total carbon entry to the tricarboxylic acid cycle was twice that of propionate. The majority of this substrate must be amino acids.

The apparent conversion of propionate to lactate in the rumen wall indicates that gluconeogenesis from propionate may not be restricted to the liver. Only small quantities of propionate are present in peripheral blood (Reid, 1950; McClymont, 1951), but lactate levels are of the order of 5–10 mg./100 ml. (Annison et al., 1963b) and recent studies have indicated that significant quantities of glucose may be synthesized in the kidney cortex (Krebs et al., 1963; Krebs and Yoshida, 1963; Newsholme and Gevers, 1967).

Steel (1970) has shown that the rate of synthesis of glucose from propionate is higher in pregnant than in nonpregnant sheep. Steel (1970) also showed that even though glucose entry rate has increased in pregnant animals fed ad libitum, the feed intake had increased roughly proportionately. It was also apparent in lactating sheep where glucose entry rates were 2 to 3 times those of nonpregnant, nonlactating sheep, but the feed intake of these animals increased approximately 2 to 3 times (Bergman and Hogue, 1967). However, in sheep on a constant intake of feed throughout pregnancy the glucose entry rate increased significantly (Steel and Leng, 1968). These studies tend to indicate that there are ample glucose precursors absorbed from the digestive tract of well-fed ruminants and that propionate supplies approximately 30 to 50% of the potential glucogenic substrate (Table VI). Thus, there is good evidence to suggest that in a feeding sheep the animal is rarely short of glucose precursors provided its feed intake is not suppressed, and it is only when the intake of a good quality feed is reduced that glucose may become limiting.

The position is not as clear in the bovine. Head et al. (1965) reported glucose entry rates of dry cows fed a diet of ad libitum hay, restricted concentrates, of 650 and 820 mg./minute (Table III) using the primed infusion and single injection techniques, respectively. The former value is probably closer to irreversible loss and the latter to total entry rate (see Section II,3). Esdale *et al.* (1968) using dry cows fed a proportion of their rations each hour, estimated the propionate production rate in the rumen to be 4.65 and 3.61 mmole/minute on a silage or hay diet, respectively. If all the propionate was converted to glucose, it would give rise to 420 and 325 mg. glucose per minute, respectively, or 65% and 50% of the irreversible loss of glucose (Head *et al.*, 1965). However, in both reports the actual quantity of feed eaten by the animals was not stated, making such calculations of dubious value.

3. GLUCONEOGENESIS FROM AMINO ACIDS

The possible association of propionate production rate, as reported, with the availability of equal amounts of other potential, glucogenic substrates is of considerable interest, especially if it is believed that these are mainly the amino acids available for degradation. A scheme for the conversion of amino acids to glucose is shown in Fig. 7.

Gluconeogenesis from amino acids in ruminants may vary widely depending on the nutrition and physiologic condition of the animal. Only a small number of studies have been made using ${}^{14}C$ labeled amino acids to estimate the extent of glucose synthesis from amino acids. Hunter and Millson (1964) estimated that about 12% of the lactose was derived from amino acids in lactating cows, but Black *et al.* (1968) pointed out that this value may be in error since it was acquired by comparing the specific radioactivity of the milk casein with lactose and that only half the amino acids in casein are glucogenic. Also, glucose is synthesized in the liver whereas casein is synthesized in the mammary gland, where the constituents and specific radioactivity of the amino acid pool may be quite different.

Black *et al.* (1968) used single injections of ${}^{14}C$ labeled amino acids to estimate their conversion to glucose in cows and goats. With alanine, 7% of the alanine flux or entry rate was converted to glucose, and this represented 6% of the glucose entry rate estimated from single injection of (U-${}^{14}C$) glucose (i.e., 950 mg. glucose per minute for a cow and 171 mg. glucose per minute for a lactating goat); on the basis of the relative proportions of other glucogenic amino acids they calculated that 30 to 50% of the glucose entry rate may be arising from amino acid carbon. Of more significance was that the rates of conversion of particular amino acids to glucose were different and the maximal peak specific radioactivity of plasma glucose was reached at different times. The authors suggested that these relationships may be physiologically advantageous since they insure a prolonged supply of glucogenic precursors.

The contribution of amino acids to glucose synthesis in sheep has

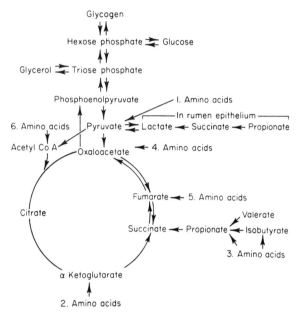

Fɪɢ. 7. Scheme showing the metabolic pathway for gluconeogenesis in the liver of ruminants and the relationship of glucose precursors that become available from the digestive tract.

Glucogenic amino acids		Ketogenic amino acids
1 cysteine	3 valine	6 isoleucine (part)
glycine	threonine	phenylalanine (part)
serine	methionine	tyrosine (part)
alanine	isoleucine (part)	lysine
2 glutamate	4 aspartate	leucine
histidine	5 tyrosine (part)	
proline	phenylalanine (part)	
arginine		

been examined by infusing a mixture of U-^{14}C labeled amino acids isolated from chlorella protein (Ford and Reilly, 1969). Although pool size and entry rates of each amino acid may be variable and the carbon from ketogenic amino acids will equilibrate in the tricarboxylic acid cycle, comparison of the specific radioactivity of circulating amino acids and glucose was taken as indicative of the contribution of amino acids to glucose synthesis. Values of 9.7 and 17.4 g. of glucose per day were estimated to be synthesized from amino acids in sheep on two different diets. Hoogenraad *et al.* (1970) adopted a different approach to this problem; ^{14}C labeled *Bacillus subtilis* and *Escherichia coli* were introduced in the abomasum of sheep and the quantities of ^{14}C flowing through the glucose pool estimated; from the known entry rates of glucose, an estimate was made of the contribution of bacterial cells to glucose synthesis. In these studies, it was assumed that the bacteria resembled the ruminal organisms closely. Approximately 16% of the glucose entry rate was calculated to arise from bacterial carbon.

The quantities of glucose that could be potentially synthesized from amino acids may be estimated from the quantity of protein passing through the abomasum of sheep per day. However, the lysis of bacteria and thus the breakdown and turnover of bacterial protein in the rumen (Jarvis, 1968; Adams et al., 1966a,b; Hoogenraad et al., 1967) suggests that the protein synthesis rate in the rumen is higher than would be indicated by the rate of passage of protein to the abomasum. In spite of the turnover of bacterial protein and the strong proteolytic activity in the rumen, the amino acid concentration of ruminal fluid is low (Annison, 1956). Amino acids are readily absorbed from ruminal fluid (Cook et al., 1965; Lewis and Emery, 1962), but absorption of amino acids from the rumen is probably low or negligible. There are no studies that measure production of amino acids in the rumen. Assuming that amino acid absorption from the rumen is negligible, relative to the amino acids available for absorption in the lower digestive tract, then the potential glucose synthesis can be calculated from the latter values by assuming that a maximum of 55 g. of glucose can be synthesized from 100 g. of protein. In the studies of Hogan and Weston (1967), approximately 100–120 g. of digestible protein passed through the abomasum of sheep given alfalfa chaff at 90% ad libitum intake (i.e., 930–1270 g. organic matter). In sheep given dried grass, 95–100 g. of digestible protein entered the duodenum (Clarke et al., 1966). These investigations suggest that a maximum of 55–66 g. of glucose could become available to sheep on a high plane of nutrition if all digestible protein was degraded and the glucogenic amino acids converted to glucose. It is of interest that the above values are close to the potential glucose synthesis rate from propionate in feeding sheep (800 g. alfalfa) (Table VI), which adds support to the suggestion that the combined glucogenic precursors available to feeding sheep is approximately twice the propionate production rate.

4. Contribution of Glycerol to Glucose Synthesis

The glycerol moiety of triglycerides is largely synthesized in adipose tissue for use in fat synthesis and since there is little or no glycerokinase in adipose tissues (Vaughn, 1961), when free fatty acids are mobilized the glycerol is released to the blood and transported to the liver where it can readily give rise to glucose. Glycerol entry rate in feeding animals

(Bergman, 1968) is low and probably approximates the slow turnover of fat of adipose tissue. In periods of fat mobilization, such as occur in undernutrition or starvation, glycerol entry rates are increased markedly (Bergman, 1968). The liver and kidney appear to be the main sites of glycerol metabolism, and, since the entry of glycerol to the gluconeogenic or glycolytic pathway is at the triose phosphate level, it is obvious that glycerol is an important glucogenic precursor when an animal is starved. The upper limit of glucose synthesis from glycerol must be controlled by the rate of glycerol release from adipose tissue, which in turn must be regulated by the rate of utilization of the free fatty acids released simultaneously from fat. Since the energy expenditure of a mature sheep is fairly constant there must be an upper limit for provision of glucose from glycerol.

Assuming that the fat of adipose tissue of sheep is largely in the triglyceride form (Body et al., 1966) with the major fatty acid constituents being 18:1, 18:0, 16:0 (Shorland et al., 1966), calculations can be made of the free fatty acids mobilized to generate the glycerol entry rates found by Bergman (1968). The calculations showed that for a glycerol entry rate of 5.2, 11.7, 17.6, and 24.8 mmole/hour the heat of combustion of the mobilized free fatty acids would be of the order of 860, 1900, 2900, and 4000 kcal/day which, except for the first value, are higher than the energy expenditure of mature animals (Blaxter, 1962).

Fatty acids that are mobilized are not necessarily oxidized, and they could be alternately converted to ketones or reconverted to fat in adipose tissue or in liver. Glucose in adipose tissue, or glucose and glucose precursors in liver, could supply the glycerol for the synthesis. This may account for fatty infiltration of the liver of undernourished pregnant ewes (Snook, 1939). Even if these assumptions overestimate the free fatty acid (FFA) production, it raises considerable concern as to the validity of the glycerol entry rate technique. In contrast, if the glycerol entry rates are correct, it raises a problem of what happens to mobilized fatty acids in these animals.

Glycerol contributed little to glucose synthesis in feeding sheep, but it contributed significantly to the synthesis in underfed and in starved pregnant sheep (Bergman et al., 1968). No values are available for the contribution of glycerol to glucose synthesis in feeding pregnant sheep, but they would presumably be low.

5. Synthesis of Glucose from Lactate and the Cori Cycle

Glycolysis is the anaerobic metabolism of glucose and occurs in all types of cells. In animal cells that become relatively anaerobic such as those of the actively working muscle, pyruvate is reduced mainly to lactate. The accumulated lactate diffuses to the blood and is carried to other more aerobic regions such as the heart, kidneys, or liver for further metabolism. The lactate in liver and kidney may be reconverted to glucose. This glucose, when liberated in the blood, may again return to the muscles to be converted to glycogen. This cyclic process is known as the Cori cycle (Cori, 1931).

The quantitative significance of the Cori cycle has not been examined in exercising sheep. Annison *et al.* (1963a) examined the contribution of lactate to glucose, and vice versa, in sheep fed and also starved for 24 hours. They showed that 15% of the glucose was coming from lactate and 40% of the lactate was being synthesized from glucose. The contribution of lactate to glucose or vice versa has not been reported in feeding ruminants. However, the Cori cycle as such would be difficult to evaluate because of the large absorption of propionate in these animals and the probably large conversion of propionate to lactate in rumen epithelium and liver (Pennington and Sutherland, 1956). Thus lactate from other sources than that produced in glucose and glycogen metabolism supplies a large proportion of the glucose to ruminants.

The recycling of glucose carbon must be of much more importance when glucogenic substrates are reduced, as during underfeeding or in starvation or where the demand for gluconeogenesis increases as in pregnancy or lactation especially in these conditions when food intake is restricted. Ballard *et al.* (1969) suggested that the fetus may convert glucose to lactate and that the lactate is then returned to the maternal liver for reutilization. Since the fetal liver can synthesize glucose from lactate (Garber and Ballard, cited by Ballard *et al.*, 1969), a proportion of this lactate may be reconverted to glucose without returning to the maternal liver.

The Cori cycle is of significance only when the supply of glucose precursors, other than lactate from glucose, is limited. In feeding ruminants, where the supply of glucose precursors is large with respect to the amount actually required, the passage of glucose carbon through lactate back to glucose occurs mainly due to a dilution of lactate in the glucogenic precursor pools. The change in Cori cycle activity in human beings during starvation is most dramatic where there is a conservation of glucose precursors (Cahill *et al.*, 1966; Cahill and Owen, 1967).

It should be noted that in the majority of studies of sheep, only the irreversible loss of glucose has been measured, and thus the actual quantity of glucose entering the body pool has not been measured; nor does this estimate include the glucose synthesized from lactate of glucose origin. Measurement of total entry rate would be of significance since it would indicate the utilization of glucose, wheres the irreversible loss may represent the amount of glucose which must be synthesized *de novo*. The actual resynthesis of glucose from lactate derived from blood glucose as a percentage of total entry rate of glucose must be higher than that reported (Annison *et al.*, 1963a).

6. OTHER SUBSTRATES FOR GLUCONEOGENESIS IN RUMINANTS

Valeric and isobutyric acids are also available glucogenic precursors but these occur only as a small proportion of the total VFA in ruminal fluid, and their combined amounts rarely exceed 2–4% of the volatile fatty acids, on a molar basis. However, they must make a small contribution to glucose synthesis (Table VII). The contribution of the ribose of nucleic acids in the rumen to glucose synthesis is unknown.

7. GLUCONEOGENESIS IN STARVATION IN SHEEP

In starvation, gluconeogenesis can occur only from mobilized body reserves, i.e., glycerol from adipose tissue and amino acids mobilized from body protein and from lactate of glycogen or glucose origin. Only animals starved 2 or more days can be considered to be receiving little glucogenic precursors from the digestive tract. The results of Steel (1970) are most interesting in this respect, as it appears that in starved (4 days) normal sheep, mobilization of body materials accounted for only 20 to 30 mg./minute (Fig. 4) whereas in pregnant sheep starved four days quantities of 40 to 50 mg./minute (Steel and Leng, 1968) were synthesized from endogenous substrate. Thus, control mechanisms of the animal appear to allow a greater mobilization of body reserves during pregnancy.

VI. Other Considerations

Glucose serves two major functions in cell metabolism. It provides "building blocks," which are used to construct the complex macromolecules of the cell, including nucleic acids, proteins, and lipids; in addition, glucose is utilized for the production of energy which is necessary for the synthesis of macromolecules, and it also may provide substrate for special purposes such as energy supply for the central nervous system. Cahill and Owen (1967) reviewed the literature on glucose metabolism in postabsorptive human beings, which may be comparable with the feeding ruminants. The authors indicated that the majority of the glucose was utilized in the brain (approximately 65% of glucose entry rate) and blood cells (15%). The brain of ruminants takes up considerable glucose (McClymont and Setchell, 1956; Setchell, 1961); however, the amount utilized by red blood cells is quite small (Leng and Annison, 1962). It is not possible to determine the proportion of the glucose entry rate by the various organs of the sheep, but the percentage of the entering glucose which is oxidized (i.e., appearing as $^{14}CO_2$) rarely exceeds 30–40% (Table

II). Where $^{14}CO_2$ production from glucose has been studied the specific radioactivity of blood or respired $^{14}CO_2$ during primed infusions of (U-^{14}C) glucose had only approximated a plateau. Therefore, the values for the contributions of glucose to energy expenditure and the quantities of glucose oxidized may be minimal. However, the data indicate that considerable glucose carbon enters other substrate pools, and some of these are potentially capable of returning carbon back to glucose. Since 40% of the glucose carbon is lost as CO_2, 60% of the glucose enters these substrate pools, and therefore these pools can potentially supply 60% of the glucose entry rate. However, equilibration of ^{14}C from glucose with fatty acids will make this carbon unavailable for glucose synthesis and will reduce this percentage. Glycerol of triglycerides, amino acids of proteins, and ribose of nucleic acids are examples of substrate pools which probably turn over slowly and are not in equilibrium with the glucose pool during the course of an experiment in which glucose entry rates are measured by isotope dilution. The synthesis of (^{14}C)ribose, (^{14}C)glycerol, or ^{14}C labeled amino acids must occur immediately and continuously during a continuous infusion or a single injection of (U-^{14}C)glucose, and they may be synthesized into macromolecules without equilibration in the circulating blood. The same substrates, produced because of the dynamic equilibrium of the body, are unlabeled since these compounds are not necessarily turned over at random in tissues; for instance, with structural components of tissues, the last molecule in may be the last one out. If, however, mixing of these pools of substrates does occur, the released substrates are labeled only to a small extent since these pools are large. The turnover of the macromolecules may take place in days rather than hours. This would suggest that irreversible loss (R. G. White *et al.,* 1969) may not include all of the compounds incorporated into macromolecules, but only those products that go through substrate pools which are confined to body fluids, such as lactate or carbon dioxide. The contribution of the substrates from macromolecules may approximate the entry rate estimated in fasted animals which is roughly 40% of that of the fed animal (Steel, 1970), suggesting that in a 35 kg. sheep with an irreversible loss of glucose of 60 mg./minute only 35 mg./minute (50 g./day) need be supplied from absorbed substrates. This amount may approximate the requirement for glucogenic precursors by the animal. The final or terminal exponent of an isotope dilution curve, following a single injection of (^{14}C)glucose, may be largely due to the turnover of these macromolecules.

VII. Control of Gluconeogenesis in Ruminants

Although the study of control of glucose metabolism has been investigated extensively, few studies have used ruminant tissues. It has been often considered that control mechanisms elucidated in rats are probably applicable to other animals. Blaxter (1968) summarized many difficulties associated with broad generalizations about mammalia as follows. "A comparison of a rat with a cow is not simply a comparison of a rodent with a herbivore or of a simple stomached species with a complex stomached one, or of a seasonally breeding animal with a non-seasonally breeding animal or of a mammal producing hapless young at birth with one producing an active species. The comparison also involves two species differing in size by a factor of 2000 or so." The differences in feeding habits could also be emphasized, the rodent, an omnivore, being predominantly a night feeder whereas the ruminant generally feeds throughout the daylight hours.

Two basic differences in the substrate availability to ruminant and monogastric animals make any generalization of similarity of control of carbohydrate metabolism appear somewhat uncertain. Maximal gluconeogenesis occurs during feeding in ruminants in contrast to monogastric animals where gluconeogenesis occurs during starvation or on low carbohydrate diets. The substrates available for glucose production by the feeding ruminant are largely propionate and glucogenic amino acids (Fig. 7), whereas they are amino acids and glycerol from mobilized body reserves of the starving rat. Normally, little glucose is absorbed from the digestive tract of ruminants, and thus the control of glucose synthesis by glucose absorption may be low. Judson (1969) has demonstrated that maximal reduction of 50% in glucose production by the feeding ruminant was effected by intravenous infusions of glucose. A further consideration is that normally gluconeogenesis by monogastric animals is stimulated in starvation, and lipogenesis is depressed and the reverse occurs on re-feeding. Generally when gluconeogenesis is high, lipogenesis is low and vice versa. However, when gluconeogenesis is high in the ruminant animal, lipogenesis may also be high and, thus, there may be a need for differences in the control of gluconeogenesis in these animals.

The pathways of gluconeogenesis and glycolysis are closely interrelated, and the mechanisms which alter the direction of flow of intermediates along the pathways are important aspects to understanding carbohydrate metabolism in animals. The individual reactions in these pathways and the enzymes catalyzing them are known in detail. The key enzymes of glucose metabolism in the liver of rats have been recognized as being pyruvate carboxylase, phosphoenolpyruvate carboxykinase, fructose-1,6-disphosphatase, and glucose-6-phosphatase in the gluconeogenic pathway; and pyruvate kinase and phosphofructokinase in the glycolytic pathway (Newsholme and Gevers, 1967). It is in these reactions that regulation of the flow of metabolites can be controlled. There are many dietary, hormonal, and physiologic factors which influence the rate of gluconeogenesis, and these have been studied extensively in monogastric animals (Krebs, 1964b; Newsholme and Gevers, 1967); it appears that conditions which create a need for increased gluconeogenesis are associated with cellular changes resulting in provision of increased quantity of all enzymes unique to gluconeogenesis, and thus an overall increase in activity of these enzymes. Enzymic activities associated with gluconeogenesis in livers of ruminants have been measured in a number of studies (Bartley *et al.*, 1966; Goetsch, 1966; Wagle and Nelson, 1966; Baird *et al.*, 1968; Ballard *et al.*, 1968, 1969; Howarth *et al.*, 1968), but it has not been shown definitely that the control of gluconeogenesis and glycolysis by enzymic activities in the ruminant is similar to that of rat liver.

Reshef *et al.* (cited by Ballard *et al.*, 1969) showed that pyruvate carboxylase is located mainly in the mitochondria of cow liver, whereas phosphoenolpyruvate carboxykinase is found in both the cytosol and mitochondria (Nordlie and Lardy, 1963; Ballard and Hanson, 1967). Because of the intracellular distribution of these enzymes in rat liver, gluconeogenesis involves carboxylation of pyruvate to oxaloacetate in mitochondria. The oxaloacetate does not diffuse to the cytosol but is transaminated to aspartate or reduced to malate which diffuses from the mitochondria and which is readily converted to phosphoenolypyruvate in the cytosol (Lardy *et al.*, 1965). In cows, the production of phosphoenolpyruvate in the liver mitochondria and cytosol and also the translocating of the latter to the cytosol, the site of gluconeogenesis, appears to reduce the significance of these steps as sites for the control of gluconeogenesis. However, Ballard *et al.* (1969) suggested that the activation of pyruvate carboxylase by acetyl CoA, propionyl CoA (Utter and Keech, 1963), and butyryl CoA (Wallace and Utter, cited by Ballard *et al.*, 1969) may be important in ruminant animals since the liver is usually provided with these substrates simultaneously.

Ballard *et al.* (1969) also postulated a control mechanism in gluconeogenesis in ruminants based on the competition for oxaloacetate in the cytosol. Oxaloacetate is produced in cytosol by direct diffusion from the mitochondria and by enzymic action from pyruvate, aspartate, and possibly malate. Cytosol oxaloacetate may enter the lipogenesis or gluconeogenesis pathways as indicated by the reaction sequence shown in Fig. 8 (after Ballard *et al.*, 1969).

Oxaloacetate would tend to be drawn into the lipogenesis pathway when malate dehydrogenase is active and an excess of NADH exists. Gluconeogenesis will compete effectively for oxaloacetate when malate dehydrogenase activity is low, NADH concentration is low, and phosphoenolpyruvate carboxykinase activity is high. Enzymic activities in cow

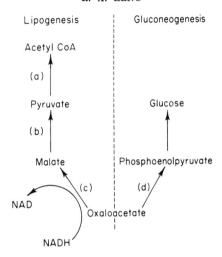

FIG. 8. Two pathways of oxaloacetate utilization in the liver. (After Ballard *et al.,* 1969.) *Enzymes:* (a) pyruvate oxidase, (b) malic enzyme, (c) malate dehydrogenase, and (d) phosphoenolpyruvate carboxykinase.

livers suggests that oxaloacetate is effectively channelled into gluconeogenesis in ruminants (Ballard *et al.,* 1969). No doubt these mechanisms will receive considerable attention in the future.

Substrate availability in the liver may be implicated in the control of glucose synthesis since production of acetoacetate from butyrate in rumen epithelium (Pennington, 1952) and its reduction to β-hydroxybutyrate in liver (Leng and West, 1969) would help maintain an oxidized redox state in the liver and facilitate gluconeogenesis.

Krebs (1966) suggested that ketonemia or ketosis in ruminants may be due mainly to excessive drain of oxaloacetate from the tricarboxylic acid cycle, blocking the entry of acetyl CoA and thus increasing their synthesis to ketone bodies. This theory has been supported (Baird *et al.,* 1968), but conflicting evidence is also provided (Ballard *et al.,* 1968).

Uptake of glucose by liver of ruminants may be low since Gallagher (1959) reported a lack of hexokinase activity in the liver of sheep, and Ballard (1965) and Ballard and Oliver (1964) have shown that, although hexokinase was present, no detectable glucokinase activity was found in the livers of ruminants. However, examinations of these enzymes in the livers of ruminants on high grain rations or in animals infused with glucose have not been made.

Studies have been made of the effects of substrate loads on glucose synthesis in sheep. The inhibition of glucose synthesis by glucose administration and the increase in glucose synthesis due to propionate load have been discussed previously. Recurrent reports showed that butyrate produced hyperglycemia in sheep (Potter, 1952; Kronfeld, 1957), but the pathway of synthesis of carbohydrate from butyrate is not significant in ruminants (see Section V). Butyrate was shown to be glycogenolytic (Phillips *et al.*, 1965), which accounts for the hyperglycemic action of injected butyrate. However, Black *et al.* (1966) suggested that butyrate may also play a role in controlling gluconeogenesis. A butyrate infusion apparently spared pyruvate oxidation, thereby conserving glucogenic precursors. These authors suggest that sparing may have been mediated by increased butyrate utilization in the liver, increasing acetyl CoA concentration which increases carbon flux toward glucose by increasing pyruvate carboxylase activity (Utter and Keech, 1963).

Ballard *et al.* (1969) cited work of Wallace and Utter, in which it was demonstrated that butyryl CoA activates pyruvate carboxylase; the latter may implicate butyrate more directly in the control of gluconeogenesis by bovine liver.

The possibility of control of gluconeogenesis through the control of pyruvate carboxylase activity in the liver is most interesting and may partially explain how nutrition effects glucose synthesis by sheep (Judson and Leng, 1968; Steel and Leng, 1968). It has long been recognized that the ruminal and omasal epithelial tissues synthesize ketone bodies, mainly acetoacetate (Pennington, 1952; Hird and Symons, 1959), from ruminal butyrate (Leng and West, 1969). However, the physiologic significance of such a process has not been discovered. Acetoacetate is reduced to β-hydroxybutyrate in the liver where it is not oxidized (Leng and Annison, 1964). If butyrate increases the concentration of butyryl CoA in the liver, then the quantity of butyrate produced in the rumen that escapes conversion to ketone bodies in the rumen epithelium and enters the portal blood may depend on the feed intake of the animal. The latter may exert some control over the rate of gluconeogenesis, since the high concentration of butyryl CoA stimulates pyruvate carboxylase and the reduction of acetoacetate lowers NADH levels in the liver and both tend to stimulate gluconeogenesis.

The conversion of propionate to lactate in ruminal epithelium (Pennington and Sutherland, 1956; Leng *et al.*, 1967) is also a means of providing substrate which may be preferentially converted to glucose by an increase in pyruvate carboxylase activity, due to an increase in the levels of acyl CoA derivatives in the liver, and the conversion of lactate to pyruvate may provide the NADH required in gluconeogenesis. As supporting evidence, Steel (1970) has shown that the percentage of the irreversible loss of glucose that arises from propionate increases as the production rate of propionate in the rumen of the sheep increases. The ruminal epithelium may thus play an important role in the regulation of metabolism in the liver by providing a variety of glucogenic substrates (propionate or lactate) or potential activators of enzyme systems (aceto-acetate lowering NADH levels, or the CoA derivatives of acetate, propionate, and butyrate stimulating pyruvate carboxylase). It is hoped that the above suggestions stimulate considerable studies of the relationship of rumen epithelial cell metabolism to liver metabolism in the intact animal.

Hormonal control of glucose metabolism of ruminants has also been explored only peripherally. However, this field is large and is beyond the scope of this review. The area appears to be one in need of much investigation in ruminants.

From the above discussion, it becomes apparent that much work is needed to increase our knowledge of the control of gluconeogenesis in ruminants. An excellent experimental animal for the study of control mechanisms in glucose metabolism would be the sheep, which synthesizes glucose during feeding. The use of experimental animals that feed at frequent intervals would remove a considerable number of variables. In any such studies, it would be desirable to study both the rumen epithelium and liver and their association in the animal.

VIII. General Discussion and Conclusion

In this review, I have discussed the investigations that have been made on glucose metabolism in sheep. In many instances, early studies which made important contributions have been criticized. Some investigators who appear now to have drawn wrong conclusions have contributed considerably by stimulating work in particular areas. Difficulties have arisen because of insufficiently detailed studies, and important contributions have accrued through more systematic investigations of glucose metabolism.

There is little value in summarizing and averaging results from different laboratories because of variations in techniques and in nutritive and physiologic conditions of the animals used by different investigators. The most important conclusions appear to be that the quality and quantity of feed eaten by the animal importantly affects the glucose synthesis rate which is probably dependent on the availability of glucose precursors absorbed from the digestive tract. This emphasises that more attention should be given to the control of glucose synthesis in ruminants. If the rate of gluconeogenesis is dependent on the feed intake of the animal, and the supply of volatile fatty acids and amino acids, there appear to be no grounds for the suggestion that ruminants are precariously balanced for glucose precursors. Evolutionary processes would seem to reduce the likelihood of this occurring in normal sheep. However, it is still possible that selection for high productivity which increases the quantitative needs for glucose, as in lactating cows or polytocous sheep, may excessively drain glucose precursors and result in metabolic disturbances under certain circumstances.

Table VII summarizes the possible sources of glucose in a 35 kg. sheep given 800 g. alfalfa chaff per day. Although only guesses may be made of some of these values, particularly of the minor substrates, the overall estimate of substrate availability for glucose synthesis is much higher than the measured irreversible loss of glucose. It could be expected that, as digestible feed intake increased or decreased, these values would increase or decrease roughly proportionately.

In order for a full understanding of carbohydrate metabolism, more studies are required on the utilization of glucose in the various organs of the body. A balance sheet of the utilization of glucose in the animals under different dietary conditions may then be completed for ruminants

TABLE VII

POSSIBLE SUBSTRATES FOR GLUCOSE SYNTHESIS IN SHEEP

Source of glucose	Potential for glucose synthesis (g./day)
Ruminal propionate[a]	90–85
Absorbed glucose[b]	5
From glycerol of fat origin[c]	6
Ruminal valeric and isobutyric acids[d]	19
Amino acids absorbed from digestive tract[e]	66–55

Total 185–170

Irreversible loss of glucose = 86 g./day

[a] Calculated from a production rate of propionate in the rumen (see Table VI) in sheep given a proportion of their ration each hour for 24 hr.

[b] Guessed at (see section on gluconeogenesis).

[c] Estimated from the work of Bergman et al. (1968) assuming that glycerol mobilized from fat in the adipose tissue is not in equilibrium with (^{14}C)glucose in plasma.

[d] The following assumptions were made: (1) Valeric and isobutyric acid concentrations were assumed to be 2 mmole/liter. (2) Valeric and isobutyric acid were each assumed to give rise to a three-carbon unit for glucose synthesis. (3) The production of these acids is related to their concentrations in ruminal fluid in a similar way to the relationship of butyrate concentration and production (Leng et al., 1968) [i.e., $Y_{but} = 0.032X_{but} + 0.085$, where Y = production (mmole/min.) and X = concentration (mmole/liter)]. This value would have a large error of approximately ±100%.

[e] Calculated from the quantity of digestible protein entering the abomasum (Clarke et al., 1966; Hogan and Weston, 1967).

as has been done for human beings (Cahill and Owen, 1967). This would lead to a fuller understanding of the role of glucose in the overall metabolism of the animal.

Future studies of quantitative metabolism in animals will be more dependent on more complete analysis of isotope dilution data, whether these studies be of lipid or carbohydrate metabolism. The important review of Baker (1969) suggests that the solution of complex biochemical interactions will depend extensively on multicompartmental computer analysis. This approach has been treated briefly in this review with regard to analysis of isotope dilution curves following administration of (U-^{14}C) glucose to sheep. The author agrees with the suggestion that there will be a further need for such an approach to pave the way for progress in the study of highly complex problems of metabolism (Baker, 1969).

ACKNOWLEDGMENTS

I wish to express my appreciation to my colleagues and students in the Department of Biochemistry and Nutrition for formulation, in discussion, of many aspects of this review. These include Professor G. L. McClymont, Messrs. J. W. Steel, R. G. White, G. J. Judson, J. V. Nolan, and Mrs. Helen Watson. I am also grateful to Mr. Frank Ball for competent assistance. I wish to thank Professor A. L. Black, Department of Physiological Sciences, School of Veterinary Medicine, University of California, Davis in whose laboratory I spent a most beneficial year and where this review was commenced.

REFERENCES

Adams, J. C., Gazaway, J. A., Brailsford, M. D., Hartman, P. A., and Jacobson, N. L. (1966a). Isolation of bacteriophages from the bovine rumen. *Experientia* **22**, 1–2.

Adams, J. C., Hartman, P. A., and Jacobson, N. L. (1966b). Longevity of selected exogenous microorganisms in the rumen. *Canadian Journal of Microbiology* **12**, 363–369.

Annison, E. F. (1956). Nitrogen metabolism in sheep. Protein digestion in the rumen. *Biochemical Journal* **64**, 705–714.

Annison, E. F. (1965). Absorption from the ruminant stomach. *Second International Symposium on the Physiology of Digestion in the Ruminant, Ames, Iowa, 1964* pp. 185–197. Butterworth, London and Washington, D. C.

Annison, E. F., and Linzell, J. L. (1964). The oxidation and utilization of glucose and acetate by the mammary gland of the goat in relation to their over-all metabolism and to milk formation. *Journal of Physiology (London)* **175**, 372–385.

Annison, E. F., and White, R. R. (1961). Glucose utilization in sheep. *Biochemical Journal* **80**, 162–169.

Annison, E. F., Leng, R. A., Lindsay, D. B., and White, R. R, (1963a). The metabolism of acetic acid, propionic acid and butyric acid in sheep. *Biochemical Journal* **88**, 248–252.

Annison, E. F., Lindsay, D. B., and White, R. R. (1963b). Metabolic interrelations of glucose and lactate in sheep. *Biochemical Journal* **88**, 243–248.

Annison, E. F., Brown, R. E., Leng, R. A., Lindsay, D. B., and West, C. E. (1967). Rates of entry and oxidation of acetate, glucose, D(−)β-hydroxy-butyrate, palmitate, oleate and stearate, and rates of production and oxidation of propionate and butyrate in fed and starved sheep. *Biochemical Journal* 104, 135–147.

Armstrong, D. G. (1965). Carbohydrate metabolism in ruminants and energy supply. *Second International Symposium on the Physiology of Digestion in the Ruminant, Ames, Iowa, 1964* pp. 272–288. Butterworth, London and Washington, D. C.

Baile, C. A., Mayer, J., Mahoney, A. W., and McLaughlin, C. (1969). Hypothalmic hyperphagia in goats and some observations of its effect on glucose utilisation rate. *Journal of Dairy Science* 52, 101–109.

Baird, G. D., Hibbitt, K. G., Hunter, G. D., Lund, P., Stubbs, M., and Krebs, H. A. (1968). Biochemical aspects of bovine ketosis. *Biochemical Journal* 107, 683–689.

Baker, N. (1969). The use of computers to study rates of lipid metabolism. *Journal of Lipid Research* 10, 1–24.

Baker, N., and Rostami, H. (1969). Effect of glucose feeding on net transport of plasma free fatty acids. *Journal of Lipid Research* 10, 83–90.

Baker, N., and Schotz, M. C. (1967). Quantitative aspects of free fatty acid metabolism in the fasted rat. *Journal of Lipid Research* 8, 646–660.

Baker, N., Shipley, R. A., Clark, R. E., and Incefy, G. E. (1959). C¹⁴ studies in carbohydrate metabolism: Glucose pool size and rate of turnover in the normal rat. *American Journal of Physiology* 196, 245–252.

Ballard, F. J. (1965). Glucose utilization in mammalian liver. *Journal of Comparative Biochemistry and Physiology* 14, 437–443.

Ballard, F. J., and Hanson, R. W. (1967). Phosphoenolpyruvate carboxykinase and pyruvate carboxylase in developing rat liver. *Biochemical Journal* 104, 866–871.

Ballard, F. J., and Oliver, I. T. (1964). Ketohexokinase, isoenzymes of glucokinase and glycogen synthesis from hexoses in neonatal rat liver. *Biochemical Journal* 90, 261–268.

Ballard, F. J., Hanson, R. W., Kronfeld, D. S., and Raggi, F. (1968). Metabolic changes in liver associated with spontaneous ketosis and starvation in cows. *Journal of Nutrition* 95, 160–172.

Ballard, F. J., Hanson, R. W., and Kronfeld, D. S. (1969). Gluconeogenesis and lipogenesis in tissue from ruminant and non-ruminant animals. *Federation Proceedings* 28, 218–231.

Bartley, J. C., and Black, A. L. (1966). Effect of exogenous glucose on glucose metabolism in dairy cows. *Journal of Nutrition* 89, 317–328.

Bartley, J. C., Freedland, R. A., and Black, A. L. (1966). Effect of ageing and glucose loading on the activities of glucose-6 phosphatase and phosphorylase of livers of cows and calves. *American Journal of Veterinary Research* 27, 1243–1248.

Baxter, C. F., Kleiber, M., and Black, A. L. (1955). Glucose metabolism in the lactating dairy cow. *Biochemica et Biophysica Acta* 17, 354–360.

Bergman, E. N. (1963). Quantitative aspects of glucose metabolism in pregnant and non-pregnant sheep. *American Journal of Physiology* 204, 147–152.

Bergman, E. N. (1968). Glycerol turnover in the non-pregnant and ketotic pregnant sheep. *American Journal of Physiology* 215, 865–873.

Bergman, E. N., and Hogue, D. E. (1967). Glucose turnover and oxidation rates in lactating sheep. *American Journal of Physiology* 213, 1378–1384.

Bergman, E. N., Reid, R. S., Murray, M. G., Brockway, J. M., and Whitelaw, F. G.

(1965). Interconversions and production of volatile fatty acids in the sheep rumen. *Biochemical Journal* **97**, 53–58.

Bergman, E. N., Roe, W. E., and Kon, K. (1966). Quantitative aspects of propionate metabolism and gluconeogenesis in sheep. *American Journal of Physiology* **211**, 793–799.

Bergman, E. N., Starr, D. J., and Reulein, S. S. (1968). Glycerol metabolism and gluconeogenesis in the normal and hypoglycemic ketotic sheep. *American Journal of Physiology* **215**, 874–880.

Berman, M. (1963). The formulation and testing of models. *Annals of the New York Academy of Sciences* **108**, 182–194.

Black, A. L., Kleiber, M., and Brown, A. M. (1961). Butyrate metabolism in the lactating cow. *Journal of Biological Chemistry* **236**, 2399–2403.

Black, A. L., Luick, J. R., Moller, F., and Anand, R. S. (1966). Pyruvate and propionate metabolism in lactating cows. Effect of butyrate on pyruvate metabolism. *Journal of Biological Chemistry* **241**, 5233–5237.

Black, A. L., Egan, A. R., Anand, R. S., and Chapman, T. E. (1968). The role of amino acids in gluconeogenesis in lactating ruminants. *In* "Isotope Studies on the Nitrogen Chain," pp. 247–263. I.A.E.A., Vienna.

Blaxter, K. L. (1962). "The Energy Metabolism of Ruminants." Hutchinson, London.

Blaxter, K. L. (1968). Chairman's opening remarks. Comparative nutrition. *Proceedings of the Nutrition Society (England and Scotland)* **27**, 120–121.

Body, D. R., Shorland, F. B., and Gass, J. P. (1966). The foetal and maternal lipids of Romney sheep. 1. Composition of the lipids of the total tissue. *Biochemica et Biophysica Acta* **125**, 207–216.

Cahill, G. F., and Owen, O. E. (1967). Some observations on carbohydrate metabolism in man. *In* "Carbohydrate Metabolism and its Disorders" (F. Dickens, P. J. Randle, and W. J. Whelan, eds.), pp. 497–522. Academic Press, New York.

Cahill, G. F., Herrera, M. G., Morgan, A. P., Soeldner, J. S., Steinke, J., Levy, P. L., Reichard, G. A., and Kipnis, D. M. (1966). Hormone-fuel interrelationships during fasting. *Journal of Clinical Investigation* **45**, 1751–1769.

Chapman, T., and Black, A. L. (1969). Personal communication. Department of Physiological Sciences, School of Veterinary Medicine, University of California, Davis, California.

Clarke, E. M. W., Ellinger, G. M., and Phillipson, A. T. (1966). The influence of diet on the nitrogenous components passing to the duodenum and through the lower ileum of sheep. *Proceedings of the Royal Society* **B166**, 63–79.

Cocimano, M. R., and Leng, R. A. (1967). Metabolism of urea in sheep. *British Journal of Nutrition* **21**, 353–371.

Cook, R. M., Brown, R. E., and Davis, C. L. (1965). Protein metabolism in the rumen. 1. Absorption of glycine and other amino acids. *Journal of Dairy Science* **48**, 475–483.

Cori, C. F. (1931). Mammalian carbohydrate metabolism. *Physiological Reviews* **11**, 143–275.

Davis, C. L., and Brown, R. E. (1962). Availability and metabolism of various substrates in ruminants. IV. Glucose metabolism in the young calf and growing steer. *Journal of Dairy Science* **45**, 513–516.

Dunn, A., and Strahs, S. (1965). A comparison of ^{3}H and ^{14}C glucose metabolism in the intact rat. *Nature* **205**, 705–706.

Dunn, A., Chenoweth, M., and Schaeffer, L. D. (1967). Estimation of glucose turnover and the Cori cycle using glucose-6-t-^{14}C. *Biochemistry* **6**, 6–11.

Esdale, W. J., Broderick, G. A., and Satter, L. D. (1968). Measurement of ruminal volatile fatty acid production from alfalfa hay and corn silage rations using a continuous infusion isotope dilution technique. *Journal of Dairy Science* **51**, 1823–1830.

Filsell, O. H., Jarrett, I. G., Atkinson, M. R., Caiger, P., and Morton, R. K. (1963). Nicotinamide nucleotide coenzymes and glucose metabolism in the livers of foetal and new born lambs. *Biochemical Journal* **89**, 92–100.

Ford, E. J. H. (1963). Glucose utilisation in pregnant sheep. *Biochemical Journal* **88**, 427–435.

Ford, E. J. H. (1965). The effect of diet on glucose utilization by sheep. *Journal of Agricultural Science* **65**, 41–43.

Ford, E. J. H., and Reilly, P. E. B. (1969). Amino acid utilization in the ruminant. *Research in Veterinary Science* **10**, 96–98.

Gallagher, C. H. (1959). Biochemical studies on ovine pregnancy toxaemia. 1. Enzymic activities of liver and brain. *Australian Journal of Agricultural Research* **10**, 854–864.

Goetsch, D. D. (1966). Liver enzyme changes during rumen development in calves. *American Journal of Veterinary Research* **27**, 1187–1192.

Gray, F. V., Jones, G. B., and Pilgrim, A. F. (1960). The rates of production of volatile fatty acids in the rumen. *Australian Journal of Agricultural Research* **11**, 383–388.

Gray, F. V., Weller, R. A., Pilgrim, A. F., and Jones, G. B. (1967). Rates of production of volatile fatty acids in the rumen. V. Evaluation of fodders in terms of volatile fatty acid produced in the rumen of the sheep. *Australian Journal of Agricultural Research* **18**, 625–634.

Gunsalus, I. C., and Shuster, C. W. (1961). Energy-yielding metabolism in bacteria. *In* "The Bacteria" (I. C. Gunsalus and R. Y. Stanier, eds.), Vol. 2, Chapter 1, pp. 1–58. Academic Press, New York.

Head, H. H., Connolly, J. D., and Williams, W. F. (1965). Glucose metabolism in dairy cattle and the effect of acetate infusion. *Journal of Dairy Science* **47**, 1371–1377.

Heald, P. J. (1951). The assessment of glucose-containing substances in rumen microorganisms during a digestion cycle in sheep. *British Journal of Nutrition* **5**, 84–93.

Hetenyi, G., Rappaport, A. M., and Wrenshall, G. A. (1961). The validity of rates of glucose appearance in the dog calculated by the method of successive tracer injections. 1. Effects of surgical hepatectomy, evisceration, and order of tracer injection. *Canadian Journal of Biochemistry and Physiology* **39**, 225–236.

Hetenyi, G., Ninomiya, R., and Wrenshall, G. A. (1966). Glucose production rates in dogs determined by two different tracers and tracer methods. *Journal of Nuclear Medicine* **7**, 454–463.

Hird, F. J. R., and Symons, R. H. (1959). The metabolism of glucose and butyrate by the omasum of the sheep. *Biochimica et Biophysica Acta* **35**, 422–434.

Hogan, J. P., and Weston, R. H. (1967). The digestion of chopped and ground roughages by sheep. II. The digestion of nitrogen and some carbohydrate fractions in the stomach and intestines. *Australian Journal of Agricultural Research* **18**, 803–819.

Holter, J. B., McCarthy, R. D., and Kesler, E. M. (1963). Butyrate metabolism in the isolated, perfused goat liver. *Journal of Dairy Science* **46**, 1256–1259.

Hoogenraad, N. J., Hird, F. J. R., Holmes, I., and Millis, N. F. (1967). Bacteriophages in rumen contents of sheep. *Journal of General Virology* **1**, 575–576.

Hoogenraad, N. J., Hird, F. J. R., White, R. G., and Leng, R. A. (1970). Utilization of ^{14}C-labeled *Bacillus subtilis* and *Escherichia coli* by sheep. *Bristish Journal of Nutrition* **24**, 129–144.

Houpt, T. R. (1968). Heat production of bovine ruminal ingesta. *American Journal of Veterinary Research* **29**, 411–419.

Howarth, R. E., Baldwin, R. L., and Ronning, M. (1968). Enzyme activities in liver, muscle, and adipose tissue of calves and steers. *Journal of Dairy Science* **51**, 1270–1274.

Hungate, R. E. (1966). "The Rumen and its Microbes." Academic Press, New York.

Hunter, G. D., and Millson, G. C. (1964). Gluconeogenesis in the lactating dairy cow. *Research in Veterinary Science* **5**, 1–6.

Jarrett, I. G., Jones, G. B., and Potter, B. J. (1964). Changes in glucose utilisation during development of the lamb. *Biochemical Journal* **90**, 189–194.

Jarvis, B. D. W. (1968). Lysis of viable rumen bacteria in bovine rumen fluid. *Applied Microbiology* **16**, 714–723.

Judson, G. J. (1969). Personal communication. Department of Biochemistry and Nutrition, School of Rural Science, University of New England, Armidale, N.S.W., Australia.

Judson, G. J., and Leng, R. A. (1968). Effect of diet on glucose synthesis in sheep. *Proceedings of the Australian Society of Animal Production* **7**, 354–358.

Judson, G. J., and Leng, R. A. (1970). Unpublished observations.

Judson, G. J., Anderson, E., Luick, J. R., and Leng, R. A. (1968). The contribution of propionate to glucose synthesis in sheep given diets of different grain content. *British Journal of Nutrition* **22**, 69–75.

Karr, M. R., Little, C. O., and Mitchell, G. E. (1966). Starch disappearance from different segments of the digestive tract of steers. *Journal of Animal Science* **25**, 652–654.

Katz, J., and Dunn, A. (1967). Glucose-2-t as a tracer for glucose metabolism. *Biochemistry* **6**, 1–5.

Kleiber, M. (1965). Metabolic body size. *In* "Energy Metabolism" (K. L. Blaxter, ed.), pp. 427–435. Academic Press, New York.

Kleiber, M. (1967). An old professor of animal husbandry ruminates. *Annual Review of Physiology* **29**, 1–20.

Kleiber, M., Black, A. L., Brown, M. A., Baxter, C. F., Luick, J. R, and Stadtman, F. H. (1955). Glucose as a prescursor of milk constituents in the intact dairy cow. *Biochimica et Biophysica Acta* **17**, 252–260.

Krebs, H. A. (1964a). The metabolic fate of amino acids. *In* "Mammalian Protein Metabolism" (H. N. Munroe and J. B. Allison, eds.), Vol. 1, pp. 125–176. Academic Press, New York.

Krebs, H. A. (1964b). Gluconeogenesis. *Proceedings of the Royal Society* **B159**, 545–564.

Krebs, H. A. (1966). Bovine ketosis. *Veterinary Record* **78**, 187–192.

Krebs, H. A. and Yoshida, T. (1963). Renal gluconeogenesis. 2. The gluconeogenic capacity of the kidney-cortex of various species. *Biochemical Journal* **89**, 398–400.

Krebs, H. A., Bennett, D. A. H., de Gasquet, P., Gascoyne, T., and Yoshida, T. (1963). Renal gluconeogenesis. 1. The effect of diet on the gluconeogenic capacity of rat kidney-cortex slices. *Biochemical Journal* **86**, 22–27.

Kronfeld, D. S. (1957). The effects of blood sugar and ketone bodies of butyrate, acetate and B-OH butyrate infused into sheep. *Australian Journal of Experimental Biology and Medical Science* **35**, 257–266.

Kronfeld, D. S. (1958). The fetal drain of hexose in ovine pregnancy toxemia. *Cornell Veterinarian* **48**, 394–404.

Kronfeld, D. S., and Raggi, F. (1964). Glucose kinetics in normal, fasting, and insulin-treated cows. *American Journal of Physiology* **206**, 109–112.

Kronfeld, D. S., and Simesen, M. G. (1961a). Glucose biokinetics in sheep. *American Journal of Physiology* **201**, 639–644.

Kronfeld, D. S., and Simesen, M. G. (1961b). Glucose biokinetics in ovine pregnancy toxemia. *Cornell Veterinarian* **51**, 478–488.

Kronfeld, D. S., Tombropoulos, E. G., and Kleiber, M. (1959). Glucose biokinetics in normal and ketotic cows. *Journal of Applied Physiology* **14**, 1026–1028.

Lardy, H. A., Paetkau, V., and Walter, P. (1965). Paths of carbon in gluconeogenesis and lipogenesis. The role of mitochondria in supplying precursors of phosphoenol pyruvate. *Proceedings of the National Academy of Sciences of the United States* **53**, 1410–1415.

Leng, R. A. (1970). Unpublished observations.

Leng, R. A., and Annison, E. F. (1962). Metabolic activities of sheep erythrocytes. 1. Glycolytic activities. *Australian Journal of Agricultural Research* **13**, 31–44.

Leng, R. A., and Annison, E. F. (1963). Metabolism of acetate, propionate and butyrate by sheep liver slices. *Biochemical Journal* **86**, 319–327.

Leng, R. A., and Annison, E. F. (1964). The metabolism of $D(-)\beta$-hydroxy-butyrate in sheep. *Biochemical Journal* **90**, 464–469.

Leng, R. A., and Black, A. L. (1970). Kinetics of glucose metabolism in goats studied by using tritium and carbon-14 labeled glucose. Unpublished observations.

Leng, R. A., and Brett, D. J. (1966). Simultaneous measurements of the rates of production of acetic, propionic and butyric acids in the rumen of sheep on different diets and the correlation between production rates and concentrations of these acids in the rumen. *British Journal of Nutrition* **20**, 541–552.

Leng, R. A., and Leonard, G. J. (1965). Measurement of the rates of production of acetic, propionic and butyric acids in the rumen of sheep. *British Journal of Nutrition* **19**, 469–483.

Leng, R. A., and West, C. E. (1969). Contribution of acetate, butyrate, palmitate, stearate and oleate to ketone body synthesis in sheep. *Research in Veterinary Science* **10**, 57–63.

Leng, R. A., and White, R. R. (1964). Possible glucogenicity of $D(-)\beta$-hydroxy-butyrate in sheep. *Nature* **201**, 78 (only).

Leng, R. A., Steel, J. W., and Luick, J. R. (1967). Contribution of propionate to glucose synthesis in sheep. *Biochemical Journal* **103**, 785–790.

Leng, R. A., Corbett, J. L., and Brett, D. J. (1968). Rates of production of volatile fatty acids in the rumen of grazing sheep and their relation to ruminal concentrations. *British Journal of Nutrition* **22**, 57–68.

Lewis, T. R., and Emery, R. S. (1962). Metabolism of amino acids in the bovine rumen. *Journal of Dairy Science* **45**, 1487–1492.

Lindsay, D. B. (1959). The significance of carbohydrate in ruminant metabolism. *Veterinary Reviews and Annotations* **5**, 103–128.

Lindsay, D. B., and Brown, R. E. (1966). Acetone metabolism in sheep. *Biochemical Journal* **100**, 589–592.

Little, C. O., Mitchell, G. E., and Reitnour, C. M. (1968). Postruminal digestion of corn starch in steers. *Journal of Animal Science* **27**, 790–792.

Luick, J. R., Black, A. L., Simesen, M. G., Kametaka, M., and Kronfeld, D. S.

(1967). Acetone metabolism in normal and ketotic cows. *Journal of Dairy Science* **50**, 544–549.

McCarthy, R. D., Shaw, J. C., and Lakshmanan, S. (1958). Metabolism of volatile fatty acids by the perfused goat liver. *Proceedings of the Society for Experimental Biology and Medicine* **99**, 560–562.

McClymont, G. L. (1949). Interrelations of the digestive and mammary physiology of ruminants. Ph.D. Thesis, University of Cambridge.

McClymont, G. L. (1951). Identification of the volatile fatty acid in the peripheral blood and rumen of cattle and the blood of other species. *Australian Journal of Agricultural Research* **2**, 92–103.

McClymont, G. L., and Setchell, B. P. (1956). Non-utilisation of acetate and utilisation of glucose by the brain of the sheep. *Australian Journal of Biological Sciences* **9**, 184–187.

MacRae, J. C., and Armstrong, D. G. (1966). Investigations of the passage of α-linked glucose polymers into the duodenum of the sheep. *Proceedings of the Nutrition Society (England and Scotland)* **25**, 33–34.

Miller, O. N., and Bazzano, G. (1965). Propanediol metabolism and its relation to lactic acid metabolism. *Annals of the New York Academy of Sciences* **119**, 957–973.

Newsholme, E. A., and Gevers, W. (1967). Control of glycolysis and gluconeogenesis in liver and kidney cortex. *Vitamins and Hormones* **25**, 1–87.

Nolan, J. V., and Leng, R. A. (1968). Contributions of protein to glucose synthesis in pregnant and non-pregnant sheep. *Proceedings of the Australian Society of Animal Production* **7**, 348–353.

Nordlie, R. C., and Lardy, H. A. (1963). Mammalian liver phosphoenolpyruvate carboxykinase activities. *Journal of Biological Chemistry* **238**, 2259–2263.

Orskov, E. R., and Fraser, C. (1968). Dietary factors influencing starch disappearance in various parts of the alimentary tract and caecal fermentation in early weaned lambs. *Proceedings of the Nutrition Society (England and Scotland)* **27**, 37A–38A.

Pennington, R. J. (1952). The metabolism of short-chain fatty acids in the sheep. 1. Fatty acid utilisation and ketone body production by rumen epithelium and other tissues. *Biochemical Journal* **51**, 251–258.

Pennington, R. J., and Sutherland, T. M. (1956). The metabolism of short-chain fatty acids in the sheep. 4. The pathway of propionate metabolism in rumen epithelium tissue. *Biochemical Journal* **63**, 618–628.

Phillips, R. W., Black, A. L., and Moller, F. (1965). Butyrate induced glycogenolysis in hypoglycemic lambs. *Life Sciences* **4**, 521–525.

Potter, B. J. (1952). Relief of hypoglycaemic convulsions with butyric acid. *Nature* **170**, 541 (only).

Ramsey, H. A., and Davis, C. L. (1965). Metabolism of n-butyrate by the adult goat. *Journal of Dairy Science* **48**, 381–390.

Reid, R. L. (1950). Studies on the carbohydrate metabolism of sheep. II. The uptake by the tissues of glucose and acetic acid from the peripheral circulation. *Australian Journal of Agricultural Research* **1**, 338–354.

Reid, R. L. (1968). The physiopathology of undernourishment in pregnant sheep, with particular reference to pregnancy toxemia. *Advances in Veterinary Science* **12**, 163–238.

Rescigno, A., and Segre, G. (1966). "Drug and Tracer Kinetics." Ginn (Blaisdell), Boston, Massachusetts.

Schambye, P. (1951a). Volatile acids and glucose in portal blood of sheep. I. *Nordisk Veterinarmedicin* **3,** 555–574.

Schambye, P. (1951b). Volatile acids and glucose in portal blood of sheep. 2. Sheep fed hay and hay plus crushed oats. *Nordisk Veterinarmedicin* **3,** 748–762.

Searle, G. L., Strisower, E. H., and Chaikoff, I. L. (1954). Glucose pool and glucose space in the normal and diabetic dog. *American Journal of Physiology* **176,** 190–194.

Searle, G. L., Strisower, E. H., and Chaikoff, I. L. (1956). Determination of rates of glucose oxidation in normal and diabetic dogs by a technique involving continuous injection of C^{14} glucose. *American Journal of Physiology* **185,** 589–594.

Segal, S., Berman, M., and Blair, A. (1961). The metabolism of variously C^{14}-labeled glucose in man and an estimation of the extent of glucose metabolism by the hexose monophosphate pathway. *Journal of Clinical Investigation* **40,** 1263–1278.

Setchell, B. P. (1961). Cerebral metabolism in the sheep. 1. Normal sheep. *Biochemical Journal* **72,** 265–275.

Shipley, R. A., Chudzik, E. B., Gibbons, A. P., Jongedyk, K., and Brummond, D. O. (1967). Rate of glucose transformation in the rat by whole-body analysis after glucose-^{14}C. *American Journal of Physiology* **213,** 1149–1158.

Shorland, F. B., Body, D. R., and Gass, J. P. (1966). The foetal and maternal lipids of Romney sheep. II. The fatty acid composition of the lipids from the total tissues. *Biochimica et Biophysica Acta* **125,** 217–225.

Skinner, S. M., Clark, R. E., Baker, N., and Shipley, R. A. (1959). Complete solution of the three-compartment model in steady state after single injection of radioactive tracer. *American Journal of Physiology* **196,** 238–244.

Snook, L. C. (1939). Fatty infiltration of the liver in pregnant ewes. *Journal of Physiology (London)* **97,** 238–249.

Steel, J. W. (1969). Personal communication. C.S.I.R.O., Division of Animal Health, McMaster Laboratories, Sydney, N.S.W., Australia.

Steel, J. W. (1970). Gluconeogenesis and glucose kinetics in pregnant and nonpregnant sheep. Ph.D. Thesis, University of New England, Armidale, N.S.W., Australia.

Steel, J. W., and Leng, R. A. (1968). Effect of plane of nutrition and pregnancy on glucose entry rates in sheep. *Proceedings of the Australian Society of Animal Production* **7,** 342–347.

Steele, R. (1964). Reflections on pools. *Federation Proceedings* **23,** 671–679.

Steele, R., Wall, J. S., de Bodo, R. C., and Altszuler, N. (1956). Measurement of size and turnover rate of body glucose pool by the isotope dilution method. *American Journal of Physiology* **187,** 15–24.

Sutton, J. D., and Nicholson, J. W. G. (1968). The digestion of energy and starch along the gastro-intestinal tract of sheep. *Proceedings of the Nutrition Society (England and Scotland)* **27,** 49A–50A.

Topps, J. H., Kay, R. N. B., and Goodall, E. D. (1968a). Digestion of concentrate and of hay diets in the stomach and intestines of ruminants. 1. Sheep. *British Journal of Nutrition* **22,** 261–280.

Topps, J. H., Kay, R. N. B., Goodall, E. D., Whitelaw, F. G., and Reid, R. S. (1968b). Digestion of concentrate and of hay diets in the stomach and intestines of ruminants. 2. Young steers. *British Journal of Nutrition* **22,** 281–290.

Tucker, R. E., Mitchell, G. E., and Little, C. O. (1968). Ruminal and post-ruminal starch digestion in sheep. *Journal of Animal Science* **27,** 824–826.

Utter, M. F., and Keech, D. B. (1963). Pyruvate carboxylase. 1. Nature of the reaction. *Journal of Biological Chemistry* **238**, 2603–2608.

Vaughn, M. (1961). The metabolism of adipose tissue *in vitro*. *Journal of Lipid Research* **2**, 293–316.

Wagle, S. R., and Nelson, P. (1966). Studies on activities of gluconeogenic enzymes in sheep liver. *Biochimica et Biophysica Acta* **121**, 190–191.

Walker, D. J., and Forrest, W. W. (1964). The application of calorimetry to the study of ruminal fermentation *in vitro*. *Australian Journal of Agricultural Research* **15**, 299–315.

Warner, A. C. I. (1964). Production of volatile fatty acids in the rumen: Methods of measurement. *Nutrition Abstracts & Reviews* **34**, 339–352.

Weinman, E. O., Strisower, E. H., and Chaikoff, I. L. (1957). Conversion of fatty acids to carbohydrate: Application of isotopes to this problem and role of the Krebs cycle as a synthetic pathway. *Physiological Reviews* **37**, 252–272.

Weller, R. A., and Pilgrim, F. V. (1953). The passage of starch through the stomach of the sheep. *Journal of Experimental Biology* **31**, 40–48.

West, C. E., and Annison, E. F. (1964). Metabolism of palmitate in sheep. *Biochemical Journal* **92**, 573–578.

West, C. E., and Passey, R. F. (1967). Effect of glucose load and of insulin on the metabolism of glucose and of palmitate in sheep. *Biochemical Journal* **102**, 58–64.

Weston, R. H., and Hogan, J. P. (1968). The digestion of pasture plants by sheep. 1. Ruminal production of volatile fatty acids by sheep offered diets of ryegrass and forage oats. *Australian Journal of Agricultural Research* **19**, 419–432.

White, R. G., Steel, J. W., Leng, R. A., and Luick, J. R. (1969). Evaluation of three isotope dilution techniques for studying the kinetics of glucose metabolism in sheep. *Biochemical Journal* **114**, 203–214.

White, R. R. (1963). Aspects of carbohydrate metabolism in sheep. Ph.D. Thesis, University of New England, Armidale, N.S.W., Australia.

Wright, P. L., Grainger, R. B., and Marco, G. J. (1966). Post ruminal degradation and absorption of carbohydrate by the mature ruminant. *Journal of Nutrition* **89**, 241–246.

The Epizootiology and Epidemiology of Foot and Mouth Disease

N. ST. G. HYSLOP*

Animal Pathology Division, Health of Animals Branch, Canada Department of Agriculture, Animal Diseases Research Institute, Hull, Quebec, Canada

* The author was Principal Scientific Officer, The Animal Virus Research Institute, Pirbright, England from 1959–1968, and is now Head of Immunology, Animal Pathology Division, Health of Animals Branch, Canada Department of Agriculture.

I. Introduction

Foot and mouth disease (FMD) has constituted a major threat to the health of livestock for at least 450 years. Although the disease has been eradicated from several of the more highly developed countries, it still remains a serious hazard to the productivity of animal populations throughout the world and, indirectly, to the well-being of human populations dependent upon them for food, motive power, and clothing.

FMD last occurred in the United States of America in 1929, in Canada in 1952, and in Mexico in 1953 (Shahan, 1962); Japan and Australia have been free of infection for more than 50 years, and there is no record of the disease in New Zealand. However, as Brooksby (1967a) remarked, "the disease continues to spread virtually unchecked and uncontrolled throughout large areas of Asia, Africa and even in some regions of South America." More recently, severe outbreaks in Northwest Europe have dispelled any complacency that may have begun to develop in those countries in which outbreaks have been absent or only sporadic for several years. Unfortunately, the epizootic characteristics of FMD are such that recurrent waves of widespread severe infection tend to occur at intervals of approximately 10 years, and so alternate with periods of only few and minor outbreaks during which economic factors may lead to the relaxation of safeguards. Although FMD is only infrequently fatal for adult stock, the productivity of recovered herds, wherever the policy of slaughter is not implemented, is reduced by at least 25%; economic losses associated with control and eradication programs may reach catastrophic proportions if the disease gains a "firm foothold" in any country.

II. Nature of the Virus

For many years, the small virus (about 20–25 millimicrons in diameter) of FMD has been regarded as one of the most infective living agents of disease.

1. Antigenic Structure, Types, and Variants

No less than 7 immunologically distinct types have been isolated (O, A, C, SAT-1, SAT-2, SAT-3, and Asia 1), and it is probable that hitherto unidentified types will be discovered in the future. The degree of antigenic differences between the types is so great that instances have been recorded of animals becoming naturally infected with virus of 3 different types within 6 months: in each type, however, recovery results in a strong immunity to reinfection with virus of the homologous strain, which frequently persists for a period of several years (Anonymous, 1937; Shahan, 1962; Cunliffe, 1964; Fagg and Hyslop, 1966). Within the types, numerous sub-type strains are being identified which exhibit an apparently infinitely variable degree of cross-protection when tested in different animal species. It is now becoming evident that the evolution of variant strains within each of the types is a dynamic process which results in the creation of a "spectrum" of sub-type strains, some of which may exhibit differences nearly as great as the differences which exist between the types themselves (Hyslop, 1965d; Fagg and Hyslop, 1966). The "new" strains emerging under experimental conditions were found to be fully infective for cattle, and continuation of such evolutionary processes may be expected to create frequent opportunities for the breaching of existing immunologic barriers under field conditions. Furthermore, steady regression of acquired immunity with the passage of time results inevitably, unless immunity is reinforced by vaccination or by exposure, in the threshold of susceptibility being reached again within the expected lifetime of the majority of animals. The potential danger of the evolution of variants is likely to be greatly diminished by the determined application of a policy of slaughtering all affected and incontact animals.

2. Pathogenicity, Invasiveness, Host Specificity

In addition to variability attributable to modification of antigenic structure, some strains of FMD virus exhibit marked differences in pathogenicity, in invasiveness, and in the specificity of their predilection for susceptible hosts. For example some, but not all, of the strains isolated during the outbreaks in Mexico, about 20 years ago, spread slowly and did not always produce disease of the generalized type among the majority of animals in exposed herds: in many cases an inapparent type of infection occurred, and this was frequently associated with resistance to deliberate reinfection by virus of the homologous strain. A special affinity for a single animal species was not observed in these outbreaks. By contrast, strains isolated in Great Britain about 25 years ago exhibited marked species-specificity, causing numerous and severe outbreaks in pigs but relatively few in cattle; elsewhere, cattle strains have been isolated which could be transferred experimentally to pigs only with some difficulty. Observations on strains manifesting species predilection were described by Brooksby (1950). However, the lability of FMD virus is such that a strain may appear to cause a smoldering type of disease in a particular host species for a period of several months, but subsequently may spread suddenly and unaccountably to other species, often causing an acute and severe syndrome in the species newly attacked.

Considerable difficulty in diagnosis may be experienced when anomalous strains exhibit virulence of a low degree and produce few typical vesicular lesions. Similarly, diagnosis may be delayed when exceptional virulence associated with high mortality is encountered, as in a recent outbreak in Tierra del Fuego during which about 30% of infected cattle died in a short period of time. These aberrant strains may remain unrecognized as FMD until major epizootics have become established.

3. Lability

Viruses of more than a single immunologic type may be recovered from the same animal in areas where 2 epizootics have coalesced; multiple infections have been produced under experimental conditions (Vallée and Carré, 1928; Cunha et al., 1958). It must be remembered that there is no valid evidence that new *types* of FMD virus have ever appeared in the field as the result of recombination from moities of pre-existing types. However, C. R. Pringle (1965, 1968) has demonstrated that hybridization may occur between distinct *strains* of the same type; the frequency of recombination (0.3%) was comparable to that of mutants of poliomyelitis virus. Although it appears that immunologic factors may be the influence most frequently responsible for selection of spontaneously evolving mutants under natural conditions, similar variations may occur in response to other adverse environmental conditions of a physical or chemical nature.

4. Survival

The viability of FMD virus propagated in tissue culture was investigated under controlled conditions of temperature, hydrogen ion concentration (pH), and the presence of chemical inactivating agents by Wesslen and Dinter (1957), Bachrach et al. (1957), Bachrach (1960), Brown et al. (1963), Bachrach (1964), Bachrach et al. (1964), Vande Woude (1967), Shafyi (1968), and by others. The virus is most stable near neutral pH. Thus, suspensions of high titer, maintained at pH 7.5, may remain infective for 18 weeks at 4°C., 11 days at 20°C., 21 hours at 37°C., 7 hours at 43°C., 1 hour at 49°C., 20 seconds at 55°C., and 3 seconds at 61°C. Inactivation occurs within a few seconds at pH 4.0; about 90% of virus is inactivated in 1 minute at pH 6.0, in 1 week at pH 9.0, and in 14 hours at pH 10.0. The observations of several workers indicate that within most populations of FMD virus, however, there may occur a small proportion of particles which possess abnormal resistance to the adverse effects of pH and temperature; such particles may occur either as mutants (C. R. Pringle, 1965, 1968) from which resistant strains may arise or, possibly, from initially mixed populations. Dimopoulos *et al.* (1959) found that very large doses (50 ml.) of high-titer viral suspensions retained some infectivity for cattle, even after being heated at 80°C. for 6 hours, but infectivity was not detected after heating at 85°C. for this period.

It is evident from the foregoing reports that, because of the probable presence of small numbers of resistant particles, it is impossible to predict that any particular combination of time, temperature, pH, etc., will render a particular viral suspension completely harmless, although, in practice, pasteurization processes (63–65°C. for 30 minutes or equivalents) are usually adequate for inactivation. The observations of Kastli and Moosbrugger (1968) and of Sellers (1969), which are described in the section on treatment of milk, provide further indication that the degree of safety afforded by some of these processes may be only marginal.

The estimates of virus survival mentioned above were all derived from experiments employing bacteria-free suspensions maintained under static and carefully controlled conditions in the laboratory. From the epizootiologic viewpoint, however, the ability of crude and usually contaminated suspensions to survive under varying ambient conditions is at least equally important. The observations of numerous investigators during the past 60 years indicate that virus secreted in the salvia of infected animals may remain viable for up to 2 days at 37°C., 3 weeks at 26°C., and for 5 weeks at 4°C., while Russian workers have claimed that virus in animal excretions may remain detectable inside a contaminated building for at least a month during warm weather and for longer than 2 months during the winter. Reports dating from the second and third decades of this century suggest that virus may occasionally survive on wood, hay, straw, etc., for about 15 weeks.

Although it is sensitive to sunlight and relatively sensitive to desiccation, the virus is resistant to many of the chemicals which are popularly supposed to kill it—notably phenol, cresols, alcohol, ether, chloroform, acetone, many other organic solvents, and detergents such as sodium dodecyl sulfate, cetylmethyl ammonium bromide, and Tween 80. Lucam *et al.* (1964) investigated the action of 21 common "disinfectants"; sublimate of mercury, potassium permanganate, sodium hydroxide, lactic acid, hypochlorite solution, and formalin were effective within 30 minutes. Sellers (1968) described comparative tests of the inactivating properties of several chemical compounds and found that solutions of sodium hypochlorite rapidly inactivated FMD virus (5 logs in 15 seconds at 20°C.), but the activity of hypochlorite was neutralized to some degree by the presence of organic matter; iodophor compounds depended on acid content for the inactivating effect, and iodophors formulated with phosphoric or sulfuric acid were less readily neutralized by organic matter than those containing hydroiodic acid. The results of Sellers confirmed previous observations that FMD virus is inactivated most rapidly by acids and alkalis. The wetting effect and penetration of acids and alkalis is increased by the addition of soaps or synthetic detergents, which may also disperse aggregates of virus. A solution containing 4% sodium carbonate and soft soap is used frequently in the field; 0.2% sodium hydroxide is more effective but is very caustic. The ability of chemical solutions to penetrate tissue fragments and other organic matter is of great importance in determining their virucidal potency.

III. Secretion and Excretion of Virus by "Natural" Host Species

An outstanding characteristic of FMD is the high titer (of the order of $10^{8.0}$ ID 50 gram) of virus which is detectable, at one time or another, in some of the tissues of animals which have contracted the disease. The virus is likely to be present in all physiologic fluids during the viremic phases. Consequently, any voided secretion or excretion must be regarded as a continuing source of infection for other animals.

1. PERSISTENCE OF VIRUS IN LESIONS

With the notable exception of the soft palate and pharynx, where it may remain detectable for long periods after apparent recovery, virus can seldom be isolated from the tissues later than a few days after the end of the acute phase. Earlier reports suggest that infection may be detected in healing foot lesions for up to 34 days, but persistence for periods as long as this is probably infrequent. Scott et al. (1966), using virus of types O, A, C, SAT-1, and SAT-2, found that the longest duration of viability within lesions was

muzzle	7 days
tongue	8 days
palate	11 days
foot	11 days

and the maximal period for which these workers were able to detect virus in the saliva was 9 days. Similar periods of viability were observed by

Afzal and Barya (1968) in lesions of buffalo calves, but Burrows (1966a) isolated virus from the tongues of cattle 23 days after infection with virus of strain A119.

Many investigators are impressed by the ability of the virus to persist in lesions for periods even as long as these. The writer has found significant titers of neutralizing antibody in the sera of cattle as early as 4 days after infection and titers increased rapidly, reaching 1/1400 and 1/8192 by day 6 and day 9, respectively. The methods employed currently for the detection of FMD antibody are not particularly sensitive, and it is possible that titers of antibody capable of inhibiting considerable amounts of virus were produced even earlier than day 4. Indeed, Litt (1967) employing guinea pig lymph nodes, stimulated with avian erythrocytes as antigen, demonstrated that small amounts of antibody may be produced in less than 8 minutes; Mosier and Cohen (1968) indicated that short exposure to immunogenic RNA from lymphoid cells resulted in rapid formation of antibody *in vitro* by mouse lymphocytes. Having regard to the early production of antibody and the high titers developed within a few days, it must be concluded that diffusion of FMD antibody into the necrotic debris of lesions is probably slow.

2. Saliva

The greatest concentration of virus occurs in the fluid of the vesicles and in the overlying epithelium, where leakage or rupture causes contamination of the saliva; further contamination may result from direct involvement of the salivary glands during the period of viremia, with subsequent proliferation of virus in the secretory cells. Waldmann and Reppin (1927) claimed that virus could be detected in the saliva before lesions appeared in the mouth, but reports of quantitative studies relating the concentration of virus in the saliva to the development of clinical signs have been remarkably difficult to find until recently. At the height of infection, viral titers of the fluid contents of vesicles and of the overlying epithelium may exceed $10^{9.0}$ID50/ml., but Hyslop (1965a) showed that virus might be excreted in the saliva of deliberately infected cattle at titers as great as $10^{2.0}$ to $10^{3.75}$ID50/ml. for several hours before clinical signs appeared. Although the titers of the saliva always remained less than that of the oral tissues, by 24 hours after inoculation the majority of fully susceptible cattle were excreting virus at titers of $10^{4.5}$ to $10^{6.0}$ in their saliva; titers in the saliva of partly immunized cattle were somewhat lower but, nevertheless, such animals would constitute a serious hazard to other stock. Peak titers detected at the height of infection were in the range $10^{5.25}$–$10^{8.5}$ mouse ID50/ml. and, because of the copious amounts of saliva secreted at this period, the total amount of virus released in the vicinity must have been great.

In addition to the risk of gross contamination of the immediate environment, Hyslop (1965a) drew attention to the probability that, when the titer reached $10^{7.0}$, small droplets ($<10\,\mu$ diam.) could be expected to contain live virus with a frequency of about 1 in 200. Droplets of this size tend to remain in aerial suspension for long periods. Evidence for airborne infection with the virus of FMD will be described later.

Although virus may persist for long periods in the tissues of the dorsal soft palate and in the pharynx and tonsils, it is important to distinguish between traces of "persistent" virus, which may be localized in cells, at these sites and the high titer virus actively secreted in the saliva during the acute phase of the disease. Virus is not detected readily in the saliva later than 10 to 14 days after the onset of clinical FMD, and Hyslop (1965a) was unable to detect its salivary excretion at 5 weeks after infection although, undoubtedly, small quantities of virus must be released into the saliva, and probably as micro-droplets or droplet-nuclei into the exhaled air, by any animals in which a pharyngeal infection occurs.

3. Urine and Feces

Blood-borne virus is soon excreted in the urine and in the feces, though titers are often variable or low. W. H. R. Hess et al. (1960) indicated that virus replicates in and is liberated from infections of the kidneys. The feces may become contaminated directly from the blood, via the bile, or as a result of development of vesicles in the alimentary tract. Virus may be detectable at least 48 hours before clinical signs are evident (Anonymous, 1931); Sellers et al. (1968) recovered virus from the rectal contents of 2 of 4 bulls at 3 to 6 days before the disease became clinically obvious. Burrows (1968a) found viable virus in 2 rectal swabs from cows on the day before vesicles were observed; in a group of 10 pigs, virus was present in the feces at a mean period of 4.2 days before the appearance of vesicles. Clearly, the less florid clinical picture of FMD in the pig and the early excretion of virus in pig feces increase the hazard that an outbreak in pigs might remain undiagnosed until the disease has spread to other stock. Russian workers have exhibited considerable interest in problems associated with fecal dissemination of the virus; Bubnov and Nauryzbaev (1966) discussed recent observations and recorded that stacked manure, when allowed to ferment normally, became free of virus after about 8 days. Gorskii and Gizatullin (1968) described treatment of manure stacks by the injection of sodium hydroxide or 5% sulfuric acid but the method appears to be expensive and its efficacy remains unconfirmed.

4. MILK

The epitheliotropic nature of FMD virus permits replication in the secretory cells of the mammary gland. Thus, in addition to passive secretion of virus carried to this organ during the viremic phase, the tissues of the udder begin to produce virus at a rate which soon leads to high concentrations in the milk (about $10^{5.0}ID50/ml.$). The hazards of milk-borne infection, often commencing during the prodromal phase, have been realized for many years (Galloway, 1931; Poppe, 1931). Burrows (1968a) isolated virus from the milk of cattle 1 to 4 days before the onset of clinical signs. Gorban (1953) emphasized the special danger of young stock becoming infected as a result of being fed on bulk milk or dairy residues from infected cows. Brooksby (1959) cited an instance in which infective milk was fed to calves in transit at Crewe, near the center of England; the subsequent distribution of these calves led directly or indirectly to 101 new outbreaks at points 150 to 300 miles from Crewe. Numerous similar instances of very widespread dissemination in dairy products have been recorded in Scandinavian countries. E. Hess (1967) reported that several outbreaks in Switzerland were attributable to these products.

There is growing evidence that man may become infected occasionally as a result of drinking infected milk; young children appear to be affected principally, but human infections are usually mild and appear to be associated with complex predisposing factors.

The titer of FMD virus in milk is greatly reduced by pasteurization processes; Kastli and Moosbrugger (1968) reported that maintenance at 65°C. for 30 seconds was adequate, but 55°C. for 10 seconds was inadequate. Sellers (1969) found that in milk at pH 6.7, 99.999% virus was inactivated in 6 minutes at 56°C., 1 minute at 63°C., 17 seconds at 72°C., and in less than 5 seconds at 80° and 85°C.; at pH 7.6 the corresponding times were 30 minutes at 56°C., 2 minutes at 63°C., 55 seconds at 72°C., and less than 5 seconds at 80° and 85°C. After treatment for these periods 0.001% virus remained viable but some decay of the residual infectivity may be expected during subsequent periods of cooling and storage.

It has been suggested that inactivation of virus may be achieved by the souring of milk, either naturally or by the addition of suitable bacillary cultures, but it has been the writer's experience that viral suspensions of high titer may be incompletely inactivated by weak acids, possibly as the result of the intracellular location of some of the viral particles and a "protective effect" caused by the presence of protein and fat. Furthermore, acid-resistant variants have been detected in several strains of FMD virus. However, Sellers (1969) found that, at 4°C., adjustment, either to pH 4.0 by hydrochloric acid or to pH 12.0 by sodium hydroxide, inactivated the virus in 2.0 and 2.5 minutes, respectively. Such severe treatment would render the milk unsuitable for consumption but might be employed to make safe large volumes of contaminated milk.

5. Coital Transmission

In addition to secreting virus in other body fluids, infected cows may liberate virus in their vaginal secretions; thus, Burrows (1968a) detected virus at titers in the range $10^{2.9}$–$10^{3.3}$ plaque forming units (p.f.u.) per sample, in the vaginas of 3 of 4 cows, at a mean period of a day before the appearance of vesicles. It must be emphasized that coital transmission has never been proved to occur in the field, nor is there much circumstantial evidence which suggests that it is a major factor in the epizootiology of the disease; nevertheless, it would seem probable that FMD may spread occasionally as a true venereal infection.

The development of extensive programs of artificial insemination (AI) in many countries, during the past 20 years, has resulted in attention being focused recently on the possibility that large numbers of female stock might become infected if semen were to be collected for AI from bulls in which the disease had entered the incubative stages. Little conclusive information is available but Cottral et al. (1968), after infecting bulls with 4 strains of virus by parenteral injection, recorded that virus was detectable in their semen within 12 to 20 hours (i.e., before vesicles appeared) and persisted for up to 10 days; 10 of 26 heifers artificially inseminated with diluted or undiluted semen developed FMD. The buffering, dilution, and freezing of semen might be expected to prolong the viability of this virus. In an experiment which also illustrated the potential dangers associated with "natural" infection of bulls in breeding establishments, Sellers et al. (1968) housed 4 bulls with 4 infected steers and, because indirect contact infection resulted in a more prolonged incubation period (5 to 10 days), virus was detected at titers to $10^{2.4}$ mouse ID50/ml. in the semen of 3 bulls at 1 to 4 days before clinical signs appeared. Spermatozoal viability decreased as a result of the disease but some libido remained even when foot lesions had rendered the animals lame. At the height of infection, viral titers up to $10^{6.2}$ ID50/ml. were encountered in the semen.

Although it is extremely unlikely that bulls exhibiting clinical signs of FMD would be employed inadvertently for breeding purposes, there can be little doubt that the possibility of dissemination of the disease by semen collected during the prodromal phase would represent a risk of such magnitude, during times of high epizooticity, that consideration should be given to restricting issues from AI Centers to samples which have been stored for periods greater than the incubation period of the disease in the donor bull.

6. MISCELLANEOUS

Tears, nasal discharge, and membranes of aborted or full-term fetuses, and their fluids, etc., are especially likely to contain virus during and immediately after periods of maximal viremia.

IV. The Carrier State among Recovered "Natural" Hosts

1. WILD STRAINS

Some 60 years ago, Loeffler (1909) stated that cattle may excrete FMD virus for up to 8 months after recovery and the subject has stimulated considerable controversy until the present time; even now, the epizootiologic importance of the carrier state remains uncertain. Well-documented outbreaks, of which carriers appear to have been the principal cause, occurred in England in 1914 and 1925, and similar outbreaks were reported in Mexico in 1945. Waldmann et al. (1931) claimed to have recovered virus from cattle at intervals up to day 246 after infection and cited circumstantial evidence for the existence of carrier animals. Similar evidence was advanced by Jerlov (1939, 1940) and by Flückiger (1943) who observed that, when lowland cattle, which had apparently recovered from FMD contracted during the winter, were moved to alpine pastures in the spring, the disease soon flared up among cattle which had remained free of infection in the alpine areas. However, there is now an indication that airborne infection may have played some part in these outbreaks. Forssman and Magnusson (1942) and Schang (1951) did not believe that carriers exerted a significant influence on the epizootiology of FMD, and this view still receives considerable support today. Indeed, only 15 years ago Voinov (1955) denied that a carrier state might exist; Fogedby (1963) believed that carriers actually transmit infection only rarely.

In the Netherlands, Dijkstra (1950) attributed 16 outbreaks, on epizootiologic grounds, to the presence of carrier cattle. The existence of carriers was established finally by the pioneer work of Van Bekkum et al. (1959) who recorded that, when samples of fluid were collected from the esophagus and pharyngeal region by means of a small metal bucket mounted on the end of a wire probang, FMD virus was regularly detectable for periods of several months. Furthermore, vaccinated cattle placed in contact with clinical cases of FMD might develop into carriers without ever showing signs of infection. Unfortunately, the reports of Dutch workers were received in several quarters with some skepticism. The veracity of this report was eventually confirmed, and the value of the probang technique was established by Sutmoller and Gaggero (1965) in South America and by Burrows (1966a) in England. Hyslop (1965c), following the renewed lead provided by Sutmoller and Gaggero, was able to isolate, in tissue culture, traces of virus of type A obtained by vigorously swabbing the pharynx and tonsillar region of recovered cattle, but it is of interest that virus was not recovered from samples of saliva collected from the same animals immediately before swabbing commenced. Wittmann and Eissner (1966) were unable to recover virus from the saliva, tonsils, or salivary glands of 6 cattle and 10 pigs at 60 to 65 days after infection.

Burrows (1966a) found that the viral titer of pharyngeal fluids might be as great as 10^3 p.f.u./ml., but generally the titer was low (about 50 p.f.u./ml. or less). Virus was recovered from 41 of 54 cattle killed for necropsy at 14 to 196 days after clinical infection; predilection sites for viral multiplication were identified as the dorsal soft palate and the walls of the pharynx, virus being recovered less frequently from the tonsillar sinus, tonsils, trachea, and esophagus. However, W. M. Henderson (1966/1967) in a valuable review of the carrier problem reported that virus may be found in the tonsillar region more consistently than elsewhere. Sutmoller and Gaggero (1965) recorded that animals in which the carrier state was detectable, at one time or another, approached 50% of all infected cattle, and virus occurred in pharyngeal scrapings despite high titers of serum antibody. Furthermore, Hyslop (1965a) observed that the saliva of recovered animals often contained inhibitory levels of a virus-neutralizing substance, presumed to be either "local" antibody or antibody originating in the serum and secreted by the salivary glands, etc. W. M. Henderson (1966/1967) reported that some carriers do not appear to produce detectable serum antibody.

The generally low virus titer of the pharyngeal fluids (Sutmoller and Cottral, 1967), the apparent periodicity of viral detection in pharyngeal fluids (several workers), the probable existence of anatomic drainage mechanisms from the oral cavity and fauces toward the esophagus (Bloomfield, 1922), and the presence of salivary antibody (Hyslop, 1965a) would seem to explain adequately the inability of numerous investigators to detect virus in the saliva of recovered cattle. Nevertheless, there can be little doubt, not only that the majority of such cattle become carriers during some part of their convalescence, but also that carrier animals may excrete virus during periods of coughing and perhaps rumination. Inapparent infection of this type is especially likely to occur in vaccinated cattle. The presence of small amounts of "carrier-virus" in the pharyngeal fluids is often masked by inhibitors, but may be revealed by treatment of the fluids with fluorocarbons (Sutmoller and Cottral, 1967).

Whether or not continuing multiplication of virus in the pharyngeal region is frequently associated with changes in the characteristics of the strain remains to be determined. However, Burrows (1966b) indicated that minor antigenic variation occurred in a strain between 14 and 17 weeks after a carrier animal first became infected. Sutmoller *et al.* (1967) showed that there might be some decrease in the infectivity of "carrier strains" for cattle, whereas infectivity for pigs was unimpaired; these observations suggest that contact between carrier cattle and pigs, or other susceptible species, could result in a flare-up of infection in the new hosts, possibly with subsequent reversion to full virulence for cattle. McVicar and Sutmoller (1969) confirmed that the presence of homologous antibody in vaccinated cattle does not materially suppress the carrier state, and they indicated that virus isolated from carriers may produce that state more efficiently than virus derived from cattle during the acute stage of FMD.

Further confirmation is necessary to establish occasional reports that virus may persist for long periods in the urogenital system and in other organs. Russian investigators have claimed that virus may even be isolated from the blood for periods of several months after apparent recovery.

Pharyngeal carriers were found among sheep (Burrows, 1968b), and the condition probably occurs in goats but has not been detected in pigs. Burrows recorded that, in contrast to his observations in cattle, virus was recovered more frequently from the tonsillar area of sheep than from the pharynx or elsewhere. The risk of spread of inapparent infection to and from the smaller ruminants, in which even the acute form of FMD is often difficult to diagnose, requires no elaboration. Therefore, when the disease is to be controlled by slaughter, it is necessary to eliminate animals of all susceptible species, including vaccinated animals, irrespective of whether or not only a single species may appear to be attacked.

The consistent results of numerous investigators now leave no doubt of the frequency with which the carrier state follows both clinical and subclinical infection; when a high proportion of animals in the population have become carriers, the probability of evolution of antigenic variants must increase; thereafter, there will exist an increasing hazard that variant strains might break through the existing herd immunity to cause a fresh wave of clinical disease.

2. Vaccine Strains

Several reports of intermittent excretion of attenuated virus, following the use of modified living strains as vaccines, were mentioned in a recent review of vaccination methods (Hyslop, 1966/1967). De Mello *et al.* (1966) indicated that periods of excretion for up to 180 days were not exceptional. Evidently, the persistence of live vaccine strains complicates still further the situation which may result from excretion of "wild" strains by convalescent animals or by exposed nonreacting vaccinates. It has been suggested (Hyslop, 1966/1967) that reasonable suspicion exists that reversion toward virulence might occur in a situation in which animals carrying persistent subclinical infection with modified strains were permitted to mingle freely with fully susceptible stock. Some degree of reversion has been observed already in at least one strain recovered from carrier cattle.

V. Living Vectors Other than "Natural" Hosts

The virus of FMD may be transmitted not only mechanically by all living animals but also cyclically, often without overt signs, by several animal species with which the disease is not popularly associated; the degree of risk to susceptible domestic livestock will depend *inter alia* on the amount of virus carried by the vector, the ambient conditions, and the degree of direct or indirect contact between vector and host.

1. MAN

Man has long been recognized as one of the principal disseminators of FMD; indeed, Moosbrugger (1960a) described human beings as "the most widely distributed, mobile, and difficult to control of all the vectors of the disease" and considered man to be of greater importance than living animals, since the dangers associated with animals are well recognized. Typical examples of the dangers inherent in the freedom of mobility and rapid transportation currently enjoyed by the human vector is revealed by the outbreak of FMD (type A) which occurred in Canada, a country hitherto free from infection (Wells, 1952; Childs, 1953; and others). Because it illustrates several important factors in the epidemiology and epizootiology of the disease, the outbreak merits description in some detail.

The virus appears to have been introduced to Canada, from a heavily infected area of Western Germany, by an agricultural worker. About 15 days after leaving the infected area in Europe, this man was employed on a farm in Saskatchewan during the first week of November 1951, *for a period of only 2 days*. His employment was terminated. About 10 days later, 7 pigs had mild illness characterized by anorexia and slight salivation. The condition passed off rapidly, causing little concern, and no further action was taken by the farmer. On November 26, cattle on the same farm developed somewhat similar symptoms but, partly as a result of aberrant reactions in horses used for differential diagnosis, the disease was diagnosed as vesicular stomatitis, an infection which was well recognized in the United States and which had been reported previously in Canada. At this stage, the signs were mild, and vesicles were not found on the feet of affected cattle. Quarantine restrictions were removed on December 8. Unfortunately, in the meantime, a few neighboring farmers had assisted with treatment of cattle on the infected premises and a mild form of the disease appeared in cattle on 2 nearby farms on or about December 10. By December 18, the disease had appeared in cattle awaiting slaughter at an abattoir, to which calves had been taken from the premises infected originally; soon afterwards, further outbreaks occurred on farms in the vicinity. In nearly all of these secondary outbreaks, transmission appears to have been mediated by the human agency, including the transfer of a farm-hand from the infected premises to a large dairy farm, on which a further outbreak occurred. The disease apparently abated during January 1952, but a recrudescence occurred with rapid reversion to characteristic virulence and invasiveness. Severe muzzle, foot, and udder lesions were reported in a high proportion of reacting animals. The condition was diagnosed provisionally as FMD on February 18 and appropriate precautions were adopted; FMD was confirmed on February 25. Full scale eradication procedures (Wells, 1952) commenced on February 29 and were completed by May 3. During the latter part of the campaign, 2 tertiary outbreaks were attributed to virus present in meat and bones which had been moved to farms from the contaminated abattoir.

Whether the virus was imported on the body of the immigrant worker, on fomites, in smuggled meat products, or as a subclinical human infection remains unknown; however, immigrants are notoriously inclined to attempt to import meat products, including local delicacies such as special sausages, among their personal effects.

Persons such as veterinarians, inseminators, livestock inspectors, and agricultural salesmen, whose occupations necessitate visits to successive farms on the same day, are especially likely to carry infection unless the most stringent precautions are adopted.

The susceptibility of man to clinical infection with the virus of FMD has been debated for many years, but there is a growing volume of evidence (Hyslop, 1970) that true infection, resulting in active excretion of virus, may occur under certain circumstances. Human excretors of virus often have a history of drinking infected milk, and young children appear to become infected more frequently than adults. Circumstantial evidence suggests that children infected by drinking milk of affected cows may have been responsible occasionally for further spread of FMD among cattle. However, clinical infection of the human adult is rare and is probably associated with an exceptional susceptibility of unknown origin. A single well-documented case was described recently by Brooksby (1967b) and by Armstrong *et al.* (1967). In this instance, as in many others, virus may have become established in the tissues of the patient as a consequence of a preexisting inflammatory condition. Clinical manifestations of human infections are usually, but not invariably, of a mild nature with a short febrile course.

2. Cats and Dogs

Galloway (1937) demonstrated that several of man's domestic pets, notably dogs and cats, may be infected with FMD virus under experimental conditions and that the disease occasionally spreads from animal to animal within these species. Epizootics among pets have never been recorded under natural conditions and cyclic transmission from them to farm livestock must be exceedingly rare. Nevertheless, such animals probably play an important part in the epizootiology of the disease, not only by wandering from infected premises to uninfected premises but also, when fed incompletely cooked scraps containing infected butchers' meat, by carrying bones, etc., to places where fully susceptible species may come in contact with such refuse. Reid (1968) cited several outbreaks during the epizootic of 1967–1968 in which circumstantial evidence tended to incriminate scavenging dogs.

3. Rodents and Other Small Mammals

Rats on infected premises are found occasionally to be clinically infected, and rats driven from their normal runways by cleaning-up operations may spread FMD mechanically. Similarly, the field vole, the gray squirrel, the Syrian hamster, and certain mice are susceptible to some extent; wild rabbits have been infected experimentally.

Hedgehogs may acquire clinical infection spontaneously on contaminated premises. Hulse and Edwards (1937) found that virus may persist in the tissues throughout the period of winter hibernation; hedgehog to hedgehog transmission occurs readily, and there is some evidence that respiratory infection may occur. Hedgehogs are frequently found in close proximity to recumbent cows, and there are strong suspicions that hedgehogs are sometimes responsible for spreading infection between contiguous premises (McLaughlan and Henderson, 1947).

The coypu (*Myocaster coypus*) may be infected by inoculation (Capel-Edwards, 1967) or by contact with infected cattle; the rapid build-up of coypu populations, as a result of escapes from nutria farms, presents an additional risk of rapid spread if FMD should occur among farm stock in the low-lying marshy areas of eastern England and elsewhere. Moles, water rats, and a wide variety of the small wild fauna of the countryside are probably equally susceptible and may play an important part in the dissemination of FMD within a limited radius from a primary outbreak.

4. Wild Game

A much greater hazard is presented in many countries by the migratory habits of the larger species of wild game, such as deer and wild pigs. In Africa, where herds of antelope may reach vast proportions, a "smoldering" type of disease may persist for long periods in infected herds, and the use of the same grazing grounds and water-holes by wild game and by cattle, sheep, and goats may result in severe outbreaks among the domestic stock. de Kock (1946) cited epizootiologic evidence for the transmission of FMD from infected game to herds of cattle which were completely isolated from other cattle by swamps and by belts of tse-tse fly country. Although Lambrechts et al. (1956) were unable to transmit FMD among kudu, cattle, and impala, their experiments were on a very small scale, and infected game were incriminated as a major source of infection in the great epizootic of type SAT-1 which occurred in South West Africa in 1961–1963 (Galloway, 1962; Viljoen, 1963, 1964; Hyslop, 1966/1967). The species principally affected in this outbreak were kudu, eland, hartebeest, springbok, steenbok, duiker, and Cape oryx, but infected impala, waterbuck, wildebeest, and sable antelope have been found during routine surveys of game. The African buffalo has been incriminated as a potent vector, frequently on purely circumstantial grounds, since lesions tend to be minimal; Lees-May and Condy (1965) during a survey of the presence of FMD antibody in game animals, found neutralizing antibody titers in the sera of 14 of 34 buffalo although FMD had not been recorded in that area for 25 years. Condy et al. (1969) found significant antibody titers in sera from 77 of 116 buffalo and in the sera of 15 of 38 other African animals. Hedger et al. (1969) recovered virus from epithelial samples collected by scraping the pharyngeal region of buffalo which were devoid of clinical signs of FMD when killed; occasionally, the virus was of a type which had not been reported among local domestic livestock for many years. The Indian buffalo is very susceptible and usually exhibits frank clinical disease. Bush pigs and warthogs also have lesions, but, in the latter species, virus may be found only in deep-seated vesicles below the thick carpal pads. Tapirs are infected occasionally.

An important factor in the dissemination of FMD in Africa is the marked tendency of many species of wild game to abandon their natural habits and grazing areas when the disease appears in their herds, and often to travel great distances, spreading infection as they move.

The disease is reported occasionally in camels, dromedaries, giraffes, and elephants (R. Pringle, 1880; Nocard and Leclainche, 1903; Urbain *et al.*, 1938), but diagnosis has usually depended on clinical observations rather than on isolation of virus. The mouflon, lama, alpaca, yak, elk and American bison are susceptible. Keane (1924) reported that North American deer were highly susceptible; in Europe, outbreaks have been recorded in deer, reindeer, bison, and in the wild descendents of escaped domestic pigs.

Although the great carnivores do not reveal clinical signs of FMD, they are capable of transferring virus mechanically and may carry a great amount of virus immediately after feeding on an infected animal of one of the "natural" host species. Carrion-eating animals and birds, especially the common crow, may spread fragments of infected carcasses over a wide area. Foxes hunt over long distances in inclement weather and have been blamed for the extension of outbreaks in England.

Snowdon (1968) found that kangaroos might transmit the disease to cattle under experimental conditions, but concluded that Australian wild fauna would be unlikely to play a major part in disseminating infection.

5. Birds

Although domestic poultry may be infected rarely by parenteral inoculation of certain strains of virus, all birds are considered to be refractory; their role in the dissemination of FMD has been the subject of discussion since Mettam (1914) first drew attention to birds as the possible vector of an inexplicable outbreak in Ireland. Stockman and Garnett (1923) were unable to exclude birds as a source of spread over long distances, and mechanical transmission over distances of a few miles is obviously likely to occur, but the evidence adduced has usually depended only on coincidence of the time of bird migration with outbreaks of the disease. Nevertheless, a quite remarkable association has been observed between outbreaks of FMD in western Europe, bird migrations to the British Isles, and outbreaks of FMD on farms (especially on the east coast) where large numbers of migratory birds have been seen. Rooks, jackdaws, lapwings, ducks, geese, and wood pigeons have been suggested as species likely to carry the disease but, because of its pasture-feeding habits, close association with grazing animals, and gregarious nature, the starling (*Sturnus vulgaris*) has attracted most attention in recent years. Idso (1943), on purely circumstantial grounds, suggested that seagulls, feeding on the dunghills of contaminated premises, might have been responsible for simultaneous outbreaks in isolated and unfrequented districts.

Bullough (1942) and Wilson and Matheson (1952), citing statistical records collected during 50 years, believed that a *prima facie* case had been established against birds, and especially against migratory starlings. Despite numerous and repeated attempts, FMD virus has never been isolated from birds captured or killed in the wild state; however, the slight probability of selecting for capture the small number of infected birds from the vast numbers presented by migrating flocks renders a negative observation almost meaningless. Although bird migration may have been the means by which FMD reached coastal regions of Britain during the major epizootic of 1952, and also on other occasions, several outbreaks having similar characteristics occurred in these areas long after migration had ceased, or even when migration in the opposite direction should have commenced. Ornithologists are exceedingly critical of some of the "evidence" purporting to incriminate birds, but perhaps not all of such criticism has been completely impartial and unbiased.

Although FMD virus was not isolated from the feathers or carcasses of 54 living and 389 dead wild birds (some of which were marked with rings or tags of Dutch or German origin) found on infected farms, and although the living birds failed to infect susceptible cattle with which they were placed in close proximity, Eccles (1939) nevertheless reported sound experimental proof that birds may carry the virus for short periods. Virus sprayed on the feathers of starlings was detectable by guinea pig inoculation 91 hours later. When birds were dosed orally with viral suspensions, virus was subsequently detectable in their feces for 26 hours. Captured starlings were placed in close contact with experimentally infected cattle at the height of their clinical reaction; in 1 of 2 experiments, susceptible cattle became infected when the contaminated birds were introduced into their looseboxes. Similarly, when about 40 pigeons, placed in contact with infected cattle, were later flown to boxes containing susceptible cattle and pigs, the cattle became infected but the pigs remained healthy. In Eccles' series of experiments, negative results were recorded more frequently than positive results; but, having regard to the differences of invasiveness and species-predilection of various strains of FMD, and also to the prevailing dependence on the guinea pig as a test animal, the results obtained are truly remarkable.

Mead (1968) recorded that birds of any species have a potential flight range of hundreds of miles in one "hop," but he was unable to correlate outbreaks of FMD in England with the arrival of birds from the Continent.

6. ARTHROPODS

Schang (1957) considered that wild animals, birds, and insects do not spread FMD frequently in South America and, until very recently, many workers on that continent believed that double-fenced paddocks were sufficient to prevent the spread of FMD between adjacent groups of experimental cattle. Nevertheless, the possibility of transmission, either mechanically or "cyclically," by "insects" has received serious consideration by European workers for many years (Roch Marra, 1908; Galloway, 1937; Waldmann and Hirschfelder, 1938). There can no longer be any serious doubt that the disease may be disseminated by arthropods; and it must be appreciated that flying species are occasionally carried thousands of miles from their normal habitat by air currents, e.g., tropical moths, probably originating in the Sahara area of North Africa, have been carried as far as the British Isles.

The period during which virus remains viable on or within the body of invertebrate hosts probably depends partly on ambient conditions. Virus may be detected in the bowel contents of houseflies fed on virus mixed with sugar, but the duration of infectivity seldom exceeds 24 hours although Rozov (1966) found that virus could be recovered for up to 48 hours. Because of the long transit time, it appears doubtful whether virus would be carried frequently over great distances by insects. It is unlikely that multiplication of virus ever occurs in the cells of invertebrates; consequently, it may be considered incorrect to employ the term cyclic to describe somatic infection of arthropods. Nevertheless, Dhennin *et al.* (1961) detected virus in the triturated bodies of flies (*Musca* and *Lucilia* species) which had settled on fragments of epithelium from bovine lesions. Similarly, virus was detected by these workers in ticks and keds, *Ixodes ricinus* and *Melophagus ovinus*, which had been allowed to feed on infected animals. Galloway (1937) observed that the tick *Argas persicus* might transmit infection; spiders failed to do so. Lukin (1963) fed *Dermacentor pictus* and *D. marginatus* on infected rabbits and was able to transmit infection to susceptible animals by means of tick bites; transovarial infection of part of the tick population was observed and virus persisted in ticks for up to 105 days after feeding. Kunetsova *et al.* (1966) found that FMD may be transmitted by adults of the species *Rhipicephalus* and *Hyalomma*, but the virus was not recovered from the eggs, nymphs, or larvae of infected adult ticks. The importance of tick-borne infection in the epizootiology of FMD remains uncertain.

It is now suggested that all ectoparasites may spread FMD from animal to animal over short distances and that biting flies such as *Stomoxys*, *Tabanus*, and *Glossina* may transmit infection over a somewhat greater area; however, the hematophagous species are unlikely to become infected unless they take a blood meal during the fairly brief periods during which viremia occurs in infected animals.

Although many of the invertebrate vectors mentioned seldom travel very far from their customary breeding areas, the development of fast international travel facilities, by airlines and by express freight services, renders necessary extreme vigilance if insect-borne diseases are to be controlled. In practice, however, the operation of the "Blocks-on" procedure, whereby insecticides are released after take-off and the cabin staff of aircraft must deliver to the Airport Health Officer, immediately on landing, an appropriate number (based on the volume of the aircraft) of empty insecticide aerosol containers, is believed to control effectively all insects which may enter at previous stops.

7. EARTHWORMS

Lumbricus terrestris, maintained in infected soil for several days by Dhennin *et al.* (1963), were washed for 30 minutes, triturated, and then inoculated intralingually in susceptible cattle; lesions of FMD developed in 2 of 3 experiments. Although transmission is thus theoretically possible, infected worms have never been found in association with field outbreaks. It appears to be just possible that during cold weather virus might persist in buried worms until the infected premises were restocked, but eradication of worm populations is clearly impossible.

VI. Dissemination in Meat, in Animal By-products, and by Inanimate Objects

1. MEAT

The importation of living animals of species susceptible to FMD is rigidly controlled in nearly all countries; in many, the importation of fresh meat is also either prohibited or controlled.

Despite routine *antemortem* examination, virus may be distributed widely in the tissues of animals inadvertently slaughtered during the incubative stages of the disease. During the past 40 years, it has become well established that virus may remain viable in the chilled or frozen carcasses of unvaccinated animals for as long as chilled meat remains marketable, and for at least 3 months in frozen meat. Virus, which is readily detectable in the musculature for up to 30 hours after slaughter, is usually killed by the release of lactic acid during "maturation" of meat at 4°C. Occasionally, and especially in carcasses which fail to "set" properly, virus may be detected for a period of about 1 month. Considerably longer periods of survival, i.e., at least 8 months, have been observed in meat which has been "quick frozen" without a period of maturation. Endocrine glands which are collected and frozen for pharmaceutical purposes may be a source of direct or indirect infection.

Processes, other than heat treatment, used for preservation of meat often tend to inhibit inactivation of virus, so that bacon, ham, and certain types of sausage may remain infective for about 2 months. However, when very protracted "pickling" processes are employed, viral viability may have disappeared by the time that the product is released for sale.

Although the musculature of carcasses presents considerable danger, by far the most serious hazard is the persistence of virus for 4 to 7 months in lymph nodes, bone marrow, and other offals stored at 1 to 4°C. All these are especially likely to be discarded with garbage. Further information on the persistence of virus in meat may be found in reports by W. M. Henderson and Brooksby (1948), Moosbrugger (1960b), Cottral et al. (1960), Cox et al. (1961), Brooksby (1962), Savi and Baldelli (1962), Wisniewski (1962), Gailiunas and Cottral (1964), and Cottral (1969). Heidelbaugh and Graves (1968) recorded, predictably, that heat processing at 155°F. or curing in citric acid–salt mixtures reduced the infectivity of virus in lymph nodes; tenderizing enzymes were ineffective. However, the observations of Dimopoulos et al. (1959), mentioned previously, indicate that complete inactivation of all virus may be difficult to achieve.

When attenuated strains of virus have been used for vaccination, the possibility of persistence of virus in meat must always remain a serious consideration; many countries prohibit importation of meat from areas in which living FMD vaccines are known to be used.

The link between infected meat and susceptible livestock is often difficult to establish with certainty. Contact with persons who have handled infected meat, chopping blocks, utensils, or wrappings has been demonstrated occasionally. More frequently, outbreaks start, often very insidiously, among pigs fed on bones, scraps trimmed from meat, or inadequately heated pig-swill originating from hotels, army camps, etc. In Great Britain the boiling of all pig-swill is prescribed by Government Order. Some years ago, in a series of 93 outbreaks in England no less than 73 started in pigs; in almost every case, raw swill had been delivered to the premises. The handling of raw swill on the premises increases greatly the chance of accidental contamination. Wilson and Matheson (1952) recorded that in 365 primary outbreaks, 223 occurred in pigs, 134 in cattle, and 8 in sheep.

Cabot (1945) reported several primary outbreaks, not always in pigs, on premises owned by butchers who regularly handled imported meat; outbreaks seldom commenced in areas where local meat production was nearly adequate for the requirements of the district. In a series of 540 primary outbreaks in Great Britain (1938–53), no fewer than 264 were attributed to the importation of meat from infected areas abroad; in a similar series from 1964–1969, 97 of 179 primary outbreaks were attributable to imported meat or meat wrappings.

The foregoing observations apply generally to meat from unvaccinated animals. The increasing use of inactivated vaccines by meat-producing countries may have modified the dangers of dissemination of FMD in beef carcasses. The recent report (Anonymous, 1966) of the Argentine–United States Joint Commission on Foot and Mouth Disease indicated that vaccination greatly reduced the probability of recovery of viable virus from lymph nodes of cattle exposed to infection 32 hours before slaughter; it was also concluded that salt-cured meat constituted very little risk. It is the writer's opinion that some caution is necessary, because the probability of complete elimination of virus may depend to some extent on the degree of antigenic similarity between the strain of virus employed in the vaccine and that to which the animal was exposed before slaughter.

Solely for reasons of economy, routine vaccination of sheep has rarely been considered sound policy in the major meat-producing countries, and FMD continues to smolder in sheep in several areas. The identification of a few infected animals on clinical grounds, during *antemortem* inspection of large flocks of sheep, may be surprisingly difficult. Circumstantial evidence (Reid, 1968) strongly suggests that the major epizootic of 1967–1968 in England may have been caused by virus present in sheep carcasses imported from South America; the Foot and Mouth Disease (Imported Meat) (No. 2) Order, 1968, provides for the licensing of distribution of sheep carcasses originating in South America. Routine vaccination of sheep is now commencing in at least one South American country.

The Northumberland Committee of Enquiry into the epizootic of 1967–1968 indicated the desirability of prohibiting importation of all but boned meat and offal processed in a manner sufficient to kill FMD virus.

2. MILK

The danger of susceptible animals coming in contact with infected milk has been mentioned previously and will not be described further. In Great Britain, the Diseases of Animals (Milk Treatment) (Amendment) Order of 1968 now requires that all milk and milk derivatives, from areas declared to be Controlled FMD Areas, shall be heat treated before being fed to animals.

3. HIDES AND SKINS

Virus contaminating the hair or wool of living animals is unlikely to remain viable for periods exceeding 4 weeks; Voinov (1968) after deliberately contaminating the body surfaces of sheep and cattle was unable to detect survival of virus for periods greater than 20 days. However, during the period of clinical infection and probably for a short period thereafter, the virus is detectable in biopsy samples of all epithelial structures, irrespective of whether or not vesicles are present. Viral titers may be as great as $10^{5.0}$ p.f.u. per gram of tissue. Gailiunas and Cottral (1967) investigated the duration of infectivity in hides preserved by 4 conventional methods. The virus remained detectable in green-salted hides for up to 90 days at 15°C. and for 352 days at 4°C.; hides cured in salt and chlorine were infective for 4 weeks at 15°C.; samples, air dried at 20°C. for 42 days, still contained virus at the end of that period; infectively was detectable in samples cured in salt for 7 days and then air dried for 21 days. Recovered virus was fully infective for cattle, and the authors noted that the periods determined by their experimental results should not be considered to be the utmost limits of survival.

4. VEHICLES

a. Road Vehicles

There are obvious possibilities of the passive carriage of virus on all road vehicles, but certain vehicles appear to possess particular dangers. This class includes vehicles used for the transport of farm livestock (special instructions for the cleansing of such conveyances exist in most countries) and those used to deliver feeding-stuffs. The infectivity of milk in the prodromal phase has been described, and milk vehicles visiting a series of farms every day are especially likely to spread infection if the driver is in the habit of dismounting to converse with farm staff, or if leakage occurs when pipe couplings are made. Modern tank vehicles operating at pressures which differ from the ambient are likely to be potent disseminators unless special precautions are adopted.

b. Railways

Outbreaks have been reported in Norway, on farms adjoining railway tracks, after the passage of animals subsequently found to have been incubating the disease. Flückiger (1956) recorded a series of outbreaks which followed the transportation of a consignment of pigs infected with virus of type C from Belgium to Switzerland; however, since some of the outbreaks in this series were diagnosed as being of types other than type C, it is probable that not all had a common origin. Pilz and Garbe (1960) described measures for the routine decontamination of railway trucks.

c. Aircraft

Aircraft are unlikely to be involved directly in the spread of FMD, but the rapidity of air travel increases the likelihood of virus being carried from one country to another by infected animals, human beings, arthropods, packing materials, or postal traffic. Attempts to disinfect travelers and their baggage are unlikely to do more than reduce the burden of infection.

5. AGRICULTURAL PRODUCTS, IMPLEMENTS, ETC.

a. Utensils

Local dissemination of FMD from farms has been reported frequently as a result of transfer of virus on buckets, tools, etc.

b. Bedding, Packing Materials

The use of imported straw, wood-shavings, etc., as bedding for farm animals is prohibited in many countries. Virus has been shown to persist for at least 46 days at room temperature on wrapping cloths from meat. All foreign packing materials must be regarded with suspicion, especially if FMD is known to exist in the country of origin.

c. Water, Fodder, Farm Produce, etc.

Water, contaminated by shreds of infected epithelium, may contain virus for as long as 67 days, though Voinov (1967) was unable to recover virus after 15 days immersion during summer and autumn.

Materials such as hay, straw, bran, flour, and sugar favor the survival of virus for long periods, and complete decontamination of the interior of bales and stacks is virtually impossible. The observations of Bedson, Maitland, and Burbury and other investigators (Series of five Reports of the British Foot and Mouth Disease Research Committee, 1925, 1927, 1928, 1931, 1937) indicated that virus may survive for many months under optimal conditions. Moosbrugger (1954) mentioned hay, straw, bran, flour, green vegetables, seeds, and peat as vehicles of infection, and reported that virus was recovered from commercial feeding-stuffs in 4 of 11 instances in which the epizootiologic picture was suggestive of infection by such products. Traub (1954) also discussed the spread of infection by contaminated plant products. Boiko (1960) recorded that virus may survive on hay for longer than 200 days. Nevertheless, Moosbrugger (1960a) considered that agricultural products, though never negligible, were unimportant factors in the dissemination of FMD.

6. BUILDINGS

At the end of an outbreak, virus may remain viable but undetected for long periods in buildings which have been cleansed inadequately. Old buildings with many structural crevices are especially difficult to decontaminate. It is customary, therefore, to restock at first with only a few "indicator" animals. The precise duration of residual infection will depend on the interaction of multiple factors, including temperature, sunlight, etc. However, Russian investigators have indicated that buildings may remain contaminated for at least a month in warm weather and for more than two months in winter.

During March–April 1968, 12 outbreaks were reported in England from farms on which infection had occurred during the major epizootic of 1967–1968 and which were restocked subsequently. However, considering the large number of outbreaks (>2,300) which resulted in the slaughter of nearly 500,000 animals during the main epizootic, the number of recurrences does not seem great.

7. PASTURES

Little convincing information is available regarding the longevity of FMD virus in the open air. Voinov (1956) recorded that virus might persist for 2 to 5 days on pastures during the summer months, and Shilnikov (1959) found that virus survived for 30 days when the average air temperature was 1.3°C. These observations should not be disparaged, but it is unwise to attempt to extrapolate figures from one set of conditions to another; these results are, at best, only a guide and probably underestimate the durability of the virus. By contrast, several investigators in South America believe that pastures become free of infection after only about 10 days. Campion and Gatto (1961) succeeded in infecting cattle only twice in eleven experiments, during which cattle were grazed on pasture vacated, only 22–95 hours previously, by clinically infected animals. However, because numerous factors in addition to survival of virus must play an important part in initiating infection, negative results have little meaning.

VII. Airborne Infection

1. EARLY FIELD OBSERVATIONS

The dissemination of FMD by air currents received little attention until recently, although there are records of several instances in which virus may have been carried for quite long distances in this way. Thus, for example, Danish investigators attributed outbreaks on the Islands of Denmark, during periods of strong S or SW winds, to airborne spread from Germany; it was impossible to exclude contact by human or other agencies, particularly birds, between the Islands and Germany, but it is interesting that during the same periods the disease advanced only slowly by contact across the land frontier to the mainland (Jutland) part of Denmark. Similarly, primary outbreaks occurred in southern Norway and Sweden, often on very isolated farms, at times when the disease was prevalent in northern Denmark; direct contact between these farms and Denmark was considered to be unlikely. However, Jerlov (1940) recorded an instance in which infection was believed to have been introduced by a German fishing boat, so the possibility of human contact cannot be excluded in every case. The importance of these early reports was confirmed by Michelsen (1968) who also described a series of outbreaks in 1966, which occurred about 3 miles down-wind from the State Veterinary Institute for Virus Research, Lindholm, Denmark, and from which virus may have been carried 40 to 60 miles across the Baltic Sea to Sweden.

2. AERIAL SPREAD ON PARTICULATE MATTER AND IN MICRODROPLETS

Poppe and Busch (1936) observed that the virus may survive for several days when adsorbed to molds, yeasts, and spores, and McLean (1938) suggested that viruses, including FMD, may be transported for long distances by air currents when adsorbed to fine particulate matter. Ludlam (1967) described the factors influencing the circulation of dusts in the air and stated that small particles may remain in the winds of the troposphere long enough to circumnavigate the hemisphere. Pitty (1968) also observed that small size was an important factor in travel of particles for long distances; particles less than 9 microns in diameter could remain airborne almost indefinitely; Pitty noted that loess found on flat surfaces in England in July 1968 was of Saharan origin, having been carried up to 35,000 feet by strong thermal currents.

It would be unwise to deduce too much from the foregoing reports because dehydration, oxidation, and the relatively intense solar ultraviolet and other radiation, to which particles would be exposed at high altitudes, would probably inactivate much of any virus which might be adsorbed to airborne dusts, etc. At lower altitudes, however, cool cloudy weather would be likely to increase the longevity of viral particles, and periods of precipitation would tend to wash out suspended virus and thus contaminate the ground beneath with small quantities of virus.

Because of differences in viability and in the rate of settling-out, it is important to differentiate between dustborne virus, virus on large drops of saliva, and virus present in microdroplets or their nuclei. Fresdorf (1949) believed droplet infection to be an important factor in the epizootiology of FMD.

The long strings of saliva which may be observed to be carried from the lips of cattle by the wind usually do not travel very far. However, Hyslop (1965b) suggested that the smacking movements of the tongue and the often foamy nature of the saliva of infected animals, during the acute phase, may result in the dissemination of large numbers of small infective droplets, almost as soon as the mucosa of the tongue begins to liberate virus. Infective droplets are certainly released during coughing or snorting and are probably released during rumination.

There have been several reports of the accidental release of virus from research institutes and from laboratories manufacturing FMD vaccines. Many of these probably resulted from failure in personal hygiene measures or from the sale of meat salvaged from infected animals. However, airborne virus may have been the cause of local outbreaks on several occasions. In January 1960, an outbreak of the type SAT-2, exotic to England, occurred on a farm at Worplesdon, Surrey. These premises were situated about 2 miles downwind from the Animal Virus Research Institute, Pirbright. After a considerable amount of investigation, it was concluded that the virus probably originated in an isolation compound containing cattle infected with type SAT-2, and that it may have been carried for at least part of the distance by the wind. At that time, the compounds were not fitted with air filtration apparatus. A further release of virus downwind occurred in 1967 (Reid, 1968) when the air filtration system of an infected cattle compound became damaged and resulted in the infection of animals in a neighboring compound; fortunately, virus was not carried to animals beyond the perimeter of the Institute. Incidents attributable to release of airborne virus have occurred in other research institutes and vaccine production plants.

3. Milking Machines, Milk Distribution Methods

In addition to the exhalations of infected animals, a large number of factors may lead to the production of infective aerosols. Maffey (1961b) agreed that exhaust air from several of the milking machines described by him (Maffey, 1961a) might well be contaminated by infective droplets whenever virus was secreted in the milk; there is also some danger from the milk-release mechanisms of some autorecorder systems. Recent observations of the high virus titers present in milk indicate that a small volume of infected milk may constitute a serious hazard even when pooled with large volumes of uninfected milk. Furthermore, investigations during the disastrous epizootic of 1967–1968 in England revealed that some of the vehicles used to collect milk from farms were equipped to siphon the milk from the farm receiver-vessels into large vehicle tanks maintained at pressures below the ambient. As the vehicles proceeded along country roads, with considerable agitation of the milk, the vacuum system operated intermittently, exhausting air to the exterior from a tank containing a large volume of potentially infected milk. Until the air exhaust systems of the vehicles were fitted with filters capable of retaining microdroplets, a serious risk of airborne infection must have existed.

4. FARM EFFLUENT AEROSOLS

Additional potential sources of airborne infection have been identified in new methods of farm sewage disposal. Instead of stacking manure, it is becoming customary on some larger dairy farms to mix urine, feces, and effluent water from the milking parlor, etc., with additional water to form a "slurry." This liquid is then pumped from the mixing tank into ditches or shallow lagoons or, alternatively, is either spread from vehicles or sprayed from high-pressure "rain guns" on agricultural land. All these methods constitute, in increasing progression, considerable hazards to other livestock because of the airborne dissemination of pathogenic organisms of many kinds.

5. EFFECTS OF PRESSURE DIFFERENTIALS IN ENCLOSED SPACES

Pressure changes in vessels, drainage systems, or buildings containing infected fluids may result in release of FMD virus to the air. Primault (1955, 1958), a meteorologist, recorded an apparent association between a fall in barometric pressure and subsequent outbreaks of FMD, though the mode of infection was not indicated.

6. THE EPIZOOTIC IN ENGLAND IN 1967–1968

The primary outbreak of the 1967–1968 epizootic was attributed to the importation of infected lamb carcasses from South America (Reid, 1968) and, because of meterologic conditions during the critical period, Hurst (1968) considered that long-distance transmission in airstreams from European foci was unlikely. Nevertheless, there are indications that the wind subsequently played an important part in the early dissemination of virus from farm to farm over distances of several miles.

Although more than a single primary focus may have occurred, FMD of type O_1 was first reported in pigs on a farm at Nantmawr near Oswestry in Shropshire. The area consists principally of intensively developed farms with a dense population of high-yielding livestock. At the time of the primary outbreaks and for several days thereafter, strong winds were blowing from the southwest. Despite the strict control of stock movement in the area and the implementation of the usual policy of slaughter on all infected premises, further foci of infection occurred in a narrow wedge-shaped zone to the northeast of the infected premises. The frequency of occurrence in the northeast quadrant diminished with increasing distance from the primary outbreak, in a manner which suggested random fall-out of infective particles from a moving airstream.

In the succeeding 5 weeks, lateral spread of tertiary and subsequent outbreaks, numbering more than 1,000 in this short period, tended to modify the picture and the greatest number occurred about a month after the first outbreak. However, in December 1967, map plots of all the infected premises notified by the Ministry of Agriculture, Fisheries and Food up to that time, still showed a well-defined wedge-shaped distribution extending from the region of Oswestry across Cheshire into Westmorland. The most distant outbreak in the series, near Carnforth in Westmorland, was attributed to the presence in the district of lamb meat originating in the Argentine; consequently the outbreak must be regarded as an additional late primary focus.

During the early phase of the epizootic, a temporary veering of the wind to a more westerly bearing was followed by the appearance of a small number of outbreaks, roughly in line, lying to the east of the main axis of the epizootic. Davies *et al.* (1968) noted that late spread to East Shropshire and Staffordshire was associated with a marked shift in wind direction to northeast and that efforts to contain the main epizootic may have been aided by two ridges of high pressure which resulted in decreased wind velocity at a critical period. In November, the disease spread, probably as a result of milk-borne infection of pigs, to three farms in Worcestershire. R. J. Henderson (1969) described the subsequent distribution of numerous additional outbreaks in which the wind apparently was the principal cause of viral dissemination over short distances. Occasionally, belts of trees may have afforded some protection by deflecting air currents, but housing of cattle only delayed the spread of the disease.

The unusual features associated with this epizootic have been attributed to unique properties of the strain, notably to a high degree of virulence and to a special ability to exist for long periods in aerial suspension, though evidence to support the latter premise is lacking. Recently, strains of virus of type O_1 had been eradicated only with considerable difficulty in Switzerland and elsewhere, and there is some indication that the Shropshire strain may have been slightly more resistant to physical and chemical agents than "older" strains of type O. Certain strains do appear to be better able to persist in the airborne state than others. Unpublished investigations, on aerosols of type SAT-1 virus maintained under conditions standardized as far as possible in small cloud chambers, revealed that the viability of strain Tur 323/62 regressed more slowly in aerial suspension than that of strain SA 13/61. However, no convincing proof has been adduced, to suggest that the strain responsible for the 1967–1968 epizootic differed markedly from other current strains of type O. Furthermore, two other outbreaks of type O_1 had occurred in Hampshire and Warwickshire during 1967; in neither instance, was airborne spread a major characteristic, although both strains of virus appeared to be identical in all other respects with that isolated in Shropshire. The most important factors in the Shropshire epizootic appear to have been:

1. The invasiveness of the strain of virus.
2. The rapid build-up of infection in a piggery.
3. The unfortunate occurrence, before diagnosis could be established, of high winds blowing toward an area containing fully susceptible livestock.
4. The overall density of the animal population in north Shropshire and Cheshire, and the housing of stock often in relatively large units.
5. Cool cloudy weather which may have contributed to the longevity of the virus.

When exposure to minimal concentrations of airborne virus occurs in circumstances such as these, a real danger of an early "silent" build-up of carrier animals, especially sheep, must exist. Experimental evidence of this hazard is described later.

More than 2,360 separate outbreaks were confirmed before the epizootic was finally eradicated, but it is likely that only a proportion of these were attributable to direct airborne spread; others may have been linked with further imported lamb carcasses. Eradication was achieved as a result of sustained efforts by the staff of the Animal Health Division of the Ministry of Agriculture, Fisheries and Food with the invaluable assistance of veterinarians from Australia, Canada, Ireland, New Zealand, U. S. A., and elsewhere. Success was achieved by traditional methods of slaughter and the control of movement; more than 440,000 animals were slaughtered and by February 1968 the cost of compensation alone had exceeded £25,000,000 ($62,000,000). The real cost of the epizootic is incalculable, though Meyer (1969) cited losses estimated to be in excess of $240,000,000.

Smith and Hugh-Jones (1969), in reviewing reports of this and 4 other epizootics, calculated an "epidemic intensity index" which was weighted less for daytime rainfall than for rainfall at night; only 15 of 280 affected farms did not lie within a rain-wind "danger sector" at a time when infection might have occurred. The observations of Sellers and Parker (1969) and annotations by Norris and Harper (1970) and by Chamberlain (1970) emphasize the importance of particle dimensions in relation to deposition on herbage and to infection by inhalation. Particles larger than about 10 microns in diameter are very susceptible to washout by rain, whereas particles in the range 2–10 microns are most readily entrapped in the respiratory tract. The relative importance of ingestion and inhalation of airborne virus remains to be established, but, because only small numbers of viral particles appear to be required to establish

FMD by inhalation, the respiratory tract probably is the most frequent portal of airborne infection.

7. LABORATORY INVESTIGATIONS

To determine whether microdroplets of FMD virus suspended in air were infective, Hyslop (1955), using an apparatus designed for studies on bovine contagious pleuropneumonia (Hyslop and Ford, 1957; Hyslop, 1963), nebulized virus within a loose box containing cattle. Two animals became clinically infected. Thorne and Burrows (1960) were able to recover viable virus from experimentally generated "aerosols" in a small glass cloud-chamber, though some of the virus was probably present in fairly large droplets which might be expected to fall out of suspension within a short-time. Thorne and Hyslop (1960), employing a Porton impinger (D. W. Henderson, 1952; May and Harper, 1957), were able to detect virus in air passing through the roof ventilators of boxes containing infected cattle. Fogedby et al. (1960) described an experiment apparently made some years previously, in which they found that susceptible cattle, when placed in an atmosphere deliberately contaminated with sterilized hay dust, became infected by an air draught directed across infected cattle which were maintained at a distance of 10 meters. From the experiments of Thorne and Hyslop and Fogedby et al., it remains a matter of opinion whether infection was airborne or dustborne. Furthermore, Traub and Wittmann (1957), who did not contaminate the atmosphere with dust, failed to transmit the disease to susceptible animals in somewhat similar experiments. Moosbrugger (1948) recorded that a calf kept in a building used for vaccine production did not become infected as a result of airborne virus but was infected by contaminated hay.

By arranging multiple impingers in parallel, Hyslop (1965b) was able to sample air at rates up to 100 cubic feet per hour within isolation boxes containing cattle reacting to virus of types SAT-1 and SAT-2; subsequently, viruses of other types were collected. Somewhat better recovery was obtained when the Porton impinger, the curved inlet tube of which was designed originally to simulate the human nasopharynx, was replaced by an impinger fitted with a straight tube projecting through a baffle. These methods were successful regularly in detecting airborne virus before clinical signs of FMD were evident. Thereafter, virus could be recovered from the air for periods up to 14 days. Less success was achieved with electrostatic virus-sampling methods similar to those described by Houwink and Rolvink (1957) and Morris et al. (1961); although the electrostatic methods may collect virus more efficiently, it appears that its viability may be impaired. Sellers and Parker (1969) reported confirmatory observations on cattle, sheep, and pigs, and noted that relative humidity greater than 70% and low temperature favored the survival of FMD virus of type O.

In preliminary transmission experiments by Hyslop (1965b), cattle were exposed to aerosols of virus by means of a face mask; in some cases, a filter capable of retaining dust and bacteria was included in the system. In an experiment with type O virus, 5 of 6 cattle became infected and, because the inclusion of filters did not affect the results, it was concluded that FMD may be caused by true aerosols of small droplets or droplet nuclei.

McKercher et al. (1966) described two experiments at the Plum Island Animal Disease Laboratory, New York, in which the air system was deliberately placed in a state of imbalance, so that air flowed from rooms housing infected cattle into rooms housing susceptible cattle. In one experiment, 4 of 10 animals developed FMD of type A₁; the results were considered to confirm preceding reports of airborne infection. Kiryukhin and Pasechnikov (1966) recovered virus from the exhaled air of 7 calves, at titers from 6.3 to 630 calf ID50/liter, at about a day after the onset of signs. Michelsen (1968) discussed further evidence for aerial transmission of FMD.

The degree of immunity against airborne infection afforded by vaccination remains to be determined, though Hyslop (1965b) showed that 2 steers vaccinated successfully, and having serum neutralization indices of 2.15 and 2.67, were resistant to respiratory infection with homologous virus of type C, whereas 2 unvaccinated steers developed generalized FMD. After investigations on a large number of fully susceptible animals, about 18 to 24 months old, some of which were exposed to respiratory tract infection by tracheotomy and tracheal intubation, the writer concluded that airborne infection often evokes a somewhat milder form of the disease than that resulting from parenteral or oral infection. The incubation period was in the range 2½ to 9 days but, unless large doses of virus were administered, periods exceeding 6 days predominated. The first clinical sign was usually transient pyrexia. The temperature generally fell and then increased again before vesicles appeared. After respiratory infection, vesicles often either appeared first on the feet, instead of on the tongue, or on the feet and in the oral cavity virtually simultaneously. These observations suggest that, after inhalation of virus, the primary site of viral multiplication may be in the organs of the thorax and not in the parts of the body usually considered to be predilection sites. Indeed, in a significant proportion of these cases, vesicles did not appear on the tongue at any stage of the disease. It is probable that the minor traumata of everyday life play an important part in determining the site at which lesions appear after virus has generalized from a primary focus in the thorax. Studies of the pathogenesis of airborne FMD revealed that virus did not multiply rapidly in the lung parenchyma, but usually was detectable first in the bronchial or mediastinal lymph nodes. Some multiplication appears to occur in the epithelial cells of the bronchi, and Korn (1957) suggested that the nasal mucosa also may be a site of replication of virus. Clinically inapparent infections, associated with seroconversion to titers exceeding 1/512, were observed on several occasions during our experiments.

Impinger-sampling of air from catheters inserted in the lower trachea and bronchi of cattle, exposed to aerosols by tracheal cannulation, indicated that adsorption and pulmonary ventilation removed virus from the tidal air by the end of the first day. By the end of the second day, however, and before clinical signs were evident, the exhaled air often contained infective virus again.

It is noteworthy that virus of type Asia 1, collected from the exhaled air of animals infected by the respiratory route, was fully infective for other cattle when resuspended as an aerosol. Thus, serial passage may occur by the respiratory route.

8. Inapparent Infections

Subclinical infection with the virus of FMD has been observed under conditions which suggest that the virus was disseminated by air currents (Hyslop, 1965c, 1967a; Fagg and Hyslop, 1966). As a typical example of inapparent infection among cattle maintained under carefully controlled conditions, 2 steers were each exposed to an aerosol containing 100 ID50 of FMD virus, type Asia 1. The animals were exposed and housed separately. One steer developed generalized FMD (confirmed by complement-fixation tests as type Asia 1), whereas the other had only slight pyrexia (103.0°F.) lasting less than a day. The latter steer did not develop visible lesions at any time but, by day 9, the viral neutralizing titer of its serum was 1/1024. At the end of the experiment, both steers were immune to reinfection by intralingual inoculation of homologous virus.

Sheep infected with FMD sometimes have only minimal clinical signs (Stockman and Minette, 1926; Geering, 1967; and others) and detection may be especially difficult when concurrent infection with *Fusiformis* spp. exists in the flock. Recently, there have been increasing grounds for suspicion that a proportion of sheep exposed to airborne virus may undergo a wholly subclinical type of infection; some of them may carry virus in the pharyngeal region for a considerable period thereafter.

In preliminary transmission experiments, 5 sheep (3 Merino and 2 Persian black-head) were exposed briefly to an aerosol of virus of type A.

Transient temperature reactions were observed in 2 Merinos but none of the sheep developed vesicles. After 4 weeks, the immunity of all sheep was challenged by intralingual inoculation of homologous virus. None developed overt lesions, whereas 2 of 3 control sheep reacted with high temperatures and small thin-walled vesicles from which FMD virus was isolated. A further experiment in which the aerosol was administered via a fine nasopharyngeal catheter produced similar results, though an exposed sheep developed clinical FMD. During subsequent investigations, a group of sheep was housed in proximity to a group of infected cattle; nearly half the sheep developed antibody and virus was recovered from the pharyngeal region; none developed clinical lesions though several had fluctuating temperatures.

Under conditions in which transient exposure to small quantities of airborne virus occurs in the field, it is probable that inapparent infections develop in cattle, whereas the present limited evidence suggests that a high prevalence of inapparent infections may be almost a characteristic of airborne FMD in sheep. Airborne virus is unlikely to cause FMD in man although a single human case was attributed to airborne infection during the outbreak in cattle described by Michelsen (1968).

9. Modification of Control Measures

The rapid establishment of a sufficiently large movement-control zone around foci of infection has received increasing attention recently. In the past, an approximately circular area, of radius about 10 to 15 miles, has been considered adequate. However, as a result of the coalescence of several zones and, recently, to facilitate more effective control during severe epizootics, much larger areas have been declared "Controlled Areas." The possibility of airborne dissemination downwind from a focus of infection necessitates careful analysis of meteorologic conditions during the critical period from 24 hours before the first appearance of lesions until completion of destruction or burial of the last slaughtered carcass. Prevalence of high winds during this decisive period would render expedient the creation of an elliptical control zone instead of a circular one. The incineration of carcasses, while strong winds are blowing, may result in dissemination of small quantities of virus in local thermal currents. Even in calm conditions, however, regular inspection of all susceptible animals, within a radius of at least 2 miles from a focus of infection, must be considered to be essential for the effective control of FMD.

VIII. The Progression of Epizootics

The distribution of the 7 types and the incidence of subtypes of FMD virus throughout the world was described by Brooksby (1959); the coexistence of several types, virtually simultaneously, in a relatively small area of the southeastern part of Southern Rhodesia was also reported. Henderson (1962) described the situation in South America; epizootics in Europe from 1937 to 1961 were described by Fogedby (1963); Mackowiak and Fontaine (1966) recorded the recent distribution of types in Europe, the Near East, and the Middle East, and Datt *et al.* (1968) gave details of the current distribution of FMD in India. Moosbrugger (1966) discussed the identification of virus of more than a single type during the course of epizootics.

As a generality, it is probably true that the most disastrous epizootics tend to occur either when virus of an exotic type is accidently imported to a new locality, or when a variant of an existing type evolves in an area in which the disease has entered a quiescent phase; thereafter, the velocity of spread is determined partly by the density of the livestock population but principally by its relative susceptibility to the particular strain.

A classic example of rapid dissemination of a type previously exotic to an area occurred when virus of type SAT-1 appeared in the Persian Gulf, at Bahrein, in December 1961. By February 1962, the disease was extending northwestward through the Gulf States, to reach Iraq, Jordan, Israel, and Syria by April. In June and July, the epizootic spread deeply into Jordan, the Asiatic part of Turkey, and Iran. In September, FMD of type SAT-1 had crossed the Bosphorus to enter Europe for the first time. On November 20, 1962, the virus was isolated from a minor outbreak near the Greco-Turkish border. At this point, the epizootic was halted by the application of rigorous control measures and the establishment, during several preceding months, of a belt of intensive vaccination along the borders between Turkey, Greece, and Bulgaria (Hyslop, 1966). The preparation and deployment of much of the vaccine and the progression of the epizootic were discussed by Hyslop (1966/1967).

It is noteworthy that, during an advance of several thousand miles through a wholly susceptible population, the strain of virus remained unchanged in all but very minor cultural characteristics. This antigenic stability of strains, when they are spreading unchecked in major epizootics, is in marked contrast to the multiplicity of strains observed in other situations. Moosbrugger *et al.* (1967) drew attention to the need for great watchfulness wherever a policy of vaccination must be adopted. Hyslop and Fagg (1965) noted that variants are likely to appear when vaccination or prolonged enzooticity cause the resistance of the population to increase; a wide range in individual immunity is especially liable to select aberrant strains.

The existence of several distinct strains in Mexico was demonstrated clearly by Galloway *et al.* (1948). Multiplicity of strains manifesting antigenic diversity within a single type, was particularly evident in an enzootic area in the valley of the River Po, Italy (Ubertini, 1951, 1953). Traub *et al.* (1966) recorded similar multiplicity of strains in an area of the Near East, i.e., Iran, where "the disease spread freely, more or less unhampered by mass vaccination and sanitary measures," and where nomadic conditions persisted.

Parenthetically, it must be remarked that nomadism is a potent factor in the dissemination of epizootic disease in many parts of Africa and Asia. Little can be done to control the extensive movements of nomadic groups, because these are dictated solely by the complete economic dependence of the human population on their herds, the progress of the latter being dominated by continuing availability of water and grazing; thus, itineraries are often determined by the vagaries of seasonal climatic factors as much as by family or tribal custom. The use of common watering points on certain routes is not infrequent.

Davie (1966) reported that although strains of subtype A_{22}, recovered from Iraq, Israel, Syria, Turkey, and Greece, were virtually homogenous in antigenic constitution, strains isolated in Iran and southern parts of the USSR gave strong evidence of variation. Hyslop (1967b) recorded studies *in vivo* and *in vitro*, which demonstrated that the antigenic difference between two of the latter strains (Iraq 24/64 and USSR 1/65) was sufficiently great to necessitate the use of vaccine of the homologous strain only.

The confusing distribution of subtypes which has resulted recently, perhaps from the development of improved techniques for the demonstration of strain differences rather than from a real increase in the multiplicity of strains, was described by Vittoz (1966).

Hedger (1968) reported the isolation of virus from up to 23% of clinically normal (carrier) cattle which had recovered from FMD of type SAT-3; several of the strains differed from the "outbreak strain" and also from a living vaccine strain which had been used in the area, thus providing further supporting evidence for the evolution of variants during the spread of virus in semi-immune cattle under natural conditions. The insidious nature of the extension of infection in enzootic areas is revealed by occasional serologic responses of a clearly anamnestic nature in animals which had been vaccinated, apparently for the first time.

Whether modification in the antigenic constitution of FMD virus is mediated solely by increasing serum or "local" antibody in the population, or whether it results from the interaction of several factors, remains unknown. However, the influence of antibody was illustrated *in vitro* (Hyslop, 1965d) by the emergence of distinct substrains when virus was propagated in monolayer cultures of pig kidney cells maintained in media containing progressively increasing concentrations of antiserum. There is little or no information relating to the extent to which immunity must decline before variants may be expected to break through and establish new epizootics. Variants seldom appear *de novo* in countries such as Denmark and Holland, where relatively high degrees of immunity are maintained by regular and properly coordinated revaccination campaigns; however, during our experiments employing serial parenteral inoculation, titers of 1/45 and 1/90 failed to suppress the evolution of the progenitors of new strains.

IX. Conclusion

The physical and biochemical properties of FMD virus permit its dissemination, either directly or indirectly, not only by a great variety of animate and inanimate objects but also, under certain circumstances, by air currents. In a "biologically temperate" environment, the virus may survive for several weeks. The role of carrier animals remains to be ascertained fully. Man becomes clinically infected, only infrequently.

Restriction of the importation of animal products is of fundamental importance for preventing the introduction of FMD to "clean" areas. Factors influencing its control and prompt eradication include (1) rapid diagnosis and determination of subtype characteristics, (2) immediate slaughter of infected and in contact animals without delays consequent to prior negotiation of compensation, (3) effective control of the movement of livestock and persons on affected premises and in peripheral zones, (4) rapid destruction of carcasses, fodder stocks, etc., without attempts to salvage anything, (5) concurrent tracing of direct and indirect contacts with infected herds, (6) complete decontamination of premises, and (7) early notification of outbreaks to neighboring countries and to international agencies, such as the Central Bureau of the Office International des Epizootics.

REFERENCES

Anonymous. (1931). "Foot and Mouth Disease Research Committee," 4th Progr. Rept. H. M. Stationery Office, London.

Anonymous. (1937). "Foot and Mouth Disease Research Committee," 5th Progr. Rept. H. M. Stationery Office, London.

Anonymous. (1966). "Studies on Foot and Mouth Disease." Report of the Argentine-United States Joint Commission on foot and mouth disease. National Academy of Sciences, Washington, D.C.

Anonymous. (1968). "N.C.D.C. Veterinary Public Health Notes." U.S. Department of Health, Education and Welfare, Atlanta, Georgia.

Armstrong, R., Davie, J., and Hedger, R. S. (1967). Foot and mouth disease in man. *British Medical Journal* 4, 529.

Afzal, H., and Barya, M. A. (1968). Occurrence and survival of foot and mouth disease virus in external lesions and discharges of experimentally infected buffalo calves. *Bulletin de l'Office international des Epizooties* **69**, 509–519.

Bachrach, H. L. (1960). The ribonucleic acid of foot and mouth disease virus. Its preparation stability, and plating efficiency in bovine tissue cultures. *Virology* **12**, 258–271.

Bachrach, H. L. (1964). Foot and mouth disease virus. Structural changes during reaction with cations and formaldehyde as deduced from absorbance measurements. *Journal of Molecular Biology* **8**, 348–358.

Bachrach, H. L., Breese, S. S., Jr., Callis, J. J., Hess, W. R., and Patty, R. E. (1957). Inactivation of foot and mouth disease virus by pH. and temperature changes and by formaldehyde. *Proceedings of the Society for Experimental Biology and Medicine* **95**, 147–152.

Bachrach, H. L., Trautman, R., and Breese, S. S., Jr. (1964). Chemical and physical properties of virtually pure foot and mouth disease virus. *American Journal of Veterinary Research* **25**, 333.

Bloomfield, A. L. (1922). The dissemination of bacteria in the upper air passages. *Johns Hopkins Hospital Bulletin* **33**, 145–149.

Boiko, A. A. (1960). Quelques problèmes de l'épizoologie de la fièvre aphteuse en URSS. *Bulletin de l'Office international des Epizooties* **54**, 20.

Brooksby, J. B. (1950). Strains of the virus of foot and mouth disease showing natural adaptation to swine. *Journal of Hygiene* **48**, 184.

Brooksby, J. B. (1959). The epizootiological picture in foot and mouth disease. *Proceedings of the 16th International Veterinary Congress, Madrid, 1959* Vol. 1, pp. 233–245.

Brooksby, J. B. (1962). International trade in meat and the dissemination of foot and mouth disease. *Bulletin de l'Office international des Epizooties* **57**, 847–852.

Brooksby, J. B. (1967a). Foot and mouth disease—a world problem. *Nature* **213**, 120–122.

Brooksby, J. B. (1967b). Foot and mouth disease in man—notes on a recent case. *Proceedings of the 71st Annual Meeting of the United States Livestock Sanitary Association, Phoenix, 1967* p. 300.

Brown, F., Hyslop, N. St. G., Crick, J., and Morrow, A. W. (1963). The use of acetylethyleneimine in the production of F.M.D. vaccines. *Journal of Hygiene* **61**, 337.

Bubnov, V. D., and Nauryzbaev, I. (1966). Destruction of foot and mouth disease virus in manure during fermentation. *Bulletin All-Union Institute for Sanitary Veterinary Science* **26**, 289–290; *Veterinary Bulletin* **37**, 368 (1967) (abstr.).

Bullough, W. S. (1942). The starling in foot and mouth disease. *Proceedings of the Royal Society* **(B)131**, 1–10.

Burrows, R. (1966a). Studies on the carrier state of cattle exposed to foot and mouth disease virus. *Journal of Hygiene* **64**, 81.

Burrows, R. (1966b). Observations on the carrier state following exposure to FMD virus. *Report to Standing Technical Committee, European Commission for the Control of Foot and Mouth Disease, Pirbright, 1966.*

Burrows, R. (1968a) Excretion of foot and mouth disease virus prior to development of lesions. *Veterinary Record* **82**, 387.

Burrows, R. (1968b). The persistence of foot and mouth disease virus in sheep. *Journal of Hygiene* **66**, 633–640.

Cabot, D. (1945). Foot and mouth disease—its epizootological aspect. *Veterinary Record* **57**, 375–377.

Campion, R. L., and Gatto, F. B. (1961). Survival of foot and mouth disease virus under natural conditions. *Gaceta veterinaria, Buenos Aires* **23**, 163–170.

Capel-Edwards, M. (1967). Foot and mouth disease in *Myocaster coypus*. *Journal of Comparative Pathology* **77**, 217–221.

Chamberlain, A. C. (1970). Deposition and uptake by cattle of airborne particles. *Nature* **225**, 99.

Childs, T. (1953). Procedures leading to the eradication of the first outbreak of foot and mouth disease in Canada. *Proceedings of the 15th International Veterinary Congress, Stockholm, 1953* Vol. 1, pp. 217–223.

Condy, J. B., Herniman, K. A. J., and Hedger, R. S. (1969). Foot and mouth disease in wildlife in Rhodesia and other African territories. *Journal of Comparative Pathology* **79**, 27–32.

Cottral, G. E. (1969). Persistence of foot and mouth disease virus in animals, their products and the environment. *Bulletin de l'Office international des Epizooties* **71**, 549–568.

Cottral, G. E., Cox, B. F, and Baldwin, D. E. (1960). The survival of foot and mouth disease virus in cured and uncured meat. *American Journal of Veterinary Research* **21**, 288–297.

Cottral, G. E., Gailiunas, P., and Cox, B. F. (1968). Foot and mouth disease virus in the semen of bulls and its transmission by artificial insemination. *Archiv für die Gesamte Virusforschung* **23**, 362–377.

Cox, B. F., Cottral, G. E., and Baldwin, D. E. (1961). Further studies on the survival of foot and mouth disease virus in meat. *American Journal of Veterinary Research* **22**, 224–226.

Cunha, R. G., Torturella, I., Saile, J. L., and Serrao, U. M. (1958). Experimental mixed infection of cattle with FMD viruses. *American Journal of Veterinary Research* **19**, 78–83.

Cunliffe, H. R. (1964). Observations on the duration of immunity in cattle after experimental infection with foot-and-mouth disease virus. *Cornell Veterinarian* **54**, 501–510.

Datt, N. S., Rao, B. U., and Sharna, G. L. (1968). Incidence and distribution of different types of foot and mouth disease virus in India. *Bulletin de l'Office international des Epizooties* **69**, 31–36.

Davie, J. (1966). Subtype strains of foot and mouth disease—the present position. *Proceedings, Meeting of the Research Group, European Commission for the Control of Foot and Mouth Disease, Pirbright, 1966.*

Davies, W. K. D., Lewis, G. B., and Randall, H. A. (1968). Some distributional features of the foot and mouth disease epidemic. *Nature* **219**, 121–125.

de Kock, G. (1946). Problems of game preservation in South Africa. *South African Journal of Science* **42**, 162–171.

de Mello, Augé P., Honigman, M. N., and Fernandes, M. V. (1966). Supervivencia en bovinos del virus modificado de la Fievre Aftosa. *Bulletin de l'Office international des Epizooties* **65**, 2091 and 2106.

Dhennin, L., Heim de Balsac, H., Verge, J., and Dhennin, L. (1961). Du rôle des parasites dans la transmission naturelle et expérimentale du virus de la fièvre aphteuse. *Recueil de médicine vétérinaire* **137**, 95–104.

Dhennin, L., Heim de Balsac, H., Verge, J., and Dhennin, L. (1963). Recherches sur le rôle éventuel de Lumbricus terrestis dans la transmission de la fièvre aphteuse. *Bulletin de l'académie vétérinaire de France* **36**, 153–155.

Dijkstra, J. M. (1950). Wat is de rol van smetstofdragers bij het mond en klauwzeer. *Tijdschrift voor diergeneeskunde* **75**, 591–597.

Dimopoullos, G. T., Fellowes, O. N., Callis, J. J., Poppensiek, G. C., Edward, A. G., and Graves, J. H. (1959). Thermal inactivation and antigenicity studies of heated tissue suspensions containing foot and mouth disease virus. *American Journal of Veterinary Research* **20**, 510–521.

Eccles, M. A. (1939). The role of birds in the spread of foot and mouth disease. *Bulletin de l'Office international des Epizooties* **18**, 118–148.

Fagg, R. H., and Hyslop, N. St.G. (1966). Isolation of a variant strain of foot and mouth disease virus (type O) during passage in partly immunized cattle. *Journal of Hygiene* **64**, 397–404.

Flückiger, G. (1943). In welchem Ausmass sind von der Maul und Klauenseuche genesene Tiere Ansteckungsträger? *Zentralblatt für Infektionskrankheiten Haustiere* **59**, 220–224.

Flückiger, G. (1956). Über die Einschleppung der Maul und Klauenseuche aus Belgien in die Schweiz und ihre Bekämpfung von Mai bis Juli 1956. *Deutsche tierärztliche Wochenschrift* **63**, 401–405.

Fogedby, E. (1963). "Review of Epizootology and Control of Foot and Mouth Disease in Europe." European Committee for the Control of Foot and Mouth Disease, F.A.O., Rome.

Fogedby, E. G., Malmquist, W. A., Osteen, O. L., and Johnson, M. L. (1960). Airborne transmission of foot and mouth disease virus. *Nordisk Veterinärmedicin* **12**, 490–498.

Forsmann, J., and Magnusson, H. (1942). In welchem Ausmass sind von der Maul und Klauenseuche genesene Tiere Austeckungsträger? *Zentralblatt für Infektionskrankheiten Haustiere* **58**, 209–225.

Fresdorf, E. (1949). The spread of foot and mouth disease. *Berliner und Münchener tierärztliche Wochenschrift* **61**, No. 3, 29.

Gailiunas, P., and Cottral, G. E. (1964). Occurrence and survival of foot and mouth disease virus in bovine synovial fluid. *Bulletin de l'Office international des Epizooties* **61**, 1.

Gailiunas, P., and Cottral, G. E. (1967). Survival of foot and mouth disease virus in bovine hides. *American Journal of Veterinary Research* **26**, 1047–1053.

Galloway, I. A. (1931). "Foot and Mouth Disease Research Committee," 4th Progr. Rept., p. 13. H. M. Stationery Office, London.

Galloway, I. A. (1937). "Foot and Mouth Disease Research Committee," 5th Progr. Rept., pp. 345–349. H. M. Stationery Office, London.

Galloway, I. A. (1962). Results of the use of two live attenuated strain vaccines in controlling outbreaks of foot and mouth disease. *Bulletin de l'Office international des Epizooties* **57**, 748–788.

Galloway, I. A., Henderson, W. M., and Brooksby, J. B. (1948). Strains of the virus of foot and mouth disease recovered from outbreaks in Mexico (6 papers). *Proceedings of the Society for Experimental Biology and Medicine* **69**, 57–84.

Geering, W. A. (1967). Foot and mouth disease in sheep. *Australian Veterinary Journal* **43**, 485–494.

Gorban, N. I. (1953). Some factors in the spread of foot and mouth disease. *Veterinariya* **30**, 22.

Gorskii, V. V., and Gizatullin, K. L. G. (1968). Chemical disinfection of manure in foot and mouth disease. *Veterinariya* (1) 98–101; *Veterinary Bulletin* **38**, 681 (1968).

Hedger, R. S. (1968). The isolation and characterization of foot and mouth disease virus from clinically normal herds of cattle in Botswana. *Journal of Hygiene* **66**, 27–36.

Hedger, R. S., Condy, J. B., and Falconer, J. (1969). The isolation of foot and mouth disease virus from African Buffalo (*Syncerus caffer*). *Veterinary Record* **84**, 516–517.

Heidelbaugh, N. D., and Graves, J. H. (1968). Effects of some techniques applicable in food processing on the infectivity of foot and mouth disease virus. *Food Technology* **22**, 120–124.

Henderson, D. W. (1952). An apparatus for the study of airborne infection. *Journal of Hygiene* **50**, 53–68.

Henderson, R. J. (1969). The outbreak of foot and mouth disease in Worcestershire. An epidemiological study: With special reference to the spread of the disease by wind carriage of the virus. *Journal of Hygiene* **67**, 21–33.

Henderson, W. M. (1962). "Foot and Mouth Disease in the Americas," Veterinary Annual, p. 17. John Wright & Sons Ltd., Bristol, England.

Henderson, W. M. (1966/1967). "Foot and Mouth Disease Carriers," Veterinary Annual, p. 136. John Wright & Sons Ltd., Bristol, England.

Henderson, W. M., and Brooksby, J. B. (1948). The survival of foot and mouth disease virus in meat and offal. *Journal of Hygiene* **46**, 394.

Hess, E. (1967). Epizootiologie der Maul und Klauenseuche. *Schweitzer Archiv für Tierheilkunde* **109**, 324–326.

Hess, W. H. R., Bachrach, H. L., and Callis, J. J. (1960). Persistence of foot and mouth disease virus in bovine kidneys and blood as related to antibodies. *American Journal of Veterinary Research* **21**, 1104–1108.

Houwink, E. H., and Rolvink, W. (1957). The quantitative assay of bacterial aerosols by electrostatic precipitation. *Journal of Hygiene* **55**, 544–563.

Hulse, E. C., and Edwards, J. T. (1937). Foot and mouth disease in hibernating hedgehogs. *Journal of Comparative Pathology and Therapeutics* **50**, 421–430.

Hurst, G. W. (1968). Foot and mouth disease. The possibility of continental sources of the virus in England. *Veterinary Record* **82**, 610–614.

Hyslop, N. St.G. (1955). Report. Chief Veterinary Research Officer, Kenya.

Hyslop, N. St.G. (1963). Experimental infection with *Mycoplasma mycoides*. *Journal of Comparative Pathology and Therapeutics* **73**, 265–276.

Hyslop, N. St.G. (1965a). Secretion of foot and mouth disease virus and antibody in the saliva of infected and immunized cattle. *Journal of Comparative Pathology and Therapeutics* **75**, 111–118.

Hyslop, N. St.G. (1965b). Airborne infection with the virus of foot and mouth disease. *Journal of Comparative Pathology and Therapeutics* **75**, 119–126.

Hyslop, N. St.G. (1965c). Unpublished observations.

Hyslop, N. St.G. (1965d). Isolation of variant strains from foot and mouth disease virus propagated in cell cultures containing antiviral sera. *Journal of General Microbiology* **41**, 135–142.

Hyslop, N. St.G. (1966). Fellowship Thesis, Royal College of Veterinary Surgeons, London.

Hyslop, N. St.G. (1966–1967). "Vaccination against Foot and Mouth Disease," Veterinary Annual, p. 140. John Wright & Sons Ltd., Bristol, England.

Hyslop, N. St.G. (1967a). Unpublished report. Animal Virus Research Institute, Pirbright, England.

Hyslop, N. St.G. (1967b). Immunogenic differences between two strains of foot and mouth disease virus (type A) originally exotic to Europe. *Proceedings of the 18th World Veterinary Congress, Paris, 1967* Vol. 1, p. 396.

Hyslop, N. St.G. (1970). Infection of man with the virus of foot and mouth disease. In press.

Hyslop, N. St.G., and Fagg, R. H. (1965). Isolation of variants during passage of a strain of foot and mouth disease virus in partly immunized cattle. *Journal of Hygiene* **63**, 357–368.

Hyslop, N. St.G., and Ford, J. (1957). Therapy of contagious bovine pleuropneumonia. Part I. Treatment of early cases with chloramphenicol. *Veterinary Record* **69**, 521.

Idso, P. T. (1943). Seagulls as carriers of infection. *Norsk Vetinaer-Tidsskrift* **55**, 84–86.

Jerlov, S. (1939). I vilken utstrackning aro djur som genomgatt mul och Klovsjuka smittforande. *Svensk Vetinärtidskrift* **44**, 295–312.

Jerlov, S. (1940). The foot and mouth outbreak in Sweden 1938–40. *Veterinary Bulletin* **11**, 511–514 (abstr.).

Kastli, P., and Moosbrugger, G. A. (1968). Inactivation of foot and mouth disease virus in dairy products by heat. *Schweizer Archiv für Tierheilkunde* **110**, 89–93.

Keane, C. (1924). Deer in California in the 1922 foot and mouth disease outbreak. *Monthly Bulletin. California Department of Agriculture* **16**, 4.

Kiryukhin, R. A., and Pasechnikov, L. A. (1966). Isolation of foot and mouth disease virus from air exhaled by infected animals. *Veterinariya* **43**, 30–31; *Veterinary Bulletin* **36**, 790 (1966) (abstr.).

Korn, G. (1957). Experimentelle Untersuchungen zum Virusnachweiss im Incubationstadium der M.K.S. und zu ihrer Pathogenese. *Archiv für experimentelle Veterinärmedizin* **11**, 637.

Kunetsova, G. M., Ikovataya, G. M., and Onufriev, V. P. (1966). The role of ticks in foot and mouth disease. *Veterinariya* **43**, 29–30.

Lambrechts, M. C., Buhr, W. H. B., and Van der Merwe, J. P. (1956). Observations on the transmission of foot and mouth disease to game and controlled transmission from game to cattle and vice versa. *Journal of the South African Veterinary Medical Association* **27**, 133–137.

Lees-May, T., and Condy, J. (1965). Foot and mouth disease in game in Rhodesia. *Bulletin de l'Office international des Epizooties* **64**, 805–811.

Litt, M. (1967). Studies of the latent period. I. *Cold Spring Harbor Symposia on Quantitative Biology* **32**, 477–480.

Loeffler, F. (1909). *Deutsche Medizinische Wochenschrift* p. 2097. Cited by Fortner, J. B. (1932). Über Virusträger und ihr Dauer Ausscheider bei Maul und Klauenseuche. *Deutsche tierärztliche Wochenschrift* **40**, 183.

Lucam, F., Dannacher, G., and Fèdida, M. (1964). Action *in vitro* de quelques desinfectants sur un virus aphteux de culture. *Bulletin de l'Office international des Epizooties* **61**, 1589–1603.

Ludlam, F. H. (1967). The circulation of air, water and particles in the troposphere. "Airborne Microbes." *17th Symposium of the Society for General Microbiology*, page 1.

Lukin, A. M. (1963). Role of ixodid ticks in the epizootology of foot and mouth disease. *Veternariya* **40**, 28–30.

McKercher, P. D., Dellers, R. W., and Giordano, A. R. (1966). Foot and mouth disease infection in cattle housed in an isolation unit. *Cornell Veterinarian* **56**, 395–401.

Mackowiak, C., and Fontaine, J. (1966). Situation de la Fièvre Aphteuse en Europe au début de l'année 1966. *Bulletin de la société des sciences vétérinaires de Lyon* **68**, 57–60.

McLaughlan, J. D., and Henderson, W. M. (1947). The occurrence of foot and mouth disease in the hedgehog under natural conditions. *Journal of Hygiene* **45**, 474.

McLean, R. C. (1938). Carriers of foot and mouth disease. *Nature* **141**, 828.

McVicar, J. W., and Sutmoller, P. (1969). The epizootiological importance of foot and mouth disease carriers. *Archiv für die Gesamte Virusforschung* **26**, 217–224.

Maffey, J. (1961a). The physical principles of milking machines. *Veterinary Record* **73**, 589–594.

Maffey, J. (1961b). Personal communication.

May, K. R., and Harper, G. J. (1957). The efficiency of various liquid impinger samplers in bacterial aerosols. *British Journal of Industrial Medicine* **14**, 287–293.

Mead, C. J. (1968). "Birds as Vectors of the Foot and Mouth Disease Virus," Veterinary Annual. John Wright & Sons Ltd., Bristol, England.

Mettam, A. E. (1914). Foot and mouth disease. *Proceedings of the 10th International Veterinary Congress, London, 1914* Vol. 2, pp. 105–107.

Meyer, N. L. (1969). Foot and mouth disease in England. *Journal of the American Veterinary Medical Association* **154**, 1226–1229.

Michelsen, E. (1968). Airborne transmission of foot and mouth disease. *Report to Meeting of European Commission for the Control of Foot and Mouth Disease, Lindholm, 1968.*

Moosbrugger, G. A. (1948). Recherches expérimentales sur la fièvre aphteuse. *Schweizer Archiv für Tierheilkunde* **90**, 176–198.

Moosbrugger, G. A. (1954). La transmission de la fièvre aphteuse par les fourrages et les produits végétaux. *Bulletin de l'Office international des Epizooties* **42**, 236.

Moosbrugger, G. A. (1960a). La prévention de l'introduction dans un Pays des types de virus qui y sont encore totalement inconnus. *Bulletin de l'Office international des Epizooties* **53**, 809.

Moosbrugger, G. A. (1960b). "Documents sur la persistance des virus de certaines maladies animales dans les viandes et produits animaux," pp. 29–37. Interafrican Bureau of Animal Health, Muguga, and Office International des Epizooties. Paris.

Moosbrugger, G. A. (1966). Les variations de type du virus aphteux en cours de Epizootie. *Bulletin de l'Office international des Epizooties* **65**, 2023–2031.

Moosbrugger, G. A., Leunen, J., Mackowiak, C., Fontaine, J., and Roumiantzeff, M. (1967). Etude sérologique et immunologique de souches de virus aphteux de type O, isolées en Europe entre 1963 et 1966. *Bulletin de l'Office international des Epizooties* **67**, 711–729.

Morris, E. J., Darlow, H. M., Peel, J. F. H., and Wright, W. C. (1961). The quantitative assay of mono-dispersed aerosols of bacteria and bacteriophage by electrostatic precipitation. *Journal of Hygiene* **59**, 487–492.

Mosier, D. E., and Cohen, E. P. (1968). Induction and rapid expression of an immune response *in vivo*. *Nature* **219**, 968–970.

Nocard, E., and Leclainche, E. (1903). "Les maledies microbiennedes Animaux," 3rd ed, p. 555. Masson, Paris.

Norris, K. P., and Harper, G. J. (1970). Windborne dispersal of foot and mouth disease virus. *Nature* **225**, 98.

Pilz, W., and Garbe, H. G. (1960). Die Eignung von Formaldehyde—Hösung zur Desinfektion MKS ,erseuchter Eisenbahn Viehtransportwagen. *Monatshefte für Tierheilkunde* **12**, 190–193.

Pitty, A. F. (1968). Particles size of the Saharan dust which fell on Britain in July 1968. *Nature* **220**, 364.

Poppe, K. (1931). Die Milch als Überträger von Krankheitserregern. *Deutsche tierärztliche Wochenschrift-Deutsche tierärztliche Rundschau* **34**, 324–328.

Poppe, K., and Busch, G. (1936). Zur Frage der Symbiose des Virus der Maul und Klauenseuche in pflanzlichen Mikroorganismen. *Zentralblatt für Bakteriologie, Parasitenkunde, Abt. I. Originale* **136**, 385–389.

Primault, B. (1955). De l'influence des variations de la pression atmosphérique sur l'apparition de la fièvre aphteuse. *Schweizer Archiv für tierheilkunde* **97**, 412.

Primault, B. (1958). Elements météorologiques agissant sur l'apparition et l'extension de la fièvre aphteuse. *Schweizer Archiv für tierheilkunde* **100**, 383.

Pringle, C. R. (1965). Evidence of genetic recombination in foot and mouth disease virus. *Virology* **25**, 48–51.

Pringle, C. R. (1968). Recombination between conditional lethal mutants within a strain of foot and mouth disease virus. *Journal of General Virology* **2**, 199–202.

Pringle, R. (1880). Foot and mouth disease in camels. *Veterinary Journal* **7**, 376.

Reid, J. (1968). "Origin of the 1967-68 Foot and Mouth Disease Epidemic." H. M. Stationery Office, London.

Roch Marra, R. (1908). Etudes sur la fièvre aphteuse. *Revue générale de médicine vétérinaire* **11**, 49–57.

Rozov, A. A. (1966). Survival of foot and mouth disease virus on and in the body of horse flies. *Trudy Vsesdyuznogo Instituta Veterinarndi Sanitarii l Ektoparazitologii* **26**, 96–103.

Savi, P., and Baldelli, B. (1962). La persistance du virus aphteux dans les viandes et dans les produits de charcuterie. *Bulletin de l'Office international des Epizooties* **57**, 891–901.

Schang, P. J. (1951). Les porteurs de virus en relation avec les plans d'immunization anti-aphteuse. *Bulletin de l'Office international des Epizooties* **35**, 672–676.

Schang, P. J. (1957). Treinta años de utilizacion de la Technica de aispamiento de focos de aftosa. *Gaceta Veterinaria, Buenos Aires* **19**, 55–56.

Scott, F. W., Cottral, G. E., and Gailiunas, P. (1966). Persistence of FMD virus in external lesions and saliva of experimentally infected cattle. *American Journal of Veterinary Research* **27**, 1531–1536.

Sellers, R. F. (1968). Inactivation of foot and mouth disease virus by chemicals and disinfectants. *Veterinary Record* **83**, 504.

Sellers, R. F. (1969). Inactivation of foot and mouth disease virus in milk. *British Veterinary Journal* **125**, 163.

Sellers, R. F., Burrows, R., Mann, J. A., and Dawe, P. (1968). Recovery of virus from bulls affected with foot and mouth disease. *Veterinary Record* **83**, 303.

Sellers, R. F., and Parker, J. (1969). Airborne excretion of foot and mouth disease virus. *Journal of Hygiene* **67**, 671–677.

Shafyi, A. (1968). pH resistance of foot and mouth disease virus. *American Journal of Veterinary Research* **29**, 1469–1478.

Shahan, M. S. (1962). The virus of foot and mouth disease. *Annals of the New York Academy of Sciences* **101**, 444–454.

Shilnikov, V. I. (1959). Survival of foot and mouth disease virus in the pre-tundra zone. *Veterinary Bulletin* **30**, 499 (abstr.).

Smith, L. P., and Hugh-Jones, M. E. (1969). The weather factor in foot and mouth disease epidemics. *Nature* **223**, 712–715.

Snowdon, W. A. (1968). The susceptibility of some Australian fauna. *Australian Journal of Experimental Biology and Medical Science* **49**, 667–687.

Stockman, S., and Garnett, M. (1923). Foot and mouth disease. *Journal of the Ministry of Agriculture (England)* **30**, 681.

Stockman, S., and Minette, F. C. (1926). Experiments on foot and mouth disease. *Journal of Comparative Pathology and Therapeutics* **39**, 231–245.

Sutmoller, P., and Cottral, G. E. (1967). Improved techniques for the detection of foot and mouth disease virus in carrier cattle. *Archiv für die gasamte Virusforschung* **21**, 170–177.

Sutmoller, P., and Gaggero, C. A. (1965). Foot and mouth disease carriers. *Veterinary Record* **77**, 968–969.

Sutmoller, P., de Mello, A. P., Honigman, M. N., and Federer, K. E. (1967). Infectivity for cattle and pigs of 3 strains of foot and mouth disease virus isolated from carrier cattle. *American Journal of Veterinary Research* **28**, 101–105.

Thorne, H. V., and Burrows, T. M. (1960). Aerosol sampling methods for the virus of foot and mouth disease and measuring of virus penetration through filters. *Journal of Hygiene* **58**, 409.

Thorne, H. V., and Hyslop, N. St.G. (1960). Cited by Thorne and Burrows (1960).

Traub, E. (1954). Produits végétaux vecteurs du virus aphteux. *Bulletin de l'Office international des Epizooties* **42**, 248–253.

Traub, E., and Wittmann, G. (1957). Experimenteller Beitrag zur Klärung der Frage Verbreitung des Maul und Klauenseuche Virus durch der Luft. *Berliner und Münchener tierärztliche Wochenschrift* **70**, 205–206.

Traub, E., Shafyi, A., Kesting, F., and Ewaldsson, B. (1966). Serological variation of foot and mouth disease virus in Iran (1963–66). *Berliner und Münchener tierärztliche Wochenschrift* **65**, 2035–2050.

Ubertini, B. (1951). Observations et recherches sur les différents virus de la fièvre aphteuse qui ont sévi dans la plaine du Pô, pendant les dix dernières années. *Bulletin de l'Office international des Epizooties* **35**, 627–643.

Ubertini, B. (1953). Observations et recherches sur l'infection aphteuse Européenne de type A de 1951 à 1952. *Bulletin de l'Office international des Epizooties* **39**, 149–153.

Urbain, A., Bullier, P., and Nouvel, J. (1938). Au sujet d'une petite epizootie de fièvre aphteuse ayant sévi sur des animaux sauvage. *Bulletin de l'academie vétérinaire de France* **11**, 59.

Vallée, H., and Carré, H. (1928). Etudes sur la fièvre aphteuse. *Annales de l'institut Pasteur* **42**, 841–869.

Van Bekkum, J. G., Frenkel, H. S., Frederiks, H. H., and Frenkel, S. (1959). Observations on the carrier state of cattle exposed to foot and mouth disease. *Tijdschrift voor diergeneeskunde* **84**, 1159–1167.

Vande Woude, G. F. (1967). The inactivation of foot and mouth disease virus at ionic strength dependent isoelectric points. *Virology* **31**, 436–441.

Viljoen, J. H. B. (1963). A brief survey of the 1961–62 epizootic of foot and mouth disease in South West Africa. *Bulletin de l'Office international des Epizooties* **60**, 869–872.

Viljoen, J. H. (1964). The successful use of attenuated and inactivated foot and mouth disease vaccine in a major epizootic. *Bulletin de l'Office international des Epizooties* **61**, 1463–1513.

Vittoz, R. (1966). Report of the director on the scientific and technical activities of the office international des Epizooties 1965–66. *Bulletin de l'Office international des Epizooties* **66**, 1425–1560.

Voinov, S. J. (1955). Carriers in foot and mouth disease. *Veterinariya* **32**, 25–28.

Voinov, S. J. (1956). Resistance of foot and mouth disease virus on pastures. *Veterinariya* **33**, 66–67.

Voinov, S. J. (1967). Survival of foot and mouth disease virus in water under Central Asian conditions. *Trudy Vsesdyuznogo Instituta Veterinarndi Sanitarii l Ektoparazitologii* **29,** 89–94.

Voinov, S. J. (1968). Persistence of foot and mouth disease virus on the hair coat of animals under Central Asian conditions. *Trudy Vsesdyuznogo Instituta Veterinarndi Sanitarii l Ektoparazitologii* **30,** 45–50.

Waldmann, O., and Hirschfelder, H. (1938). Die epizootische bedeutung der Ratten, des Wildes, der Vögel und der Insekten für die Verbreitung der Maul- und Klauensenche. *Berliner tierärztliche Wochenschrift* **46,** 229–234.

Waldmann, O., and Reppin, K. (1927). Die Dauer der Infectiosität der Mundschleimhaut bei der Maul- und Klauenseuche des Rindes. *Archiv für wissenschaftliche und praktische Tierheilkunde* **55,** 407–409.

Waldmann, O., Trautwein, K., and Pyl, G. (1931). Die Persistenz des Maul- und Klauenseuche Virus in Körper durchgeseuchter Tiere und seine Ausscheidung. *Zentralblatt für Bakteriologie, Parasitenkunde, Abt. I. Originale* **121,** 19–32.

Wells, K. F. (1952). Foot and mouth disease control and eradication measures in Canada. *Proceedings 56th of the Annual Meeting of the United States Livestock Sanitary Association, Louisville, 1952* p. 166.

Wesslen, T., and Dinter, Z. (1957). The inactivation of foot and mouth disease virus by formalin. *Archiv für die Gesamte Virusforschung* **7,** 394–402.

Wilson, W. W., and Matheson, R. C. (1952). Bird migration and foot and mouth disease. *Veterinary Record* **64,** 541–548.

Wisniewski, J. (1962). Teneur en virus aphteux des tissus de bovins. *Bulletin de l'Office international des Epizooties* **57,** 902–907.

Wittmann, G., and Eissner, G. (1966). "Die Ausscheidung des MKS Virus durch MKS kranke Rinder sowie durch immune Rinder und Schweine nach der experimentellen Neuinfektion. *Berliner und Münchener Tierarztliche Wochenschrift* **79,** 105–109.

Canine and Feline Neoplasia

ROBERT S. BRODEY*

*Department of Surgery and the Tumor Clinic, University of Pennsylvania
School of Veterinary Medicine, Philadelphia, Pennsylvania*

Neoplastic diseases, although common in both the dog and cat, received very little attention from the veterinary medical profession until the early 1950's. Most observations prior to this time were restricted to case reports or to microscopic descriptions of neoplastic lesions with little, if any, clinical correlation. Collections of tumors, largely derived from biopsy material submitted from veterinary practitioners, were made in several areas (Mulligan, 1949; Cotchin, 1951, 1952). These collections, while contributing much to our knowledge of neoplasia, had serious deficiencies. One could not determine breed, age, and sex predilections, as the animals with tumors could not be related among the populations from which they were derived. Second, the clinical, surgical, and necropsy

* The author is Professor of Surgery and Director of the Tumor Clinic, University of Pennsylvania School of Veterinary Medicine, Philadelphia, Pennsylvania.

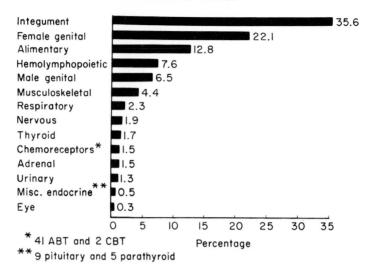

Fig. 1. Site distribution of 2917 canine neoplasms. ABT: aortic body tumor; CBT: carotid body tumor. (Brodey and Riser, 1969.)

findings and follow-up information were often poorly documented or not recorded at all. Third, the tissue submitted was sometimes inadequately fixed or poorly representative of the tumor in question.

Interest in small animal neoplasms was awakened in the late 1940's and early 1950's. The veterinary medical literature since that time has

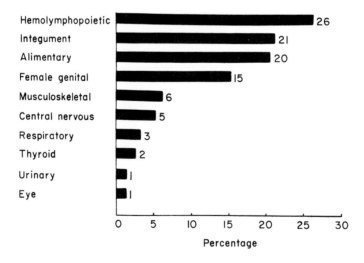

Fig. 2. Site distribution of 395 feline neoplasms. (Engle and Brodey, 1969.)

contained an increasing number of articles dealing with various phases of neoplasia. Reasons for this increase were primarily twofold. First of all, the clinical aspects of neoplasia assumed greater importance because of the increasing proficiency of small animal practitioners and the greater proportions of older animals being presented to the veterinarian as a result of decreased mortality from other diseases in early life. Therefore, it was essential that the clinician learn more about the diagnostic features, biologic behavior, prognosis, and treatment of these neoplastic lesions. Second, the great increase in both the scope and sophistication of human cancer research prompted further investigation of spontaneous canine and feline neoplasms. Because of the high frequency of spontaneous neoplasia among both dogs and cats and the close association of these animals with man, the importance of comparative research in this area was obviously considerable.

I have not attempted to review all the known facts about neoplasia in the dog and cat. Rather, I have indicated the general state of our knowledge and, more particularly, have tried to suggest directions for future studies. I have chosen to discuss certain neoplasms under the organ systems involved and the species affected. Where possible, I have relied primarily on case material seen at the University of Pennsylvania Veterinary Hospital, particularly in surveys of 2917 canine tumors seen from 1952 to 1964 (Fig. 1) and of 395 feline neoplasms seen from 1952 to 1967 (Fig. 2). These cases were derived either from our hospital population or from biopsy or necropsy specimens submitted to our pathology department by private practitioners.

I. Skin Neoplasms

The skin constitutes by far the commonest site for neoplasia of the dog. In our hospital, 35.6% of 2,917 tumors were of cutaneous origin (Fig. 1). A compilation of the histologic types of 984 canine skin tumors removed in our surgical clinic from 1952 to 1960 appears in Table I. Many more skin neoplasms were observed than are listed, but for one reason or another, usually because the tumor seemed benign and thus of no clinical concern, surgical treatment was not carried out.

The skin is an important site for neoplasia of cats (21% of 395 tumors), being second in importance only to lymphosarcoma (Fig. 2) (Engle and Brodey, 1969). The histologic diagnosis of these 83 skin neoplasms is listed in Table II. As benign skin tumors appear far less common in cats than in dogs, we usually recommend that all feline skin tumors be surgically removed.

The proportions of epithelial, mesenchymal, and melanomatous neoplasms in the 2 species were remarkably similar (Table III). The major

TABLE I

HISTOLOGIC DIAGNOSES OF 984 CANINE SKIN NEOPLASMS[a]

Type	Number
I. *Epithelial*	
Adnexal	205
Perianal	180
Squamous cell carcinoma	35
Papilloma	25
	445
II. *Mesenchymal*	
Mast cell tumor	210
Lipoma	85
Fibrosarcoma	58
Fibroma	31
Hemangiopericytoma	31
Hemangioma	30
Histiocytoma	25
Hemangiosarcoma	15
Liposarcoma	4
	489
III. *Melanoma*	
Benign and malignant	50

[a] University of Pennsylvania, Small Animal Surgical Clinic, 1952–1960.

cutaneous neoplasms of the dog and cat will be discussed under these three headings.

1. EPITHELIAL NEOPLASMS

a. Adnexal

(1) *Dog.* Neoplasms arising from the skin adnexae, i.e., hair follicles, sebaceous glands, and sweat glands, are extremely common in dogs (Table I). Tumors arising from perianal glands, which are modified sebaceous glands, and those arising from mammary glands, which are modified apocrine sweat glands, are discussed separately.

Because these adnexal lesions of old dogs are so common, often multiple, and almost invariably benign, many of them are not removed surgically. Breed, age, sex, and site incidences of dogs with hair follicle, sweat gland, and sebaceous gland tumors were compiled in our surgical clinic from 1952 to 1960 (Table IV). Although the results of this chart are somewhat artificial, because some tumors designated as one particular type actually contained a variable mixture of glandular components,

TABLE II
HISTOLOGIC DIAGNOSES OF 83 FELINE SKIN NEOPLASMS[a]

Type	Number
I. *Epithelial*	
Adnexal	30
Squamous cell carcinoma	16
	—
	46
II. *Mesenchymal*	
Fibrosarcoma	10
Fibroma	10
Mast cell tumor	6
Lipoma	5
Hemangioma	2
Hemangiosarcoma	1
Liposarcoma	1
Hemangiopericytoma	1
	—
	36
III. *Melanoma*	
Malignant	1

[a] University of Pennsylvania, 1952–1968. Reprinted courtesy of the Journal of the American Animal Hospital Association.

certain generalizations can be made. There were no sex differences except for those tumors of sebaceous gland type. The average ages of dogs with all 3 types were quite similar. The Cocker Spaniel was the dominant breed with all 3 tumors, whereas the Kerry Blue appeared over-represented in the hair follicle tumor group and the Boston Terrier figured prominently in sebaceous neoplasms. Site predilections were very similar for the hair follicle and sebaceous types, as would be expected by their anatomic juxtaposition, with most tumors arising from the head and neck. In contrast, sweat gland tumors were more evenly distributed over the body, with the majority occurring on the trunk.

The causes of these tumors are unknown. Certainly, breed predilection,

TABLE III
TYPE DISTRIBUTION OF 1067 CANINE AND FELINE SKIN NEOPLASMS[a]

Species	Number of tumors	Epithelial	Mesenchymal	Melanomas
Dog	984	445 (45%)	489 (50%)	50 (5%)
Cat	83	46 (55%)	36 (43%)	1 (2%)

[a] University of Pennsylvania.

TABLE IV

CLINICAL FEATURES OF DOGS WITH CUTANEOUS NEOPLASMS[a]

| Tumor type | Number of tumors | Male to female ratio | Average age (years) | Breed (%) | | Site (%) | | |
				Tumor population	Total hospital population	Head and neck	Trunk	Extremities
Hair follicle	50	1.4:1	8.4	Cocker Spaniel 18	9.5	62	28	10
Sebaceous	81	2.1:1	9.6	Kerry Blue 12	0.2	60	26	14
				Cocker Spaniel 21	9.5			
				Boston Terrier 7	2.3			
Sweat gland	24	1:1	8.7	Cocker Spaniel 35	9.5	36	47	27
Papilloma	19	5.3:1	5.3	No breed predilection	—	44	33	23
Squamous cell carcinoma	33	1.8:1	10.7	No breed predilection	—	19	31	50
Fibroma	31	1.4:1	8.0	Boxer 31	7.2	12	44	44
Fibrosarcoma	58	1.1:1	8.8	Cocker Spaniel 16	9.5	10	34	56
Hemangiopericytoma	31	1:1.4	10.3	Boxer 21	7.2	6	55	39
				Cocker Spaniel 18	9.5			
Mast cell tumor	210	1.5:1	7.5	Boxer 40	7.2	10	50	40
				Boston Terrier 13	2.3			
Histiocytoma	30	1.1:1	1.9	Boxer 34	7.2	28	28	43
Lipoma	85	1:2.3	7.9	Cocker Spaniel 16	9.5	4	88	8
Melanoma	32	1:1.3	8.4	Boxer 13	7.2	50	22	28

[a] University of Pennsylvania, Small Animal Surgical Clinic, 1952–1960.

e.g., of the Cocker Spaniel, is a factor of some importance. Pedigree analyses may indicate that certain families of Cocker Spaniels have a much higher incidence of adnexal tumors than do others. In general, the Cocker Spaniel is predisposed to develop various types of skin neoplasms, e.g., adnexal and perianal, as well as being commonly affected with seborrheic dermatitis. Interestingly, the Boxer, a breed commonly afflicted with many types of neoplasms, is not predisposed to adnexal tumors. Long-term cutaneous absorption of air pollutants may play a role in the genesis of these neoplasms, but this likelihood has not been determined.

Such terms as trichoepithelioma, trichocarcinoma, hair matrixoma, sebaceous gland adenoma and carcinoma, sweat gland adenoma and carcinoma, and basal cell carcinoma have been used to denote neoplasms of the various components of skin adnexae. Furthermore, some adnexal tumors have a mixture of glandular patterns, thus further compounding the problem of terminology. In order to simplify the nomenclature, we now employ the term adnexal tumor, to denote this entire range of neoplasms. This approach seems justified as the biologic behavior of the vast majority of these tumors appears to vary little with the type of histologic differentiation. Using this simple classification, the pathologist can, if he wishes, mention the type(s) of cellular differentiation that is present. A few adnexal tumors show "histologic evidence" of malignancy, but the biologic behavior of such lesions is usually benign. On rare occasions, however, adnexal tumors will exhibit widespread metastases.

(2) *Cat.* Adnexal tumors are quite important, the 2 most important sites appearing to be the region of the external ear canal and the trunk. The fact that metastases have been observed in several cats suggests that feline adnexal tumors are much more malignant than their canine counterparts.

b. Perianal Neoplasms

These tumors are peculiar to the dog and constitute one of the most common forms of skin neoplasia. Of 188 tumorous dogs operated on in our hospital from 1952 to 1960, there was an 8.8:1 male to female ratio. The average age was 11.3 years and the mode was 10 years. Only 4% of the dogs were under 6 years of age. Cocker Spaniels constituted 26% of the tumor population, as contrasted to 9.5% of the total hospital dog population.

The biologic behavior of these neoplasms is well known. The vast majority are classified as adenomas. Generally, they grow very slowly and often persist for many months or several years without causing clinical signs. Histologically, they closely resemble normal perianal glandular tissue. The lesions are often multicentric, particularly in the perianal area. They may also arise in the dorsal and ventral tail root areas, rarely from the dorsal lumbar and preputial skin. Infrequently, they become locally invasive and recur postoperatively. In rare instances, metastasis to the iliac lymph nodes develops.

A number of treatments have been suggested. They range from surgical excision and irradiation to castration and the oral and parenteral administration of synthetic or natural estrogens. A carefully designed prospective study is clearly indicated to clarify the value of these treatments. Such a study must utilize randomly selected cases which would then be treated by one or more of the previously mentioned methods. Until this type of investigation is carried out, it will be impossible to know with certainty what effects various forms of therapy may have on what is essentially a very benign process.

Recent histochemical studies have suggested that the perianal (hepatoid) glands may have an endocrine function, as they appear to produce secretory granules. These glands arise as buds from compound hair follicles and enlarge rapidly after birth (Baker, 1967). Because perianal adenomas occur primarily in old male dogs, it has long been postulated that testicular androgen plays an important role in their development. In females, it has been suggested that androgens of adrenal cortical origin may promote the growth of the perianal gland (Baker, 1967). Endocrinologic and histologic studies of affected dogs and appropriate controls are necessary to validate these hypotheses. Progressive hyperplasia of the perianal gland area is a common finding, particularly among aging male dogs. It is logical to assume that adenomatous change represents further progression of this hyperplastic state in some dogs.

c. Papilloma and Squamous Cell Carcinomas (SCC)

(1) *Dog.* Some clinical features observed in dogs with papillomas and SCC are recorded (Table IV).

The number of papillomas is undoubtedly underrepresented, as most papillomas are small pedunculated inocuous lesions which are usually only removed for cosmetic reasons. This group of cutaneous papillomas excludes the papillomas (verruca vulgaris) of viral origin, occasionally observed in the oral cavities of young dogs. There is no clinical evidence that skin papillomas are precancerous lesions. Papillomas and SCC differ in their sites of origin and in the age and sex of dogs affected (Table IV).

SCC is the only consistently malignant epithelial tumor of the dog's skin. It is locally invasive in most cases and is often characterized by superficial ulceration with ragged indurated edges. While regional and distant spread have been observed, ulceration usually occurs rather late in the course of the disease. Recurrence on one or more occasions has been observed in several animals without any subsequent metastasis. An important site for SCC is the digital region. Here, the tumor often invades the adjacent phalanges, causing marked osteolysis which is readily visualized radiographically. In one advanced case, all the bones up to the midshaft of the tibia were almost completely destroyed, and recurrence and metastasis developed several months after amputation. Recently, metastasis was reported in 2 of 5 dogs with digital SCC (Liu and Hohn, 1968). Malignant melanoma, which is even more likely to spread to regional nodes or lungs, or both, than SCC, is another important digital neoplasm. Both SCC and melanoma must be differentiated from chronic paronychia. Biopsy and exfoliative cytologic studies are important diagnostic aids. In the absence of inoperable metastasis, early diagnosis should be followed by digital amputation. SCC rarely affects light-skinned, exposed, relatively hairless areas, as it does in cats, and thus does not appear related to exposure to sunlight.

(2) *Cat.* Cutaneous papillomas are rare, but SCC is relatively more common than in dogs. SCC most commonly affects the head region, particularly the tips of the pinnae, and seems to be most prevelant in white cats. The eyelids are another fairly frequent site for this tumor. Unicentric or multicentric origin can occur. SCC often develops insidiously from a small nonhealing ulcer to a crusted invasive tumor. Radical excision is often curative. Solar irradiation appears to be an important predisposing factor.

2. MESENCHYMAL NEOPLASMS

a. Mast Cell

(1) *Dog.* Without question, the mast cell tumor, also referred to as mastocytoma and, if malignant, as mast cell sarcoma, is the most important cutaneous neoplasm of the dog. The clinical features of 210 mast cell tumors are summarized in Table IV. The 3 most common sites of the tumor were thigh (35), thoracic region (34), and scrotum (23).

Many investigators have pointed out the predilection of this lesion for Boxers and Boston Terriers. Over 50% of our cases occurred in these 2 breeds, a clear indication of their marked susceptibility. It has been postulated that common ancestral configuration of these 2 breeds may explain their increased relative risk to mast cell tumors (Peters, 1969). Further investigation relative to genetic susceptibility would be rewarding, particularly if pedigree analyses were carried out.

The clinical and pathologic features of these tumors have been reviewed (Hottendorf and Nielsen, 1969), and a few general comments seem warranted. The use of differential stains to demonstrate metachromatic mast cell granules is common. We were unable to get positive granule staining in formalin-fixed tissue of a few tumors but were able to observe it in touch smears of appropriately stained fresh tumor tissue. While the diagnosis of mast cell tumors can be confused with inflammatory and reactive skin lesions associated with secondary mast cell proliferation, a good clinical history coupled with careful histologic examination will usually differentiate these processes. It is sometimes impossible to determine histologically whether or not the tumor should be designated as benign or malignant unless tissue infiltration is present. Well-differentiated tumors have been known to recur and metastasize. In general, the owner is given a guarded prognosis for any mast cell tumor, and periodic re-examination is advised. Some investigators have stated that 50% of mast cell tumors are malignant or potentially malignant. In most clinics, adequate postsurgical follow-up material is not available. In some instances, only those tumors known to have recurred or metastasized are reported, whereas cases, in which follow-up information is absent, are assumed not to have caused any further problem. In a study of 300 surgically excised mast cell tumors, 15.3% recurred (Hottendorf and Nielsen, 1969). However, follow-up of all cases was not possible, and this figure is undoubtedly somewhat low.

Mast cell tumors have a wide range of behavioral patterns; some grow insidiously for many months or years and are of minimal clinical significance; others grow slowly for a while and suddenly undergo exacerbation of growth and become obviously malignant. The third type appears clinically malignant, either when first observed or shortly thereafter. Careful clinicopathologic correlation of many more affected dogs will be mandatory to gain a better insight of the behavior of these neoplasms.

In most cases, mast cell tumors of lymph nodes and viscera are thought to be related to metastasis but, in a few instances, tumors that appeared to be of multicentric origin (systemic mastocytosis) have been reported. In these cases, mast cell infiltration of spleen, liver, and bone marrow has been prominent. In some dogs, multicentric skin involvement was present with the number of tumors ranging from a few to several hundred or more.

Considerable biochemical study of the heparin–histamine complex found in the mast cell granules has been carried out (Hottendorf et al., 1965). Increased bleeding tendencies have been reported, e.g., prolonged clotting times of patients with mast cell tumors. In my experience, uncontrollable bleeding has not presented a major problem in surgical removal of these lesions. In a few dogs, usually those with extensive mast cell tumors, gastroduodenal ulcerations, presumably attributable to the increased levels of circulating histamine of tumorous origin, has been observed (Carrig and Seawright, 1968; Brodey, 1969). Histamine is known to increase the release of gastric hydrochloric acid.

A characteristic vasculitis has been seen in mast cell tumors. It appears to begin as an inflammatory process with medial infiltration by eosinophiles and to progress to fibrinoid degeneration and, finally, to sclerosis of small vessels characterized by concentric rings of collagen around vessels with the neoplasms. The latter finding, "onion ring" sclerosis, has been observed in human spleens affected with systemic lupus erythematosis. It has been suggested that dogs with mast cell tumors might be utilized as experimental models to study collagen diseases (Hottendorf and Neilsen, 1968).

The cause of cutaneous mast cell tumors has yet to be demonstrated, although 2 spontaneous canine mast cell leukemias were proved to be of viral etiology (Lombard *et al.*, 1963; Post *et al.*, 1967; Rickard, 1968). A transplantable mast cell tumor was experimentally induced in the skin of a 16-month-old male mouse by the repeated topical application of methylcholanthrene (Dunn and Potter, 1957). It would be of great interest to know if the long-term application of such a carcinogen to the skin of a Boxer or Boston Terrier would induce mast cell neoplasia.

(2) *Cat.* Mast cell tumors are comparatively rare in this species. In a recent report, 6 mast cell tumors were observed among a group of 83 skin tumors (Engle and Brodey, 1969). They were located as follows: trunk (3) and eyelid, neck, and limb (1 each). Very little is known of the biologic behavior of these tumors. Some are localized, and cured by surgical removal; others may begin as a focal lesion but soon disseminate, or develop multicentricity throughout the skin and internal organs. Gastroduodenal ulceration has been reported in a cat with several hundred cutaneous mast cell tumors, infiltration of the liver and spleen, and terminal mast cell leukemia. Increased circulating histamine content, presumably of tumoric origin, was thought to play a primary role in the genesis of the ulcer, which subsequently perforated (Seawright and Grono, 1964).

Involvement of the liver, spleen, bone marrow, and occasionally the blood of a few cats has indicated multicentric involvement similar to that seen with various forms of malignant lymphoma. This type of mast cell disease is more properly referred to as mastocytosis or mast cell reticulosis.

The increasing frequency of isolation of oncogenic viruses from cats, and the fact that 2 canine mast cell leukemias were proved to be of viral origin, should stimulate search for viruses in feline mast cell neoplasms.

b. Histiocytoma

Because this tumor is small, rarely exceeding 2–3 cm. in diameter, well circumscribed, and primarily confined to young dogs, affected animals are not as likely to be referred to a university clinic as are the obvious malignancies usually seen in older dogs. Some clinical features of 30 dogs with histiocytoma are summarized in Table IV.

Although histiocytoma and transmissible venereal tumor (TVT) bear close resemblance histologically, a recent study of 520 histiocytomas clearly indicated that these tumors represent distinct entities on morphologic, biologic, and epizootiologic ground (Taylor *et al.*, 1969). Cytogenetic studies have shown that the number of chromosomes in TVT from Pennsylvania and Japan is consistently reduced from the normal diploid number of 78 to 59 (Weber *et al.*, 1965). Similar karyotyping should be carried out with histiocytoma.

Pure-bred dogs, particularly Boxers and Dachshunds, had an excess risk rate whereas poodles appeared to have a reduced rate. The most important site was the skin of the head, particularly the pinna. This tumor was unique, as it reached its peak incidence in young dogs (50% occurrence before 2 years of age) and rapidly decreased in incidence as the population aged (Taylor *et al.*, 1969). This observation is in marked contrast to those on all other canine neoplasms.

Most authors consider histiocytoma to represent a true neoplasm. On clinical grounds, however, this view may be questioned. Recurrence is rare, and metastasis has yet to be reported. Almost invariably the lesions are surgically removed a short time after they are first observed, so there is almost no knowledge of their behavior in untreated dogs. Histiocytoma may be a self-limiting lesion which may undergo spontaneous regression if surgery is not performed.

The cause of this histiocytic proliferation has not been defined. Microbiologic, tissue culture, and transmission studies have been negative. Electron microscopy and development of experimental transmission techniques appear to be important areas for research.

Of great comparative oncologic interest is the Yaba monkey tumor pox virus. It causes localized benign cutaneous histiocytomas in Asian monkeys in West Africa. Experimentally, intravenous inoculation of Yaba virus may produce miliary histiocytomas in many tissues. These miliae are thought to be due to viral infection of multiple sites rather than to metastasis of tumor cells (Fenner, 1968).

c. Lipoma

(1) *Dog.* Lipomas are extremely common in the subcutaneous tissues, particularly of the trunk and especially of the chest. This is the only skin tumor of the dog which has been far more common in females than males (Table IV). Lipomas may be solitary or multiple. Growth is usually slow and expansile rather than infiltrative. Because of their extreme benignancy, removal is often not advised; thus, the numbers of lipomas

listed in Table I is rather small. In rare instances, lipomas have infiltrated striated muscle, and radical surgery has been required for cure.

There is no evidence that lipomas predispose to liposarcomas. While lipomas are exceedingly common, liposarcomas are rare and appear malignant from their onset.

(2) *Cat*. While fatty neoplasms are very common in dogs, they appear to be quite uncommon in cats. We observed 5 lipomas and 1 liposarcoma in 395 cats with tumors (Engle and Brodey, 1969). While liposarcoma appears to be a rare spontaneous feline neoplasm, it was induced recently in 5 kittens given injections of feline leukemia virus (Rickard, 1969).

d. Fibroma, Fibrosarcoma, and Hemangiopericytoma

(1) *Dog*. These 3 neoplasms are closely related histogenically and biologically. In some instances, well differentiated fibroblastic tumors may be designated histologically as benign, yet they may infiltrate locally, recur, and, in rare instances, even metastasize. The ultimate decision as to the tumor's classification as benign or malignant should rest on its clinical behavior rather than on its histologic features.

In general, these neoplasms (Table I) have been slow-growing subcutaneous lesions which have certain features in common (Table IV). No sex predilection was apparent. Hemangiopericytomas appeared to affect somewhat older dogs than the other 2 types. Boxers appeared overrepresented in the fibroma and hemangiopericytoma groups, whereas Cocker Spaniels appeared overrepresented in the hemangiopericytoma and fibrosarcoma groups. These 3 tumors arose far more frequently from the integument of the trunk or extremities in contrast to the adnexal tumors which arose most commonly from the head and neck region. In a few instances, metastasis of fibrosarcomas has been observed. Although some hemangiopericytomas were very invasive and tended to recur repeatedly, metastasis was not reported (Mills and Nielsen, 1967).

(2) *Cat*. Fibromas and fibrosarcomas are important skin tumors of cats, but hemangiopericytomas are rare. The prognosis of most of these lesions appears to be good, although we did observe local recurrence and regional node metastasis in a cat with fibrosarcoma (Engle and Brodey, 1969). As in the dog, the histologic differentiation between fibroma and fibrosarcoma has been difficult in the absence of metastasis, unless the tumor was locally invasive or tumor emboli were present in vascular or lymphatic channels.

Multiple subcutaneous fibrosarcomas were observed recently in a 2-year-old cat (Snyder and Theilen, 1969; Dienhardt *et al.*, 1970). Electron microscopy revealed many budding C-type particles similar to those of the cat leukemia virus. Cell-free transmission was readily accomplished in neonatal kittens, puppies, and marmosets. Further studies are needed to determine if this virus will produce fibrosarcomas in other species and if this virus is a variant of the feline leukemia virus or represents an as yet unidentified sarcoma virus. Many more feline fibroblastic tumors should be examined for the presence of virus.

3. Melanotic Neoplasms

a. Dog

The biologic behavior of these neoplasms appears to vary considerably with their site of origin. Melanomas of the distal portions of the extremities, particularly the digits, the skin or mucocutaneous junction of the lips and cheeks, and the scrotum are often malignant, whereas those arising from the trunk or other sites on the head and neck are usually benign. Cutaneous melanomas, just as oral melanomas, arise primarily in heavily pigmented breeds. Some skin tumors appear heavily pigmented, but cut section of the lesion may reveal that the pigment is confined solely to the overlying epithelium. In other instances, the entire lesion may be pigmented but may not be a true melanoma histologically, i.e., it may represent a fibroma or adnexal tumor which is infiltrated by melanin.

Almost nothing is known about the cause of melanomas. Passey (1938) produced melanomas of the skin of several Airedales after long-term topical applications of carcinogenic tars. This result was unusual, as such applications usually cause the development of papillomas and squamous cell carcinomas. The experiments should be repeated in other heavily pigmented breeds.

b. Cat

Little is known of the biology of feline melanomas. We observed only one melanoma in a study of 83 skin neoplasms (Engle and Brodey, 1969). This tumor arose from the skin of the tail base of a black cat and metastasized to its iliac lymph nodes.

II. Respiratory Tract Neoplasms

1. Nose and Paranasal Sinuses

a. Dog

Tumors of the respiratory tract comprised 66 (2.3%) of the 2917 canine neoplasms (Fig. 1). The tumors were nearly equally divided between the nasal and paranasal sinuses, and the lungs. Tumors of the larynx and trachea were rare.

Twenty-one tumors were of nasal origin and 9 arose from the para-nasal sinuses (frontal and maxillary). Carcinomas, mostly adenocar-cinomas, but also epidermoid and undifferentiated types, comprised 75% of the tumor types. The male to female ratio was 3.3:1. The average age was 9.2 years, with 75% of the dogs ranging from 7 to 11 years. Large breeds appeared overrepresented in the tumor population, and mixed breeds appeared underrepresented.

The important clinical signs were sneezing, nasal discharge, or epistaxis (unilateral or bilateral), nasal obstruction and, in advanced cases, facial bone deformities, nasolachrymal duct obstruction, and ocular proptosis. Radiographic findings in more advanced cases were unilateral or bilateral obliteration of normal nasal architecture owing to invasion and lysis of adjacent bone, as well as erosion, displacement, or destruction of the median nasal septum. Sometimes, obstruction to normal drainage from the frontal sinus(es) resulted in the accumulation of mucus or mucopus, which was often seen radiographically.

One of the major clinical problems is that of making a diagnosis early enough to effect possible cure. Usually, by the time obvious radiographic signs are evident, the lesion is too extensive for complete surgical removal. In early cases, the clinical signs of nasal cancer may be indistinguishable from those of rhinitis or sinusitis, or both. A technique is needed for nasal cavity irrigation to permit subsequent cytologic examination of the irriga-tion fluid for neoplastic cells. Such a technique might permit earlier diagnosis. Cytologic suspicion of malignancy would then be followed by thorough surgical exploration of the affected cavity.

Although nasal carcinomas are very invasive locally, they rarely pro-duce regional or distant metastasis.

Sarcomas, primarily osteosarcoma and chondrosarcoma, also arise in the nasal region, usually of large breeds. In most cases, osteosarcomas arise from the nasal or surrounding facial bones. Hardy *et al.* (1967) reported that 12 of 33 skull osteosarcomas were of facial bone origin. In contrast, chondrosarcomas arise intranasally, e.g., from the cartilage of the turbinates. While the nasal region was unimportant as a site of osteo-sarcomas (approximately 2% of 194 cases), it constituted the second most common site for chondrosarcomas (30% of 23 cases). Both osteosarcoma and chondrosarcoma, however, are best considered as bone tumors and not as primary nasal tumors (Brodey, 1969).

b. Cat

Tumors of the respiratory tract comprised 8 (3%) of 395 neoplasms (Fig. 2). Five of these neoplasms arose from the nasal cavity or para-nasal sinuses; all of them were carcinomas. None of the tumors was

operable. The clinical and radiographic signs in the cat were essentially
the same as in the dog. Of 19 osteosarcomas, 2 arose from the maxillae
and 2 from the orbital bones.

Nothing is known of the etiologic factors of canine or feline nasal
cancer. Whether air pollutants play a role is not known. Epizootiologic
studies might help to resolve the problem.

2. LUNG

Many facets of primary pulmonary neoplasia need clarification; however, some preliminary information has been gathered. A vexing problem
concerns the incidence of the disease in various parts of the world and
whether or not the increased number of cases diagnosed in the past decade
reflects a true rise per se or simply mirrors the greater sophistication in
diagnostic methodology (bronchoscopy, exfoliative cytology, radiography,
and surgery) that has developed in the last decade. In our hospital, we
diagnosed 9 lung carcinomas from 1952 to 1958 as compared to 20 between 1959 and 1965. This increase in numbers of cases being diagnosed
annually is continuing. Improved diagnostic techniques plus increased
clinical awareness would seem to be the major factors. Most canine
tumors tend to arise from peripheral portions of the lung. In contrast,
most lung tumors of man originate near the hilus and are thus much more
readily visualized by bronchoscopy than their canine counterparts.

It is essential to employ strict criteria in arriving at a final diagnosis
of primary lung neoplasia. Detailed clinical, radiographic, and pathologic
studies, including necropsy, are essential to distinguish primary tumors,
which are quite uncommon, from metastatic lung tumors, which are very
common. Obviously, no analysis of a population of dogs with lung tumors
will have validity unless the diagnostic criteria are strictly enforced.

Another controversial point concerns the histogenesis of these tumors.
Some authors have reported that most canine lung tumors are of bronchiolar origin, with a small number of bronchial origin (Nielsen and
Horava, 1960). These authors observed that most bronchiolar carcinomas
did not metastasize, whereas the few bronchial carcinomas did spread.
In a study of 29 lung tumors seen at our hospital, we concluded that it
was impossible to determine their histiogenesis with any certainty (Brodey
and Craig, 1965). There is no proof that bronchial, bronchiolar, or
alveolar epithelium represent immutable cell lines, and thus there would
seem to be little justification for assuming that a tumor containing
epithelium resembling bronchiolar mucosa actually arose within a bron-
chiole. We therefore used a simple histologic classification which avoided
speculation on the cellular locus of origin. Tumors were classified in order
of frequency as adenocarcinoma, squamous cell carcinoma, and anaplastic

carcinoma. In about a third of the cases, more than one histologic type was observed in a single tumor. Undoubtedly, the number of composite tumors would have increased if a larger number of sections from each tumor had been studied.

Metastasis was far more common in our case material than in that of Nielsen and Horava (1960). The major reason for the disparity probably lay in the sources of material of the 2 studies. In the report of Nielsen and Horava (1960), many of the tumors were detected incidentally at necropsy and thus were often small and well localized. Our study, however, utilized cases primarily diagnosed clinically and then subjected to pathologic examination. We therefore observed tumors that were far larger, more invasive, and more commonly associated with metastasis. In 18 dogs with metastases, 17 affected the lung. This propensity of primary lung tumors to spread to other portions of the lung has caused considerable diagnostic confusion. Because of the central position of the lung in the circulatory system, hematogeneous and lymphatic metastases and transmigration of tumor cells through the air spaces all result in a redistribution of the tumor within the lung parenchyma. In a few instances, the tumors became disseminated throughout the lung and were of similar size, making it difficult to determine the lobe of origin, assuming it to be a primary lung carcinoma, or whether or not the lung nodules were secondary to some primary extrapulmonary tumor. In a few cases, it was impossible to be certain which interpretation was correct.

Our study revealed that the Boxer breed had a marked predisposition to lung carcinoma. The disease was not observed in dogs under 7 years of age and the average age of affected dogs was near 11 years. No sex predilection was detected among dogs in contrast to human beings where males were far more frequently affected than females (Ackerman and del Regato, 1954). This predilection may, in part, be related to the smoking habits of the human population.

The most important clinical sign in the dog is chronic nonproductive cough. Any persistent cough in an older dog should prompt detailed clinical and radiographic examinations. A large, clearly defined lung mass, with or without smaller pulmonary densities, constitutes important radiographic evidence of lung carcinoma, particularly in the absence of other extrapulmonary malignancies. Bronchoscopy and cytologic examination of bronchial washings are other valuable diagnostic techniques. If metastasis is not apparent clinically or radiographically, exploratory thoracotomy is indicated. Hypertrophic osteoarthropathy (HPO) was observed in 5 of 29 dogs with primary lung carcinomas. This syndrome may precede or follow the respiratory signs induced by the lung lesion. Removal of the lung tumor is usually followed by rapid regression of the

HPO. Because of the marked similarity of HPO in dogs and man, the dog has proved to be a valuable experimental model of the human disease (Holling and Brodey, 1961).

Too few canine lung tumors have been resected to allow accumulation of significant postsurgical data. In general, however, after clinical signs have developed, the tumor has either metastasized or will do so shortly after excision of the primary tumor. The main hope for cure would appear to be the radiographic detection of the tumor before clinical signs have appeared. This would involve radiographic chest screening procedures which are not economically feasible, in view of the low incidence of primary lung neoplasia.

Little is known of the etiology of lung tumors in dogs. Experimentally, carcinoma of the canine bronchus has been induced by weekly intrabronchial instillation of a carcinogen (DMBA) over a period of 2 to 14 months (Staub *et al.*, 1965). Epizootiologic studies of urban and rural dog populations and a large group of dogs with lung cancer might yield important new information. Because of the short life span of the dog as contrasted to man, dogs have limited geographic mobility. This allows a more meaningful analysis for unusual urban/rural distribution.

III. Thyroid Neoplasms

Thyroid neoplasms are not common in either dogs or cats. They comprised 2% of 395 feline neoplasms (Fig. 2) and 1.7% of 2917 canine tumors (Fig. 1). Although the percentages of thyroid tumors in both species were similar, neoplasms of thyroid origin were of clinical importance only in dogs.

Undoubtedly, many canine thyroid neoplasms are mistaken for other lesions and, thus, are frequently undiagnosed. Thyroid neoplasms were commonly observed in dogs in highly goiterous areas of Sweden, Switzerland, Germany, and the Great Lakes region of the U. S. A., earlier in this century. Recently, however, studies of tumor collections from England, U. S. A., and South Africa have suggested that thyroid neoplasia is far less common now than it was formerly. Only 2 of 57 thyroid tumors studied in our hospital were found concomitantly with hyperplasia or goiter (Brodey and Kelly, 1968). It was suggested that while hyperplasia probably predisposes to canine thyroid neoplasia, it is not a necessary prelude.

Of the 57 thyroid neoplasms, there were approximately equal numbers of adenomas and adenocarcinomas. In 35 dogs, thyroid tumors (22 carcinomas and 13 adenomas) were detected clinically; the remaining 18 adenomas and 4 carcinomas were discovered at necropsy. There was no sex predilection for either type. The average age of dogs with adenomas or carcinomas was approximately 10 years. Only 1 of the 57 dogs was under 5 years of age. Boxers accounted for 40% of the thyroid tumor population, although they represented only 7.2% of the total hospital population. The Boxer breed was thus significantly overrepresented ($P < 0.001$). Clinical duration of the thyroid tumor often ranged over many months; in a few instances, the tumor had been observed for 1 or 2 years. Bilateral thyroid neoplasia was observed in 3 of 29 dogs with adenomas as contrasted to 10 of 28 dogs with carcinomas. Adenomas were well circumscribed and readily excised. Carcinomas were usually very invasive locally, and commonly extended to adjacent veins and metastasized to the lungs. Successful surgical removal of most carcinomas was usually not possible. Clinical signs of thyroid hypofunction or hyperfunction were not detected. Studies are underway to determine plasma thyroxine levels of dogs with thyroid neoplasms (Siegel, 1969).

The adenomas consisted of flattened or cuboidal well-differentiated thyroid cells in solid and follicular groupings. Hemorrhage, calcification, and fibrosis were common. Hemorrhage was often marked and frequently left only small areas of tumor tissue for uncomplicated histologic assessment. Nodules of well-differentiated thyroid epithelium were present in the capsule in 7 adenomas. Such foci might be mistaken for carcinomatous invasion of the capsule.

The 25 carcinomas consisted of varying mixtures of solid, follicular, and columnar groups of well-differentiated cells. Three of the tumors were solidly anaplastic. Papillary carcinoma, so common in the human thyroid gland, was absent in the canine material. There was often considerable discrepancy between the microscopic appearance of primary and metastatic tumors from the same dog. Invasion of adjacent tissues, veins, and lymphatics was common.

A transplantable canine thyroid tumor, derived from a Boxer, was maintained in serial passage through 30 generations of mixed breed puppies (Allam *et al.*, 1956).

IV. Bone Neoplasms

1. OSTEOSARCOMA

a. Dog

Musculoskeletal neoplasms comprised 4.4% of 2917 tumors (Fig. 1); approximately 80% were osteosarcomas and 10% were chondrosarcomas. Most of the remaining tumors consisted of such uncommon lesions as fibrosarcoma, hemangiosarcoma, and plasma cell myeloma. Benign neoplasms were very uncommon.

The clinicopathologic and radiographic features of osteosarcoma of the dog and man are similar in most respects (Brodey *et al.*, 1963; Brodey and Riser, 1969). The predilection toward osteosarcoma by the large canine breeds is well known; we observed that only 4% of 194 dogs with osteosarcoma weighed under 25 pounds (Table V). A study of man, based on this knowledge about dogs, revealed that children with osteosarcoma were of greater bone stature than were matched control children with nonosseous malignancies (Fraumeni, 1967). Osteosarcoma of man developed most commonly in the metaphyses during the period of active bone growth and reconstruction of adolescence and early youth; in dogs and cats, the tumors develop in the metaphyses, usually long after metaphyseal growth has ceased. This striking intraspecies difference needs to be investigated. Osteosarcoma primarily arises in the major weight-bearing bones, the radius, humerus, femur, and tibia of the dog and the femur and tibia, primarily the knee joint area, of man. Interestingly, site

TABLE V

CLINICAL FEATURES OF CANINE CHONDROSARCOMA AND OSTEOSARCOMA

Clinical features	Chondrosarcoma	Osteosarcoma
Number of tumors	23	194
Breed	No giant breeds, i.e., St. Bernard, Great Dane 9% weighed under 25 lb. Boxers, 22% German Shepherd, 17%	24% occurred in giant breeds 4% weighed under 25 lb. Boxers, 23% German Shepherd, 10%
Age (years)	Average, 5.9 Mode, 6 Median, 6 13%, 2 years or less	Average, 7.7 Mode, 9 Median, 7 10%, 2 years or less
Male to female ratio	1:1.5	1.2:1
Site	100% in flat bones (ribs, 10; head, 8; pelvis, 3; etc.)	23% in flat bones (head, 26; ribs, 11; pelvis, 3; etc.) 77% in long bones (primarily radius, humerus, tibia, and femur)
Average duration of clinical signs	16 weeks	9 weeks
Biologic behavior	Metastasis infrequent (4 of 23 dogs) Surgical treatment often curative if tumor is of rib origin	Early hematogenous metastasis, particularly to lungs Postsurgical results in 41 dogs: 56% dead in 4 months 85% dead in 8 months

[a] University of Pennsylvania, 1952–1968.

distributions vary significantly among the major breeds of dogs affected, e.g., about 70% of osteosarcomas in Great Danes involve the distal radius as compared to 10% in Boxers; flat bone involvement is much commoner in Boxers than in Great Danes, St. Bernards, Collies, and German Shepherd dogs (Brodey *et al.*, 1963). These and other breed differences in sites of predilection may be related to growth and weight-bearing stresses on the metaphyses of the forelimb and hind limb during locomotion. These observations should be expanded.

Relatively few dogs with osteosarcoma have been treated by amputation, so comparison of canine to human survival rates is somewhat difficult. Further complicating such comparison is the great difference in longevity between man and dog. In a study of 41 surgically treated dogs with osteosarcoma of the long bones, 56% died or were euthanatized due to lung metastasis, recurrence, or both within 4 months after amputation and 85% were dead within 8 months. Of the remaining 15%, only one was considered to be cured, as it was clinically free of disease 6 years postoperatively. Another dog lived almost 3 years after amputation, and 2 others, which were euthanatized for causes unrelated to osteosarcoma, one at 18 months, the other at 6 months postsurgery, had no evidence of osteosarcoma at necropsy. Another dog, which was destroyed 6 months after surgery because of a lumbar intervertebral disc protrusion, had only one tiny osteosarcomatous lesion, a 1 mm. lung nodule (Brodey, 1964; Brodey and Riser, 1969). In man, 5 year survival rates following amputation have ranged from 10 to 20% in most studies. In a recent report, 30 human patients of a total of 300 with osteosarcoma had exceptionally long survival times. The authors could find no characteristics, i.e., age, sex of patient, site and duration of tumor, histologic features, etc., of the long-term survivors that distinguished them from the 270 patients who did not fare so well (O'Hara *et al.*, 1968). Obviously, survival was linked primarily to host-tumor factors which have only been superficially investigated. Dogs with osteosarcoma should serve as excellent models of the human disease and greatly facilitate research on treatment, etiology, and host-tumor relationships.

High titers of osteosarcoma antibodies were demonstrated recently by immunofluorescence in the serums of human patients with osteosarcoma, and in their close relatives and friends; in sharp contrast, control patients had low or negative titers. The presence of antibody reactivity to osteosarcoma in a few controls suggests that an infectious agent, presumably an oncogenic virus, had produced unrecognized infection (Morton and Malmgren, 1968). These findings in man and the isolation of a murine osteosarcoma virus (Finkel *et al.*, 1966) suggest that attempts should be made to isolate viruses from osteosarcoma or chondrosarcoma in dogs.

b. Cat

It was observed that 21 (6%) of 395 tumors arose from the skeleton (Engle and Brodey, 1969). Of these, 19 were osteosarcomas. The cats ranged from 3 to 18 years with a mean age of 10.5 years. The male to female ratio was 3.5:1. No pure-bred cats were affected.

Long bones, humerus (4), femur (4), and tibia (3) were affected in 11 cats while flat bones, maxilla (2), orbit (2), vertebra (2), scapula (1), and mandible (1) were involved in 8 cats. This distribution indicates that osteosarcomas are more likely to affect flat bones in the cat than in the dog where only 23% of 194 osteosarcomas arose from flat bones. However, the Boxer breed had a much greater tendency toward flat bone involvement, e.g., the ratio of long bone to flat bone involvement having been 2:1 as contrasted to 3:1 for Irish Setter and German Shepherd dogs and 26:1 and 19:0 for the Great Dane and St. Bernard, respectively (Brodey and Riser, 1969).

We have recently observed osteosarcomas in 2 cats suffering from severe chronic osteodystrophies related to excessive feeding of liver (Riser and Brodey, 1968; Brodey, 1969). The resultant destructive and reparative bony changes induced by this diet, which is exceedingly high in vitamin A and phosphorus and deficient in calcium, may predispose to ultimate neoplasia. The significance of this preliminary observation needs further evaluation. An association has long been known between Paget's disease and bone sarcomas of man. It has been estimated that 7.5% of all people with Paget's disease eventually develop osteosarcoma (Ackerman and del Regato, 1954).

The biologic behavior of feline osteosarcomas has not been as thoroughly studied as that of their canine counterparts. It would appear that the cat tumors tend to grow more slowly, as evidenced by the duration of clinical signs in the 2 species. Of 194 dogs, 75% had signs for 1 to 9 weeks whereas of 9 cats, 6 had signs for 2 to 5 months. Metastases were observed in 23 of 49 untreated dogs and 4 of 11 untreated cats.

The fact that feline lymphosarcoma is of viral origin and that a feline fibrosarcoma virus has recently been isolated (Snyder and Theilen, 1969) should spur efforts to find oncogenic viruses in feline as well as canine osteosarcoma.

2. CHONDROSARCOMA

a. Dog

This neoplasm is a clinicopathologic entity distinct from osteosarcoma. In the early literature, many osteosarcomas were incorrectly designated as chondrosarcomas, primarily because insufficient tissue was examined microscopically. Many sections of any tumor-containing areas of cartilage should be examined before concluding it is a chondrosarcoma and not an osteosarcoma. Even though a tumor may contain predominantly carti- laginous tissue, it should be designated as an osteosarcoma if osteoid is being directly produced by the sarcomatous cells, no matter how small the focus (Brodey et al., 1963). It is not always possible to distinguish a benign from a malignant cartilaginous tumor by its histologic appearance, even if it is carefully correlated with the clinical history and radiographic findings. It would appear that most canine cartilaginous tumors are ma- lignant or potentially malignant.

Many clinical differences in dogs with osteosarcoma and chondrosar- coma are evident (Table V). The differential diagnosis is important be- cause the biologic behavior and, hence, the prognosis of these 2 tumors often varies so greatly.

b. Cat

We observed only one chondrosarcoma in a group of 21 bone neo- plasms. It arose from the scapula of a 4-year-old female Siamese cat. Since few chondrosarcomas have been reported, little is known of their clinicopathologic features.

V. Hematopoietic Neoplasms

In domestic animals (fowl, cattle, horses, swine, dogs, and cats) spontaneous lymphoid neoplasia, primarily lymphosarcoma, predominates, and myeloid neoplasia has been rarely observed. Marked differences in the frequency of lymphosarcoma exist in the 2 species. In cats, lympho- sarcoma was the most common and comprised about 26% of 395 tumors (Fig. 2). In the dog, however, lymphosarcoma comprised only 5.3% of 2917 neoplasms (Fig. 1). The characteristic clinicopathologic picture in the dog was generalized superficial lymphadenopathy, often with hepato- splenomegaly (Moulton, 1961), whereas in the cat, peripheral adenopathy was less frequent and visceral involvement, particularly of the cranial mediastinum, small intestine and mesenteric lymph node, and the kid- ney, are common (Holzworth, 1960). Although characteristic syndromes occurred in both species, highly atypical cases were also observed. It would appear that the types of syndromes seen in cats varied markedly in Philadelphia and Scotland. In Philadelphia (Engle and Brodey, 1969), the mediastinal form appeared to be most common, whereas in Scotland it was the least common form (Crighton, 1965). The mediastinal form affected a much younger group of cats than did the other forms of lymphosarcoma, and pure-bred cats, particularly Siamese, seemed to be more susceptible. Lymphocytic leukemia was infrequent in both species. Final diagnosis was usually based on lymph node or tissue biopsy and less frequently on bone marrow aspirates.

Although occasional reports on therapy have been published, many more cases need to be studied. We must have a clearer idea of the biologic behavior of these tumors in untreated patients, before we can hope to evaluate the results of therapy.

The etiology of lymphoid tumors in cats has been greatly clarified in the past few years. The observations of Jarrett *et al.* (1964) have been expanded and confirmed by workers in New York, i.e., Rickard *et al.* (1967), Rickard (1968), Hardy *et al.* (1969), and in California, Kawakami *et al.* (1967). Many investigators have experimentally transmitted lymphosarcoma to kittens using cell-free material derived from tumor tissue or blood of clinical cases. It is now clear that at least some, if not all, cases of feline lymphosarcoma are caused by C-type viral particles, morphologically and biophysically almost identical to other known avian and murine leukemia viruses. In a series of experimental transmissions, in New York State, several kittens inoculated with cat leukemia virus (FeLV) also developed liposarcoma, a rare spontaneous feline neoplasm (Rickard, 1969). These observations suggest the FeLV may have a wide spectrum of oncogenic activity similar to that already shown for different strains of the avian leukosis and mouse leukemia viruses. A spontaneous feline fibrosarcoma, containing many budding C-type viral particles, similar to those of the FeLV, has just been described (Snyder and Theilen, 1969). Cell-free material from this tumor produced fibrosarcomas when injected subcutaneously in puppies and kittens. Whether this virus represents a new agent or is merely a strain of the FeLV is not known. Variations in the age and genetic constitution of the host, the amount of virus, its route of infection, and other external factors (irradiation, hormones, carcinogens) can markedly affect the latent period and type of neoplastic end result.

It has been demonstrated that the FeLV and murine leukemia viruses possess a common group specific antigen, a relationship that needs further clarification (Geering *et al.*, 1968). Little is known about the natural spread of FeLV. Is the virus spread through the mother's milk or the placenta, or via the ovum and sperm as in the mouse? The reports of Schneider *et al.* (1967) and Engle and Brodey (1969) and current clinical observations suggest that aggregations of cases in related and nonrelated cats are relatively common and that both vertical and horizontal transmission may be important. The latter could be accomplished by virus-contaminated urine and feces or particularly saliva, as cats commonly scratch and bite one another. Recently, FeLV antigen has been detected by immunodiffusion studies, in the salivary glands of leukemic cats (Hardy et al., 1969). The Siamese breed, particularly certain highly inbred strains, appears to be more susceptible to lymphosarcoma than mixed breeds, but further statistical studies are needed.

Seroepidemiologic techniques are vital for elucidating the natural history of lymphosarcoma in cats and the relationship of the feline disease to other avian and mammalian leukemias. The use of the gel diffusion technique (Ouchterlony) or the development of other serologic techniques such as complement fixation, fluorescent antibody, or hemagglutination inhibition should allow the screening of various cat populations for the presence of the FeLV. FeLV antigen was demonstrated in 25 of 33 cats with lymphosarcoma using an immunodiffusion technique (Hardy et al., 1969). Serologic techniques are simpler, faster, more economic and often more precise than electron microscopic preparations. It is clear that serologic studies will greatly enhance our knowledge of the disease in a short time. If feline leukemia is similar to that of the mouse, as it appears to be, one would expect to find evidence of the FeLV in clinically normal cats. In general, the model systems used in murine leukemia are excellent guides for investigation of feline leukemia. Hardy et al. (1970) observed budding C-type particles, identical to those of FeLV, from a histologically normal cervical lymph node of a 5-month-old Abyssinian cat. Immunodiffusion Ouchterlony studies of the same lymph node revealed the presence of FeLV antigen. Five months after this finding, the cat was still clinically normal. It was from a household which had already lost 2, and probably 3, cats from lymphosarcoma.

The cat is prone to develop a number of leukoproliferative disorders. While most of these are lymphoproliferative, other proliferative diseases, i.e., reticuloendotheliosis and mastocytosis, have been described. Reticuloendotheliosis is characterized by proliferation of reticulum cells in the liver, spleen, bone marrow, lymph nodes, and blood (Gilmore et al., 1964). This reticulum cell proliferation, which is classified by some as lying between the lympho- and myeloproliferative types, may represent an unusual variant of lymphosarcoma. Particles morphologically identical to FeLV have been observed in a cat with reticuloendotheliosis and in another with granulocytic leukemia; these particles have yet to be evaluated biologically or antigenically (Theilen, 1969). Systemic mastocytosis is characterized by infiltration of mast cells into the liver, bone marrow, blood stream, and, in particular, the spleen. Metachromatic staining is required to differentiate mastocytosis from lymphosarcoma and reticuloendotheliosis. Proliferative disorders affecting lymphocytes, reticulum cells, mast cells, and myeloid cells all cause diffuse progressive parenchymal infiltration. It appears more and more that some of these diseases may be virally induced. Should this be the case it will be necessary to determine whether or not they have a common viral etiology or are due to different oncogenic viruses.

Another feline disease, infectious fibrinous peritonitis, is now thought to be of viral origin (Zook et al., 1968). FeLV antigen was demonstrated in 5 of 13 cats with peritonitis (Hardy et al., 1969). It is possible that active infection with the infectious peritonitis virus may activate a latent leukemia virus.

C-type particles have been propagated in tissue culture, using suspensions of neoplastic feline lymphocytes (Theilen, 1969). These particles, when inoculated in susceptible kittens, produced lymphosarcoma, indicating that the virus grown in the cell suspension culture was indeed FeLV. This tissue culture technique appears to provide a reliable source of large amounts of virus which can then be utilized to prepare antibody for a variety of seroepidemiologic investigations.

The demonstration that lymphosarcoma of the cat is caused by a virus opens further the possibilities that other mammalian lymphomas and leukemias (human, canine, bovine, etc.) which bear strong clinical and pathologic similarities are also viral in origin. The close contact relationship of cats to man, mouse, dog, and cattle provides further impetus to such speculation.

Whole cell transmissions have been accomplished using cell suspensions from the spleen of a dog with spontaneous lymphosarcoma as well as cells from a tissue culture line of canine lymphosarcoma. However, cell-free filtrates derived from spontaneous tumors or tissue culture material failed to induce lymphosarcoma in puppies (Friedman et al., 1968). Electron microscopic studies of a limited amount of canine lymphosarcoma material have shown preliminary but not conclusive evidence of viral content (Chapman et al., 1967).

Splenic tumors, primarily hemangioma and hemangiosarcoma, are important surgical lesions of dogs. The clinicopathologic features of the canine tumors have been described (Brodey, 1965). They appear rather rarely in cats; only 2 of 395 feline neoplasms were splenic hemangiosarcomas (Engle and Brodey, 1969), and thus little is known of their biologic behavior.

VI. Testicular Neoplasms

Tumors of the testes constitute an important clinical entity of dogs (Fig. 1). All 3 tumor types, Sertoli cell tumor (SCT), seminoma (SEM), and interstitial cell tumor (ICT), were commonly represented. In general, the type of study, e.g., primarily surgical or postmortem, has determined which neoplasm was most common. Generally, ICT is a small inconspicuous tumor which is commonly undetected clinically, whereas SCT and SEM often become large, and the former may be associated with a feminization syndrome. The latter 2 neoplasms therefore would be more commonly represented in a study of surgically removed tumors.

Canine testicular tumors as a group are usually benign. We have never observed an ICT which metastasized. SEM, while histologically similar to malignant seminomas in man, only rarely extended along the vas deferens or metastasized internally. The SCT, however, metastasized in approximately 10% of our cases, particularly to the iliac or sublumbar lymph nodes and occasionally to other lymph nodes, spleen, liver, and kidney (Brodey and Martin, 1958).

It has been repeatedly shown that cryptorchidism of man predisposes to testicular neoplasia. Furthermore, a cryptorchid testis, brought into the scrotum surgically (orchiopexy), is still more likely to become neoplastic than a normally descended testis. This observation suggests that cryptorchidism per se may not be the essential tumorigenic factor, but may be only one of many signs of developmental disturbances, perhaps mediated by hormones, which under certain situations can lead to testicular neoplasia (Vechinski et al., 1965). For this reason, many surgeons now advise orchidectomy rather than orchiopexy.

Human cryptorchidism is associated with an 11% prevalence of pseudohermaphroditism. Two canine SCT arising from cryptorchid testes have been observed in male pseudohermaphrodites, phenotypically females but genotypically males, i.e., both gonads were testes (Frey et al., 1965; Brodey, 1969).Undoubtedly, this association is more common than is generally realized.

Recent canine studies by Reif and Brodey (1970) have established the following facts:

1. There is a highly significant association between cryptorchidism and SCT, and SEM ($P < 0.001$), whereas ICT rarely develop in undescended gonads.

2. SCT or SEM arising from cryptorchid testes were diagnosed in a younger group of dogs than those with SCT or SEM arising from scrotal testis. In SCT, this association of earlier age at diagnosis with cryptorchid tumors is highly significant ($P < 0.001$).

3. Feminization, which occurs in approximately 30–40% of dogs with SCT, has been significantly more common in association with SCT of an undescended testis than in SCT of a scrotal testis ($P < 0.001$). Feminization occurred in 17% of dogs with scrotal SCT, 50% of those with inguinal SCT, and 70% of those with abdominal SCT. One explanaton for this

association may lie in the fact that in dogs with cryptorchid, particularly abdominal SCT, various features of the feminization syndrome (hair loss, attraction of males, gynecomastia) rather than obvious testicular swelling, brings the owner to the veterinarian. In contrast, some dogs with obvious scrotal SCT may be brought in for treatment before feminization has had time to develop. It is also possible that hormonal production, from a cryptorchid SCT, may differ both quantitatively and qualitatively from that of a scrotal SCT. It is well known that hyperplasia of Sertoli cells is common in the atrophic seminiferous tubules of dogs with cryptorchidism. Whether this hyperplasia predisposes to SCT is not known. A recent electron microscopic study of normal and neoplastic Sertoli cells in man revealed many similarities (Able and Lee, 1969).

Having established the relationship of SCT and SEM to cryptorchidism by retrospective methods, prospective studies must be designed with cryptorchid dogs and breed-matched control populations to learn the relative risk of testicular neoplasia in each group. Breed should also be taken into consideration as the Boxer may have a higher incidence of testicular tumors than other breeds.

Of the 3 canine testicular tumors, most attention has focused on SCT, primarily because 30 to 40% of the tumors are associated with a striking clinicopathologic syndrome, characterized by feminization, i.e., gynecomastia, attraction of males, atrophy of the scrotal nonneoplastic testicle, symmetrical alopecia, squamous metaplasia of prostatic epithelium, and atrophy of the prepuce. Feminizing signs regressed after removal of the SCT in 2 dogs but recurred a few months later (Coffin et al., 1952; Brodey and Martin, 1958). In both instances, metastases, presmuably functional, were present in the sublumbar lymph nodes. Repeated administration of a synthetic estrogen, i.e., diethyl stilbesterol, had been shown to cause changes similar to those observed in feminized dogs having SCT (Mulligan, 1947). Assays of several primary SCT and of spermatic and jugular vein plasma in dogs with feminizing SCT failed to show the presence of excessive amounts of the common highly active estrogens, estradiol-17β and estrone (Siegel et al., 1967). Work is needed to determine whether or not this feminization is induced by an estrogen of unknown structure.

Testicular tumors are exceedingly rare in cats. We failed to observe any tumors of the testis among 395 feline tumors. An important reason for this negative finding is that many cats in this country are castrated during the first year of life, whereas castration of young dogs in far less common. It would be valuable to determine the prevalence of testicular tumors in a large population of intact older male cats.

VII. Female Genital Tract

1. MAMMARY GLAND

a. Dog

Tumors of the female genital tract were second in frequency only to those of the integument. In our hospital, they comprised 776 (22.1%) of 2917 neoplasms (Fig. 1). The site distribution in bitches was mammary gland (687), vagina and vulva (56), ovary (24), and uterus (9).

Much empiricism, misinformation, and confusion surrounds the subject of mammary neoplasms and their relationship to various phases of the estrual cycle. Statements made without proof of accuracy have dominated much of the thinking and surgical treatment for decades. Only recently have some of these statements been challenged. While much more work is needed, certain preliminary statements can be made.

A study of estrual histories in 161 bitches with mammary tumors and 244 age- and breed-matched controls revealed no relationship of irregular estrus or number of pregnancies to mammary tumor development. It did, however, indicate significantly fewer episodes of pseudopregnancy in bitches with mammary tumors than in the control bitches ($P < 0.001$). Furthermore, there were no significant differences in age of mammary tumor onset or in the histologic type distribution of tumors between bitches with one or more pseudopregnancies and those with no reported episodes (Fidler et al., 1967). It had been thought that one or more pseudopregnancies, irregular estrual cycles, or failure to have puppies, would predispose a bitch to develop mammary tumors. It has been suggested that kennel bitches which are regularly bred may have a decreased prevalence of mammary neoplasms, an observation that needs clarification.

Pseudopregnancy is thought to be a normal metestrual phenomenon of the bitch. However, the intensity of the associated changes varies greatly from animal to animal and at different metestrual periods of the same bitch. The variation in intensity is presumably related to the degree or duration, or both, of luteal stimulation or possibly to the sensitivity of the target tissues (mammary gland, endometrium) to progestational compounds. Thus, while the histologic changes of pseudopregnancy, mammary secretion, and endometrial glandular hyperplasia probably occur to some degree in all bitches in metestrum, only those with more severe changes actually exhibit clinical pseudopregnancy. Further contributing to the awareness of this syndrome is the perspicacity of the owner or veterinarian, or both. Further clarification of pseudopregnancy will be possible when definitive steroid assays are carried out on bitches in various phases of metestrum. Such assays could be correlated with vaginal cytologic examinations and endometrial biopsies.

Also needed is comparison of pathologic findings of the ovaries and uteri of bitches with mammary tumors with those of age- and breed-matched controls. Present statements concerning the increased frequency of cystic endometrial hyperplasia, pyometra, and ovarian cysts and neoplasms in bitches with mammary tumors are open to considerable question. I believe that controlled studies will reveal that such ovarian and uterine changes are associated with increasing age, i.e., an increased number of estrual cycles, rather than with the presence or absence of mammary neoplasms.

For years, ovariectomy at the time of mastectomy has been recommended empirically but proof of its efficacy has been lacking. Proponents of this procedure have suggested that ovariectomy reduced the possibility of recurrence and metastasis as well as inhibiting the development of mammary tumors in the remaining glands. The relationship of ovariectomy to the later development of mammary tumors has been clarified (Fidler et al., 1967). Bitches spayed prior to 2 years of age rarely developed mammary tumors, whereas those spayed at 5 years or older developed, not infrequently, mammary tumors or increased growth of preexisting mammary tumors, or both. Thus, it would appear that the development of mammary neoplasms may be determined by the time the bitch is 2 or 3 years of age. I have ovariectomized approximately 20 bitches with inoperable mammary cancer and observed no regression of the primary or metastatic lesions. A well-designed prospective study using standardized procedures for the preoperative, surgical, pathologic, and postoperative findings is essential to clarify the confusion in this area. Random selection, using a random table of numbers, should be used to designate bitches for each group, e.g., mastectomy alone or mastectomy combined with ovariectomy. The study must be open-ended at the beginning until the differences in median survival times of each group is known, e.g., if there is a 50% difference, only 20 bitches are needed in each group but if there is only a 10% difference, which seems far more likely, 100 bitches would be required in each group. Even then, these numbers would give only a 75% assurance of arriving at a significant result (Abt, 1969).

Since approximately 50% of all surgically removed mammary neoplasms are benign (Frye et al., 1967; Cotchin, 1958), only the remaining 50% with malignant tumors would be suitable for the proposed study. Furthermore, some bitches with mammary malignancies would have to be excluded because of inoperable local invasion, distant metastasis, severe organic diseases, i.e., cardiac or renal failure, or client refusal to permit surgery. Assuming a 10% difference in median survival time, and the other exclusion factors just mentioned, one would need to draw the 200 bitches with mammary cancer for the proposed study from a base population of approximately 500 to 600 bitches with mammary neoplasms. Few hospitals have a clinic population large enough to make such a study feasible. A well-coordinated project involving a group of hospitals is clearly indicated.

In the meantime, the surgeon must balance the nebulous value of ovariectomy at the time of mastectomy against the mortality and morbidity associated with abdominal surgery in an old dog. In my opinion, ovariectomy at the time of mastectomy should be discontinued unless future study indicates it to be of value.

When the metabolism of estrogen and progestogens is elucidated, these hormones or their metabolites could be assayed in the plasma or urine of bitches with and without mammary tumors, and correlated with estrual histories, vaginal cytologic changes, and the gross and microscopic changes in the ovaries, uterus, vagina, and mammary glands.

The relationship of adrenal cortical and pituitary hormones to canine mammary tumor growth is largely unknown. The results of adrenalectomy or hypophysectomy, or both, on primary and metastatic canine mammary cancer have to be determined. It is well nown that some breast carcinomas of women initially respond dramatically to ovariectomy, adrenalectomy, and hypophysectomy.

Little is known of the evolution of malignant mammary lesions in dogs. Do they begin as malignancies from their inception or do they evolve from benign to malignant processes? The intensity and duration of the oncogenic stimulus, the hormonal environment, and the genetic resistance of the host may play a major part in determining whether or not the end result is a benign or malignant neoplasm. It would be highly informative to study the histology of mammary tumors during various phases of growth. Generally speaking, these tumors appear to follow 3 main clinical patterns. Group I: their growth is slow and often persists for many months or years without harming the host. Group II: growth is slow at first, often for months or years; then suddenly there is a growth spurt, and the tumor becomes invasive and metastatic, e.g., sudden acceleration of growth was noted in 71 of 85 bitches with malignant tumors as compared to 17 of 67 with benign tumors (Fidler et al., 1967). Group III: growth is quite rapid from the time tumors are first detected and they appear malignant very early after their onset. Faced with this variation in growth patterns and the inability to predict accurately the behavior of tumors which appear to be in Group I or the early phase of Group II, it is often difficult for the clinician to give the owner a sound recommendation as to the ultimate need or value of surgical removal.

Opinions differ as to the reasons for the formation of mucoid, chondroid, or osseous tissue in many canine mammary tumors. These mixed tumors, so common in dogs, are rare in cats and in man. The main theories are that (1) myoepithelial cells, often spoken of as "interposed cells," may produce a mucoid or chondroid matrix which may be subsequently ossified; (2) fibroblasts may undergo metaplasia to osteoblasts or chondroblasts; (3) the neoplastic epithelium may induce stromal metaplasia; it was shown experimentally that mammary epithelium implanted in the sheath of the rectus abdominis muscle could induce bone formation (Cotchin, 1958). Electron microscopy and tissue culture studies should help to clarify the problem.

The histologic criteria of malignancy must be correlated with the clinical behavior of the tumor in arriving at final assessment of a given tumor's growth potential. Much more clinical and surgical follow-up is necessary before the percentage of mammary tumors that are biologically malignant can be determined. Present studies suggest that close to 50% are histologically malignant; however, disparities undoubtedly exist among pathologist's criteria for malignancy. The recent attempts by the World Health Organization to standardize diagnostic terms used to evaluate the morphologic appearances of mammary tumors should go a long way toward solving this basic problem. Most published reports have derived their material primarily from surgically removed tumors. Generally, one would expect that tumors removed surgically would be larger and more aggressive than those which are either ignored or go unnoticed. Thus, review of findings on a large number of purely necropsy cases should result in a much lower percentage of mammary malignancies than has been reported, as tiny benign nodules are common in the mammary glands of older bitches.

We studied 56 bitches treated surgically for malignant mammary tumors, after excluding 29 other bitches with mammary cancer because of lung metastasis or inoperable local involvement. Of the 56 bitches, 48% died or were euthanatized because of recurrence, metastases, or both, with a median time of 4 to 8 months after surgery (Fidler et al., 1967).

No experimental method of inducing canine mammary tumors has been developed. In one instance, the long-term administration of stilbesterol, with or without progesterone, produced hormonally dependent ovarian carcinomas but no mammary neoplasia (Jabara, 1962). The experiment should be repeated using a natural estrogen, such as estradiol, to see if it would induce the same lesions as the synthetic stilbesterol. Of considerable interest is the report of a male Boxer with a large feminizing cryptorchid Sertoli cell tumor that developed several mammary adenomas (Walker, 1968). This case suggests that a hormonal product of the testicular neoplasm, presumably an estrogen of some type, may play a role in the induction of the mammary tumors. Obviously, further studies are needed to test this hypothesis. In addition, electron microscopic search for possible oncogenic viruses, tissue culture studies, and a variety of other laboratory investigations represent important areas for future research.

b. Cat

In our hospital, tumors of the female genital tract comprised 59 (15%) of 395 tumors (Fig. 2). Of these, 56 arose from the mammary gland and 3 from the ovaries.

The histologic appearance and biologic behavior of feline mammary neoplasms have been much more constant and predictable than those of the dog. Approximately 80% were histologically diagnosed as adenocarcinomas; mixed tumors were rare. The carcinomas usually grew rapidly, and ulceration, local invasion, and metastasis were often present. All 4 mammary glands were more or less equally affected, whereas in the dog, tumors were far more common in the 2 most caudal mammary glands. Mammary carcinomas occurred in cats whose average age was 12.6 years; tumors were not observed in cats under 6 years of age.

Almost nothing is known about the relationship of ovarian function to feline mammary tumorigenesis. Pseudocyesis is extremely rare in this species. It is not known whether a higher percentage of young cats than dogs is spayed. This factor is obviously important as it is known that dogs spayed prior to the first year or 2 of life almost never develop mammary tumors. It has been estimated that intact female cats have a sevenfold higher relative risk of mammary cancer than neutered females (Dorn et al., 1968b).

The results of mastectomy on 15 cats indicated that most of them eventually died of recurrent or metastatic disease or both. A remarkable exception, a 13-year-old cat, has survived 5 operations for recurrent and regionally metastatic mammary carcinomas over a 5-year period. While recurrent nodules are still present, the cat remains in good health and apparently free of pulmonary metastases. Its 5-year-old daughter has just developed a mammary nodule which consisted of an orderly hyperplasia of ducts and fibrous stroma. Immunologic studies of such patients may be of considerable value. The cat will be observed closely to see if other mammary nodules develop. Both cats received biannual injections of medroxyprogesterone to prevent estrus for 4 to 5 years. With observations on only 2 cats it is impossible to speculate what, if any, relationship there is between the progestational compound and the mammary tumors.

Out of 24 domestic short-hair cats from a single household, 4 all un-
spayed and 9, 12, 12, and 13 years of age have developed mammary
carcinomas since September 1966. Two of them were sisters, whose neoplasms developed within 2 months of each other. Both of these cats are
still alive, although one had recurrence 18 months after operation. The
2 unrelated cats were euthanatized because of extensive recurrence, 16
and 19 months postsurgery (Brodey, 1969).

The case histories just described suggest the possibilities of vertical
or horizontal transmission, or both, of an infective agent, presumably a
virus. Electron microscopic studies of these neoplasms should be carried
out, as cats may carry a mammary tumor virus similar to the Bittner
virus of mice. Immature budding C-type particles, similar to the cat
leukemia virus, have been observed in 2 of 6 feline mammary carcinomas
(Gross and Feldman, 1969). Whether this virus is etiologically related
to the mammary tumors or is a passenger virus, is unkown.

2. Vaginal and Vulvar

Ninety-six neoplasms of the vulva, vagina, and uterus were described in 90 bitches seen in our hospital by Brodey and Roszel (1967).
It was estimated that 1 of every 375 bitches examined had a neoplasm
in one of these 3 sites.

In 70 of the 90 bitches, the tumors were designated leiomyomas.
Histologically, they were classified as leiomyomas, although the amount
of vascularity and hyalinization and of fibrous proliferation varied from
tumor to tumor, and in different sections of the same tumor these microscopic variations did not seem to be related to their biologic behavior.
The leiomyomas were confined to the vulva or vagina of 66 bitches and
to the uterus of 10 bitches. The ages of the 66 with leiomyomas ranged
from 5 to 16 years and averaged 10.8 years. Boxers comprised 16.2% of
the tumor population, as contrasted to 7.2% of the overall hospital
population; this is significant at the 5% level. The duration of clinical
signs varied greatly depending on the extraluminal or intraluminal growth
pattern of the tumor. In 12 bitches with extraluminal leiomyomas, the
average duration of signs was 24 weeks, whereas in 26 bitches with
intraluminal leiomyomas, the average duration was only 7 weeks. The
shorter duration was primarily related to the owner's concern when a
mass suddenly prolapses through the vulvar labia. Most leiomyomas
arose in the vestibule of the vulva rather than in the vagina. They grew
extraluminally, particularly from the roof of the vestibule, or intralumi-
nally, where they appeared as solitary, predunculated, firm lesions which
often prolapsed through the labia. Surgical excision was almost always
curative. The role of estrogenic stimulation in the development of these

tumors is unknown. It is possible that ovariectomy may retard growth of a recurrent tumor, but this relationship has to be explored.

Uterine leiomyomas, although relatively infrequent in dogs, are thought to affect 20% of all women over 30 years of age (Willis, 1960). In contrast, vaginal leiomyomas which are common in dogs are rare in women. Furthermore, although cystic glandular hyperplasia of the canine endometrium is common, endometrial and cervical carcinomas are exceedingly rare. In women, however, cervical and to lesser extent, endometrial carcinoma are important neoplasms. Neoplasms of the feline genital tract, excluding the mammary glands, are rare; a few uterine adenocarcinomas and vaginal leiomyomas have been reported. These marked intraspecies differences need to be investigated further, with particular emphasis on the endocrine status of each patient. Whether there is any correlation between abnormalities in the estrual cycle and the development of genital leiomyomas in dogs is unknown. In all probability, no significant differences would occur between bitches with these tumors and matched controls. It have never observed a vulvovaginal leiomyoma in a bitch spayed prior to 2 years of age; hence, spaying prior to this age would appear to have a highly significant sparing effect. Suggestions that cystic endometrial hyperplasia, pyometra, and mammary neoplasms are more frequent in bitches with vulvovaginal leiomyomas need to be explored further, as all of these lesions are common in older bitches.

Other neoplasms occasionally observed in the vulva and vagina are transmissible venereal tumors, lipomas, and leiomyosarcomas (Brodey and Roszel, 1967). Squamous cell carcinoma, an important neoplasm of the human vaginal vulvar mucosa, appears to be rare in both the dog and cat.

VIII. Digestive Tract Neoplasms

1. MOUTH, PHARYNX, AND SALIVARY GLANDS

In the dog, alimentary tract (including liver and pancreas) tumors comprised 12.8% of 2917 tumors (Fig. 1), whereas 20% of 395 tumors of cats were of alimentary tract origin (Fig. 2). In both dogs and cats, neoplasia (excluding lymphosarcoma) appears far more commonly in the mouth and pharynx than in the stomach and intestines. Part of this disparity is due to the ease with which oral and pharyngeal tumors can be detected and the difficulties involved in diagnosis of gastrointestinal tumors Most of the oral and pharyngeal (OP) tumors of cats were squamous cell carcinomas; fibrosarcomas were less frequent and melanomas exceedingly rare. The 2 commonest OP tumors of dogs were squamous cell carcinomas and malignant melanomas. Fibrosarcomas, while third in frequency of occurrence, are important OP tumors of the dog. Site frequencies varied greatly between dogs and cats. The most important sites in dogs in the Philadelphia area in order of frequency were (1) gingiva, (2) tonsil, (3) buccal and labial mucosa, (4) hard palate, and (5) tongue (Brodey, 1960, 1961; Cohen et al., 1964). In the cat, the gingivae were by far the commonest site for neoplasia with the frenulum of the tongue, a second important site (Engle and Brodey, 1969).

Cocker Spaniels were predisposed to OP melanomas. Breed predilections were not detected for the other OP malignancies. Male dogs were more commonly affected than females with tonsillar carcinoma (3:1), OP melanomas (4.3:1), and OP fibrosarcomas (2:1). The one exception to this observation was gingival carcinoma which affected males and females equally.

Canine tonsillar carcinomas and almost all OP melanomas were invasive locally, and recurrence with regional and distant metastases were common. Gingival carcinomas and fibrosarcomas of dogs, while invasive locally, metastasized infrequently. Gingival and lingual carcinomas of cats were invasive, but little has been learned of their metastatic potential.

Diagnosis of all OP neoplasms is greatly aided by cytologic examination of scrapings from the surface of the lesion, unless it is covered by intact mucosa. In some dogs with obvious carcinoma of one tonsil, combined cytologic and histopathologic examination of the supposedly normal tonsil has revealed that it too was carcinomatous. The fact that both tonsils are neoplastic in some cases provides one explanation for the bilaterality of regional lymph node metastases; it further compounds attempts at therapy, which have been futile.

No precancerous lesion such as oral leukoplakia of man has been observed in the mouths of dogs and cats. Cytologic studies of the oral mucosa and tonsillar epithelium of older dogs and cats, with and without OP neoplasia, may alter this opinion. If such a precancerous lesion could be identified, it would greatly contribute to studies of etiology, pathogenesis, and treatment.

While tongue tumors are quite uncommon in dogs, they are important OP tumors of cats. Melanomas, carcinomas, and fibrosarcomas occur on the tongue of dogs. The first 2 usually involve the dorsum, whereas fibrosarcomas are more likely to involve the body of the tongue. In contrast, almost all feline tongue neoplasms are squamous cell carcinomas which almost invariably arise from the frenulum.

The treatment of OP cancer of dogs is usually highly unsatisfactory for a variety of reasons. First of all, most of these neoplasms are characterized by early invasion of soft and bony tissues, with or without regional node or distant metastasis, making curative surgical treatment highly unlikely. Diagnostic delays in some cases further contribute to the already poor prognosis. Cure or good palliation is primarily possible for gingival squamous cell carcinoma if extensive bony invasion has not occurred, as this lesion is quite radiosensitive and usually only metastasizes late in its course. In tonsillar carcinoma and all OP fibrosarcomas and melanomas, the results of surgical and irradiation therapy are usually poor. Almost nothing is known concerning the treatment of feline OP tumors. As most of these tumors are squamous cell carcinomas, irradiation therapy combined with earlier diagnosis will undoubtedly improve results somewhat. Almost no information is available on the value of chemotherapy for treatment of OP malignancies in either species.

It has been suggested that industrial and automative air pollution may play a role in the genesis of tonsillar carcinoma in dogs. A survey of 2 university veterinary clinics revealed that tonsillar carcinoma was statistically far less common in Pullman, Washington, a primarily rural area (Ragland and Gorham, 1967) as compared to Philadelphia, a primarily urban area (Cohen et al., 1964). Further epizootiologic data from other areas need to be analyzed to test this hypothesis.

The occurrence of such tumors as tonsillar carcinoma and primary lung carcinoma might be used to monitor the severity of air pollution over a long period and its possible effects on man. Clinical observation suggests that male dogs would be more valuable since tonsillar carcinoma occurs 3 times as commonly in males as in females. All breeds could be used, as no breed predilection has been observed. Dogs, because of their relatively short life spans and close association with man's environment, would serve as excellent experimental models.

Salivary gland tumors would appear to be relatively more frequent in cats than in dogs. Engle and Brodey (1969) observed 4 parotid and 2 mandibular gland tumors in 395 feline tumors as compared to 6 parotid and 1 mandibular gland tumor in 2917 dogs. The tumors in both species were adenocarcinomas except for a benign mixed tumor in a dog. Neoplasia of the sublingual gland was not observed in either species.

2. ESOPHAGUS

The dog develops osteosarcoma and fibrosarcoma of the thoracic esophagus in areas where *Spirocerca lupi*, the esophageal worm, is enzootic particularly in the southeastern U. S. A. (Bailey, 1963), in East Africa (Murray, 1968), and in other areas of the world that have been less thoroughly investigated. The highly cellular loose granulation tissue in the worm-induced granulomas is similar to fibrosarcoma, and neoplastic transformation is not unusual. Whether *Spirocerca lupi* induces neoplasia secondary to its secretions or metabolic products or by carrying an oncogenic virus is unknown. Electron microscopic and tissue culture studies may clarify this situation. Leiomyomas are occasionally observed in the esophagogastric area, but they rarely become large enough to cause clinical signs.

Cats in England have been reported to develop carcinoma of the cranial thoracic esophagus (Cotchin, 1952), a disease almost unknown, or unreported, in other parts of the world. Furthermore, tonsillar carcinomas appear to be far more common in English than in American cats.

3. STOMACH AND INTESTINE

Gastric carcinoma, while considered to be infrequent in dogs, is being recognized more and more frequently when careful clinical and radiographic observations are correlated with surgical and necropsy results. The findings associated with canine gastric carcinoma are typical of the leather bottle (linitis plastica) type of human scirrhous gastric carcinoma (Brodey and Cohen, 1964). Present evidence indicates a declining incidence of this tumor in man. Gastric carcinoma has not been reported in cats.

The 2 most common intestinal neoplasms of dogs and cats are adenocarcinomas and lymphosarcomas (Brodey and Cohen, 1964). The former is more common in the large intestine, particularly the rectum, of dogs, and the latter most often affects the small intestine of cats. Adenocarcinomas tend to be scirrhous annular stenosing lesions, with early mucosal ulceration and progressive luminal obstruction. Metastases to regional nodes, liver, and lungs are common. In many dogs, the disease is too advanced for a surgical cure to be affected. Lymphosarcoma is best considered as a hematopoietic neoplasm. Even though the most conspicuous lesions may be confined to the intestine and mesenteric lymph nodes, examination of other tissues and organs will usually reveal disseminated lesions, which suggest multicentric or metastatic origin, or both. Surgical treatment, therefore, offers almost no hope of cure.

IX. Discussion

An outstanding difference between feline and canine neoplasms was that approximately 80% of all feline tumors were malignant (Engle and Brodey, 1969). The percent, while not known for the dog, is obviously far lower. The biggest reason for the overall difference was that canine skin tumors, which constituted 35.6% of the total, were mostly benign with a few notable exceptions, particularly mast cell sarcoma. In contrast, hematopoietic tumors, mostly lymphosarcomas, the commonest neoplasms of cats and which constituted 26% of the total, were almost invariably malignant. Hematopoietic tumors of dogs were usually malignant, with the exception of splenic hemangiomas, but they constituted only 7.6% of all canine tumors. Mammary neoplasms further illustrated this difference. Fifty percent or less of canine tumors were malignant, as compared to 80% of the feline tumors. Testicular tumors which were common in dogs, i.e., 6.5% of the total, with the exception of a few SCT, were benign. Another major difference between canine and feline neoplasia, excluding site and type incidences, was that multiple tumor types appeared to be far more common in dogs, particularly Boxers, than they were in cats (Brodey, 1969).

It is difficult to evaluate all of the factors which bear on high prevalence of canine neoplasms and the relatively small number of feline tumors seen in our hospital. Several explanations, other than those of inherent species difference(s), are suggested when the total hospital population is analyzed. From 1963 to 1968, we treated 26,489 dogs and 4,168 cats, a more than sixfold difference. Furthermore, 34% of all dogs treated were over 5 years of age as contrasted to only 19% of all cats. Thus, many more dogs than cats were in the cancer-prone age groups.

In a survey of animal neoplasms in Alameda County, California, the estimated annual incidence rates for cancer from all sites were 381.2 per 100,000 dogs and 155.8 per 100,000 cats (Dorn et al., 1968b). From 1966 to 1968, our observed prevalence rate for neoplasia of all types was 633.1 per 10,000 dogs and 266.8 per 10,000 cats. These rates are much higher because our baseline population was derived from a referral hospital, whereas the baseline California population was derived from a canine census sample from a county.

Tumor site and type prevalence figures vary tremendously from one hospital to another because of many factors which must be understood if such information is to be meaningfully interpreted. First, one must know the type of hospital practice, i.e., whether it is of general or referral type. Baseline populations of various breeds need to be more critically evaluated, particularly as to their age and sex characteristics, to determine what percentage of a particular breed is at risk for the tumor in question, e.g., a 10-month-old female Cocker Spaniel would hardly be at risk for perianal adenoma. The particular interests of a clinician or pathologist may lead to the collection of certain types of neoplasms in unusually large proportions, thus giving a false impression of significant geographic association. The types of case recording and data retrieval systems being used and the thoroughness with which the case material is studied play an important role in the resultant data. One of the hindrances to the collection of information has been the almost universal lack of modern data retrieval systems. This deficiency is being corrected by many, but not all institutions. While these systems are of tremendous value to the oncologist, the data secured are only as good as the quality of information obtained and recorded for each case.

The concept of the natural history or biologic behavior of a neoplasm is essential to determination of its prognosis and for supplying baseline data for the evaluation of various treatments. It is often difficult to evaluate the results of treatment if the behavior of the neoplasm in the untreated animal has not been determined. For example, a few dogs with lymphosarcoma will live a year or more without treatment. If a clinician does not know this, he may falsely ascribe long survival to the drug he is using, without taking into account the natural history of the disease. Such problems can only be resolved by carefully designed and controlled research, employing random methods of patient selectivity.

The problem of comparing ages of man to equivalent ages in dogs can be resolved by studying the canine life charts prepared by Lebeau (1953). After maturity, dogs age 4 times faster than human beings. If a dog matures at 2 years and a man at 24 years, then a 10-year-old dog would be equivalent in age to a 56-year-old woman. Thus, the relative peak ages at which mammary cancer develops in both species are similar. However, the peak age for osteosarcoma in man is from 10 to 25 years, whereas in dogs it is 7 to 8 years which is equivalent to 44 or 48 years in man.

Breed predilections are important in the incidences of many canine tumors. The Boxer breed stands out above all others in this regard. Boxers have been shown to have more multiple unrelated tumors and a significantly greater incidence of neoplasms than other breeds $P < 0.005$ (Howard and Nielsen, 1965). Specifically, Boxers show predilections, of varying degrees, to mastocytomas, histocytomas, lymphosarcomas, osteosarcomas, aortic body tumors, gliomas, and hemangiomas, as well as thyroid, lung, and testicular neoplasms. In contrast, Cocker Spaniels have predilection toward oral melanomas, cutaneous adnexal tumors, and tumors of the perianal glands. The Beagle, commonly used as a research animal, has low spontaneous frequency of all types of neoplasia. While breed predilections to various neoplasms have been studied to a degree, almost nothing is known about family or strain susceptibilities within a particular breed, e.g., whether certain families of Great Danes develop osteosarcoma with higher frequency than does the breed as a whole. By locating such strains through carfeul pedigree analysis, it might be possible to produce inbred strains of dogs with specific neoplasms, thus affording excellent animal models for comparative studies.

Unfortunately, the emphasis in most large institutions is on making a diagnosis rather than on in depth study of a disease. Such an approach is usually dictated by heavy work loads and teaching and research commitments. If a disease like cancer is to be studied, clinical, radiographic, and pathologic studies must be done in great detail; in some cases, serial sectioning of tissues and lymph nodes, etc., may be necessary, to understand certain facets of metastasis. Until such in-depth studies can be carried out, we will have only inadequate knowledge of many aspects of neoplasia.

Research on the geographic aspects of cancer in animals is still in its infancy. The availability of more uniform standards of diagnosis throughout the world will open the way to gather data of great epizo-ootiologic value. A few of the suggested geographic differences already suspected are (1) the relatively frequent occurrence of tonsillar and esophageal carcinomas in English cats in contrast to their rarity or absence in North American cats; (2) the apparent correlation of canine tonsillar carcinomas with areas of high air pollution, usually large industrial areas. Initially tonsillar carcinoma was thought to be primarily confined to England; however, subsequent studies in the U. S. A. revealed carcinomas to be important tonsillar neoplasms among Philadelphia dogs and probably those of other areas of the industrialized Eastern seaboard. Thus, underreporting or failure to report a disease may contribute to the erroneous idea that a neoplasm is common in one area and rare or nonexistent in another; (3) in Alabama almost 10% of all dogs with spirocercosis also had osteo- and fibrosarcomas of the esophagus. The association of this parasite with esophageal sarcomas appears far less common in Kenya, but this finding may be related to the type of dog population under study. Additional enzootic areas of *S. lupi* infection need to be investigated to determine more accurately the relationship of esophageal granuloma to sarcoma. Once the various geographic differences in animal cancer distribution are outlined, each of these situations can be closely investigated using an epizootiologic approach in the hope that one or more etiologic clues can be discovered. This method of study has already yielded important results in human cancer.

Many of the answers needed, both on clinical and research bases, will be forthcoming only when a well-planned attack on the whole problem is made. Individuals or small groups working on their own will continue to make significant contributions. Nevertheless, important advances in knowledge will be made more rapidly and efficiently if a broadly interdisciplinary approach is employed, both nationally and internationally. An excellent example of a well-designed epizootiologic study is being carried out in 2 countries in the San Francisco bay area (Dorn *et al.*, 1968a,b).

Standardized histopathologic criteria, such as those now being developed by the World Health Organization for canine and feline mammary neoplasms, are a necessary basis for further studies. However, these criteria will need to be modified from time to time to encourage the uniformity of reporting so essential to proper interpretation of data.

Clinical research has a vital role to play in understanding the riddle of cancer although some scientists feel that the major problems of cancer can be solved only by working with pure substances and highly inbred animals. Most naturally occurring diseases occur under complex environmental situations, far removed from controlled laboratory environments. Shimkin and Friolo (1969) in a review of chemical carcinogenesis stated, "If we are interested in the effect of alcohol on carcinogenesis for example, perhaps we should start with alcoholic beverages that are actually consumed rather than with chemically pure ethanol. After all, coal tar is a dirty mess and so is tobacco tar. So, too, for that matter, is cancer."

REFERENCES

Able, M. E., and Lee, J. C. (1969). Ultrastructure of a sertoli-cell adenoma of the testis. *Cancer* **23**, 481–486.

Abt, D. (1969). Personal communication. University of Pennsylvania, School of Veterinary Medicine, Philadelphia, Pennsylvania.

Ackerman, L. V., and del Regato, J. A. (1954). "Cancer, Diagnosis, Treatment and Prognosis." Mosby, St. Louis, Missouri.

Allam, M. W., Lombard, L. S., Stubbs, E. L., and Shirer, J. F. (1956). Transplantability of a canine thyroid carcinoma through thirty generations in mixed-breed puppies. *Journal of the National Cancer Institute* **17**, 123–129.

Bailey, W. S. (1963). Parasites and cancer: Sarcoma in dogs associated with spirocerca lupi. *Annals of the New York Academy of Sciences* **108**, 890–923.

Baker, K. P. (1967). The histology and histochemistry of the circumanal hepatoid glands of the dog. *Journal of Small Animal Practice* **8**, 639–647.

Brodey, R. S. (1960). A clinical and pathological study of 130 neoplasms of the mouth and pharynx. *American Journal of Veterinary Research* **21**, 787–812.

Brodey, R. S. (1961). A clinico-pathological study of 200 cases of oral and pharyngeal cancer in the dog. *In* "The Newer Knowledge About Dogs," pp. 5–11. Gaines Dog Res. Center, New York.

Brodey, R. S. (1964). Surgical treatment of canine osteosarcoma. *Journal of the American Veterinary Medical Association* **147**, 729–735.

Brodey, R. S. (1965). "Spleen. Canine Surgery," 1st Archibald ed., pp. 700–705. Am. Vet. Publ., Santa Barbara, California.

Brodey, R. S. (1969). Personal observations. University of Pennsylvania, School of Veterinary Medicine, Philadelphia, Pennsylvania.

Brodey, R. S., and Cohen, D. (1964). An epizootiologic and clinicopathologic study of 95 cases of gastrointestinal neoplasms in the dog. *Scientific Proceedings of the 101st Annual Meeting of the American Veterinary Medical Association* pp. 167–179.

Brodey, R. S., and Craig, P. H. (1965). Primary pulmonary neoplasms in the dog. A review of 29 cases. *Journal of the American Veterinary Medical Assoviation* **147**, 1628–1643.

Brodey, R. S., and Kelley, D. F. (1968). Thyroid neoplasms in the dog. A clinico-pathologic study of fifty-seven cases. *Cancer* **22**, 406–416.

Brodey, R. S., and Martin, J. E. (1958). Sertoli cell neoplasms in the dog: The clinicopathological and endocrinological findings in thirty-seven dogs. *Journal of the American Veterinary Medical Association* **133**, 249–257.

Brodey, R. S., and Riser, W. H. (1969). Canine osteosarcoma. A clinico-pathologic study of 194 cases. *Clinical Orthopaedics and Related Research* **62**, 54–64.

Brodey, R. S., and Roszel, J. F. (1967). Neoplasms of the canine uterus, vagina and vulva: A clinicopathologic survey of 90 cases. *Journal of the American Veterinary Medical Association* **151**, 1294–1307.

Brodey, R. S., Sauer, R. M., and Medway, W. (1963). Canine bone neoplasms. *Journal of the American Veterinary Medical Association* **143**, 471–495.

Carrig, C. B., and Seawright, A. A. (1968). Mastocytosis with gastro-intestinal ulceration in a dog. *Australian Veterinary Journal* **44**, 503–507.

Chapman, A. L., Bopp, W. J., Brightwell, A. S., Cohen, H., Nielsen, A. H., Gravelle, C. R., and Werder, A. A. (1967). Preliminary report on virus-like particles in canine leukemia and derived cell cultures. *Cancer Research* **27**, 18–25.

Coffin, D. L., Munson, T. O., and Scully, R. E. (1952). Functional sertoli cell tumor with metastasis in a dog. *Journal of the American Veterinary Medical Association* **121**, 352–359.

Cohen, D., Brodey, R. S., and Chen, S. M. (1964). Epidemiologic aspects of oral and pharyngeal neoplasms of the dog. *American Journal of Veterinary Research* **25**, 1776–1779.

Cotchin, E. (1951). Neoplasms in small animals. *Veterinary Record* **63**, 67–72.

Cotchin, E. (1952). Neoplasms in cats. *Proceedings of the Royal Society of Medicine* **45**, 671–674.

Cotchin, E. (1958). Mammary neoplasms of the bitch. *Journal of Comparative Pathology and Therapeutics* **68**, 1–22.

Crighton, G. W. (1965). Lymphosarcoma or lymphatic leukemia of the dog and cat. Ph.D. Thesis to faculty of Medicine, University of Glasgow.

Dienhardt, F., Wolfe, L. G., Theilen, G. H., and Snyder, S. P. (1970). ST-feline fibrosarcoma virus; induction of tumors in marmoset monkeys. *Science* **167**, 881.

Dorn, C. R., and Taylor, D. O. N., Frye, F. L., and Hibbard, H. H. (1968a). Survey of animal neoplasms in Alameda and Contra Costa Counties, California. I. Methodology and description of cases. *Journal of the National Cancer Institute* **40**, 295–305.

Dorn, C. R., Taylor, D. O. N., Frye, F. L., and Hibbard, H. H. (1968b). Survey of animal neoplasms in Alameda and Contra Costa Counties, California. II. Cancer morbidity in dogs and cats from Alameda County. *Journal of the National Cancer Institute* **40**, 307–318.

Dunn, T. B., and Potter, N. (1957). A transplantable mast cell neoplasm in the mouse. *Journal of the National Cancer Institute* **18**, 587–601.

Engle, C. G., and Brodey, R. S. (1969). A retrospective study of 395 feline neoplasms. *Journal of the American Animal Hospital Association* **5**, 21–31.

Fenner, F. (1968). "Biology of Animal Viruses," Volume 2, pp. 644–645. Academic Press, New York.

Fidler, I. J., Abt, D. A., and Brodey, R. S. (1967). The biological behavior of canine mammary neoplasms. *Journal of the American Veterinary Medical Association* **151**, 1311–1318.

Finkel, M. P., Biskis, B. O., and Jinkins, P. B. (1966). Virus induction of osteosarcomas in mice. *Science* **151**, 698–701.

Fraumeni, J. F. (1967). Stature and malignant tumors of bone in childhood and adolescence. *Cancer* **20**, 967–973.

Frey, D. C., Tyler, D. E., and Ramsey, F. K. (1965). Pyometra associated with bilateral cryptorchism and Sertoli's cell tumor in a male pseudohermaphroditic dog. *Journal of the American Veterinary Medical Association* **146**, 723–727.

Friedman, M., Moldovanu, G., Moore, A. E., and Miller, D. G. (1968). The transplantation of tumors in higher animals. *Progress in Experimental Tumor Research* **10**, 1–21.

Frye, F. L., Dorn, C. R., Taylor, D. O. N., and Hibbard, H. H. (1967). Characteristics of canine mammary gland tumor cases. *Animal Hospital* **3**, 1–12.

Geering, G., Hardy, W. D., Jr., Old, L. J., de Harven, E., and Brodey, R. S. (1968). Shared group—specific antigen of murine and feline leukemia viruses. *Virology* **36**, 678–680.

Gilmore, C. E., Gilmore, V. H., and Jones, T. C. (1964). Reticuloendotheliosis, myeloproliferative disorder of cats. A comparison with lymphocytic leukemia. *Pathologia Veterinaria (Basel)* **1**, 161–183.

Gross, L., and Feldman, D. G. (1969). Virus particles in guinea pig leukemia and in cat mammary carcinoma. *Proceedings of the American Association of Cancer Research* **10**, 33.

Hardy, W. D., Jr., Brodey, R. S., and Riser, W. H. (1967). Osteosarcoma of the canine skull. *Journal of the American Veterinary Radiology Society* **7**, 5–16.

Hardy, W. D., Jr., Geering, G., Old, L. J., de Harven, E., Brodey, R. S., and McDonough, S. (1969). Feline leukemia virus; occurrence of viral antigen in the tissues of cats with lymphosarcoma and other diseases. *Science* **166**, 1019–1021.

Holling, H. E., and Brodey, R. S. (1961). Pulmonary hypertrophic osteoarthropathy. *Journal of the American Medical Association* **178**, 977–982.

Holzworth, J. (1960). Leukemia and related neoplasms in the cat. I. Lymphoid malignancies. *Journal of the American Veterinary Medical Association* **136**, 107–121.

Hottendorf, G. H., and Nielsen, S. W. (1968). Pathologic report of 29 necropsies on dogs with mastocytoma. *Pathologia Veterinaria (Basel)* **5**, 102–121.

Hottendorf, G. H., and Nielsen, S. W. (1969). Canine Mastocytoma—a review of clinical aspects. *Journal of the American Veterinary Medical Association* **154**, 917–924.

Hottendorf, G. H., Nielsen, S. W., and Kenyon, A. J. (1965). Canine Mastocytoma. I. Blood coagulation time in dogs with mastocytoma. *Pathologia Veterinaria (Basel)* **2**, 129–141.

Howard, E. B., and Nielsen, S. W. (1965). Neoplasia of the boxer dog. *American Journal of Veterinary Research* **26**, 1121–1131.

Jabara, A. G. (1962). Induction of canine ovarian tumours by diethylstilbestrol and progesterone. *Australian Journal of Experimental Biology and Medicine* **40**, 139–152.

Jarrett, W. F. H., Crawford, E. M., Martin, W. B., and Davie, F. (1964). Leukemia in the cat: A virus-like particle associated with leukemia (lymphosarcoma). *Nature* **202**, 567–568.

Kawakami, T. G., Theilen, G. H., Dungworth, D. L., Mann, R. J., and Beall, S. G.

(1967). "C" type viral particles in plasma of cats with feline leukemia. *Science* **158**, 1049–1050.

Lebeau, A. (1953). L'age du chien et celui de l'homme, essai de statistique sur la mortalité canine. *Bulletin de l'académie vétérinaire de France* **26**, 229–232.

Liu, S. K., and Hohn, R. B. (1968). Squamous cell carcinoma of the digit of the dog. *Journal of the American Veterinary Medical Association* **153**, 411–424.

Lombard, L. S., Moloney, J. B., and Rickard, C. G. (1963). Transmissible canine mastocytoma. *Annals of the New York Academy of Sciences* **108**, 1086–1105.

Mills, J. H. L., and Nielsen, S. W. (1967). Canine haemangiopericytomas—a survey of 200 tumours. *Journal of Small Animal Practice* **8**, 599–604.

Morton, D. L., and Malmgren, R. A. (1968). Human osteosarcomas: Immunologic evidence suggesting an associated infectious agent. *Science* **162**, 1279–1281.

Moulton, J. E. (1961). "Tumors in Domestic Animals," pp. 89–92. Univ. of California Press, Berkeley and Los Angeles, California.

Mulligan, R. M. (1947). Some effects of chronic doses of stilbesterol in female dogs. *Experimental Medicine and Surgery* **5**, 196–205.

Mulligan, R. M. (1949). "Neoplasms of the Dog." Williams & Wilkins, Baltimore, Maryland.

Murray, M. (1968). Incidence and pathology of spirocerca lupi in Kenya. *Journal of Comparative Pathology* **78**, 401–405.

Nielsen, S. W., and Horava, A. (1960). Primary pulmonary tumors of the dog—a report of sixteen cases. *American Journal of Veterinary Research* **21**, 813–830.

O'Hara, J. M., Hutter, R. V. P., Foote, F. W., Miller, T., and Woodard, H. Q. (1968). An analysis of thirty patients surviving longer than ten years after treatment for osteogenic sarcoma. *Journal of Bone and Joint Surgery* **50**, 335–354.

Passey, R. D. (1938). Experimental tar tumours in dogs. *Journal of Pathology and Bacteriology* **47**, 349–351.

Peters, J. A. (1969). Canine mastocytoma: Excess risk as related to ancestry. *Journal of the National Cancer Institute* **42**, 435–443.

Post, J. E., Noronha, F., and Rickard, C. G. (1967). "Mast Cell Leukemia in the Dog," Report, pp. 57–58. New York State Veterinary College, Ithaca, New York.

Ragland, W. L., III, and Gorham, J. R. (1967). Tonsillar carcinoma in rural dogs. *Nature* **214**, 925–926.

Reif, J. S., and Brodey, R. S. (1970). The relationship between cryptorchidism and canine testicular neoplasia. *Journal of the American Veterinary Medical Association,* **155**, 2005–2010.

Rickard, C. G. (1968). Experimental leukemia and cats and dogs. *In* "Experimental Leukemia," pp. 173–189. Appleton, New York.

Rickard, C. G. (1969). Personal communication. New York State Veterinary College, Ithaca, New York.

Rickard, C. G., Barr, L. M., Noronha, F., Dougherty, E., 3rd, and Post. J. E. (1967). C-type virus particles in spontaneous lymphocytic leukemia in a cat. *Cornell Veterinarian* **57**, 302–307.

Riser, W. H., and Brodey, R. S. (1968). Osteodystrophy in mature cats: A nutritional disease. *Journal of the American Veterinary Radiology Society* **9**, 37–46.

Schneider, R., Frye, F. L., Taylor, D. O. N., and Dorn, C. R. (1967). A household cluster of feline malignant lymphoma. *Cancer Research* **27**, 1316–1322.

Seawright, A. A., and Grono, L. R. (1964). Malignant mast cell tumour in a cat with perforating duodenal ulcer. *Journal of Pathology and Bacteriology* **87**, 107–111.

Shimkin, M. B., and Friolo, V. A. (1969). History of chemical carcinogenesis: Some prospective remarks. *Progress in Experimental Tumor Research* **2**, 1–20.

Siegel, E. T. (1969). Personal communication. University of Pennsylvania, School of Veterinary Medicine, Philadelphia, Pennsylvania.

Siegel, E. T., Forchielli, E., Dorfman, R. I., Brodey, R. S., and Prier, J. E. (1967). An estrogen study in the feminized dog with testicular neoplasia. *Endocrinology* **80**, 272–277.

Snyder, S. P., and Theilen, G. H. (1969). Transmissible feline fibrosarcoma. *Nature* **221**, 1074–1075.

Staub, E. W., Eisenstein, R., Hass, G., and Beattie, E. J. (1965). Bronchogenic carcinoma produced experimentally in the normal dog. *Journal of Thoracic & Cardiovascular Surgery* **49**, 364–372.

Taylor, D. O. N., Dorn, C. R., and Luis, O. H. (1969). Morphologic and biologic characteristics of the canine cutaneous histiocytoma. *Cancer Research* **29**, 83–92.

Theilen, G. H. (1969). Personal communication. University of California, School of Veterinary Medicine, Davis, California.

Theilen, G. H., Kawakami, T. G., Rush, J. D., and Munn, R. J. (1970). Replication of cat leukemia virus in cell suspension cultures. *Nature* (to be published).

Vechinski, T. O., Jaeschke, W. H., and Vermund, H. (1965). Testicular tumors; an analysis of 112 consecutive cases. *American Journal of Roentgenology, Radium Therapy and Nuclear Medicine* **95**, 494–514.

Walker, D. (1968). Mammary adenomas in a male dog—probable oestrogenic neoplasms. *Journal of Small Animal Practice* **9**, 15–20.

Weber, W. T., Nowell, P. C., and Hare, W. C. D. (1965). Chromosome studies of a transplanted and primary canine venereal sarcoma. *Journal of the National Cancer Institute* **35**, 537–547.

Willis, R. A. (1960). "Pathology of Tumours," 3rd ed. Butterworth, London and Washington, D. C.

Zook, B. C., King, N. W., Robison, R. L., and McCombs, H. L. (1968). Ultrastructural evidence for the viral etiology of feline infectious peritonitis. *Pathologia Veterinaria (Basel)* **5**, 91–95.

Veterinary Medicine in Indonesia

JOSEPH W. SKAGGS, M. MANSJOER, AND
SOERATNO PARTOATMODJO*†

*Kentucky State Department of Health, Frankfort, Kentucky; Padjadjaran
State University, Bandung, Indonesia; College of Veterinary Science, Institute
of Agricultural Sciences, Bogor, Indonesia*

It has not been easy to collect authorative information on any subject in Indonesia for the past decade. Communication and transportation problems in this vast tropical arphipelago are not modern. There is a paucity of scientific journals, and those which remain in publication are poorly financed and restricted in distribution. Local and national funds for research are almost nonexistent due to recurrent economic crises which have plagued the nation. Despite these deterrents, veterinary medicine in Indonesia has a rich history of accomplishment and a firm foundation on which to build. The need for further improvement in veterinary education and the development of meaningful programs of research are the goals of Indonesia's leading veterinarians (Mansjoer, 1965a). They look proudly at the past, realistically at the present, and optimistically to the future of veterinary medicine in Indonesia.

I. History of Veterinary Medicine in Indonesia

The first graduate veterinarians in Indonesia came from The Netherlands as military assignees to the Dutch East Indies Company (Schoute, 1937). Their professional activities were restricted to the animals owned by the Company itself. The first civilian veterinarian, Dr. Coppieters, came to Indonesia from Holland in 1820. Then, and even today, the

* Dr. Skaggs is Acting Director, Office of Communicable Diseases, Kentucky State Department of Health, Frankfort, Kentucky. Dr. Mansjoer is Director, Zoonoses Laboratory, Padjadjaran State University, Bandung, Indonesia. Dr. Partoatmodjo is Chairman, Bacteriology Section, College of Veterinary Science, Institute of Agricultural Sciences, Bogor, Indonesia.
† Dr. James H. Steele has served as Coordinator of this article.

Indonesian culture was rich with a plethora of pagan beliefs and super-stitions concerning the care and breeding of animals and the origin and treatment of their ills (Dieben, 1939; Kraneveld, 1957a,b,c, 1958; Seyffers and Van Dulken, 1941).

The difficulty of attracting veterinarians from Holland stimulated the Dutch East Indies Government to establish an institute of veterinary education at Surabaja, East Java, in 1860. Only eight Indonesians had successfully completed the two-year course of study, and only two students were currently enrolled by 1869. Support of this school was with-drawn, and it closed in 1875. The Civil Veterinary Service consisted of a total of seven veterinarians in 1879. A large outbreak of rinderpest on the islands of Sumatra and Java in the 1880's stimulated the colonial government to bring in nine Dutch veterinarians. They, along with a large contingent of nonprofessional personnel, were successful in even-tually eradicating rinderpest by a program of wholesale slaughter of all suspected animals.

A medical research laboratory, later called the Eykman Institute, was established in Djakarta in 1888. A Dutch veterinarian, Dr. J. K. F. De Does, a member of the Institute staff, persuaded the colonial author-ities to establish a veterinary research laboratory at Bogor in West Java in 1907. It was placed under the administrative authority of the newly founded Department of Veterinary Service of the Ministry of Agriculture, Industry and Commerce. Attached to the laboratory was a clinical and educational facility. To this day, a college of veterinary medicine has continued, and Bogor is the center for veterinary education, research, diagnostic service, and biologics production for the nation.

The cities of Surabaja, Semarang, and Djakarta established the first veterinary public health programs in Indonesia in 1911. Every major municipality had followed suit by 1940. The content of the local veter-inary public health programs was established by a Dutch Governmental Decree to the municipal governments (Ressang, 1962). Such programs continue under loose direction of the Ministry of Home Affairs. Orig-inally, the programs concentrated solely on meat hygiene. Eventually, they included dairy sanitation and milk hygiene. In some cities, the municipal public health veterinarians also assumed responsibility for the supervision of processing and marketing of other foods. They were also responsible for zoonoses control, in cooperation with the district veterinarians of the Ministry of Agriculture.

The Dutch Colonial Government also became interested in animal husbandry research in Indonesia early in the twentieth century. Large numbers of Holstein-Friesian cattle had already been imported for milk production, but little, if any, attention had been directed to upgrading native breeds of livestock and poultry. A limited number of such breeding experiments were conducted prior to the Japanese occupation of the islands during World War II.

II. Current Status of Veterinary Medicine in Indonesia

Indonesia, with approximately 108,000,000 people, is now the fifth most populous nation of the world. The most recent livestock census (1957) revealed almost 20,000,000 animals distributed by species as follows:

Cattle	5,059,346
Buffalo	2,888,211
Goats	7,173,910
Sheep	2,781,563
Horses	584,294
Swine	1,469,224

Total quantity of meat marketed in Indonesia was estimated at 275,000,000 kilograms per year. Annual slaughter (heads) estimates by species were:

Cattle and buffalo	1,100,000
Sheep and goats	3,900,000
Swine	1,200,000
Chickens	10,000,000
Ducks	10,000,000

Total milk production estimate was about 25,000,000 kilograms per year. Total annual egg production, both of chickens and ducks, was approximately 1,250,000,000.

There are now approximately 750 veterinarians in Indonesia. About a third are engaged in teaching, primarily at the five existing colleges of veterinary medicine. Another third are employed by the Ministry of Agriculture, or indirectly by the Ministry of Home Affairs as municipal public health veterinarians. The remainder are in other kinds of endeavor as will be indicated.

The Ministry of Agriculture is organizationally divided into three functional units: agriculture, forestry, and animal husbandry. Under the Directorate General of Animal Husbandry is the Veterinary Service, the Institute of Animal Diseases at Bogor, the Institute of Animal Virus Diseases at Surabaja, and the Institute of Animal Husbandry, also at Bogor. In every province throughout Indonesia, there is a Ministry of Agriculture veterinary officer working in governmental financed programs of regulatory veterinary medicine, animal husbandry, research, or combinations thereof.

Every major municipality has at least one veterinarian engaged in veterinary public health activities under the Ministry of Home Affairs. There is no organized veterinary public health program within the Ministry of Health.

The remaining 250 veterinarians are either in the Indonesian Army, working at one of the few zoologic gardens, engaged in private practice (a relative rarity today due to the poor economic situation), or pursuing nonveterinary endeavors.

Since declaring independence from the Dutch in 1945, Indonesia's most significant advances have been in the field of public education. The professional course in veterinary medicine now consists of a 5- or a 6-year post high school curriculum (Ressang *et al.*, 1959). Colleges of veterinary medical science now exist at the following universities:

1. Institute of Agricultural Sciences, Bogor, West Java, founded in 1907; it has 558 graduates; enrollment is 325 veterinary students.
2. Gadja Mada State University, Jogjakarta, Central Java, founded in 1945; it has 100 graduates; enrollment is 450 students.
3. Udayana State University, Denpasar, Bali, founded in 1962; the first class graduated in 1968; enrollment of veterinary students is 135.
4. Brawidjaja State University, Malang, East Java, founded in 1962; its first class graduated in 1969; enrollment is 300 veterinary students.
5. Sjiah Kuala State University, Darussalam, North Sumatra, founded in 1962; one veterinarian has graduated; enrollment is 98 veterinary students.
6. State University of Djambi, Djambi, Sumarta, established in 1962; there were no graduates and it closed in 1967.

It is generally agreed that sufficient facilities and equipment for a satisfactory school are available only at Bogor and Jogjakarta. These longer established colleges have received much more technical and financial assistance than the others, chiefly through USAID, Ford Foundation, and Rockefeller Foundation programs.

Veterinary medicine and animal husbandry were more or less combined curricula in Indonesia before 1963; eleven separate colleges offering 5-year degree programs in animal husbandry have been established since then. Over 1500 students are enrolled at these university-based colleges. Despite the formal separation of curricula, the coordination and cooperation between professional veterinarians and trained animal husbandrymen continues (Tojib, 1962).

Also of interest is a vocational school for veterinary technical assistants at Malang, East Java. Most of its graduates are eventually employed by the Veterinary Service to work under the direction of district veterinarians.

III. Facilities for Veterinary Medical Research

In addition to the two well-staffed and well-equipped colleges of veterinary medicine at Bogor and Jogjakarta, there are other facilities suitable for meaningful veterinary research in Indonesia. These are as follows:

1. Institute of Animal Diseases at Bogor, also known as the Central Veterinary Institute: Its facilities, originally established in 1907, are under the administrative direction of the Ministry of Agriculture and are an essential part of the General Agricultural Experiment Station. In addition to routine diagnostic procedures and the production of selected biologic products for the control of anthrax, hemorrhagic septicemia, blackleg, rabies, Newcastle disease, etc., the staff is engaged in basic and applied research on infectious diseases of animals, e.g., rinderpest, bovine pleuropneumonia, malignant catarrhal fever, surra, anthrax, hemorrhagic septicemia, piroplasmosis, anaplasmosis, tuberculosis, brucellosis, leptospirosis, salmonellosis, blackleg, listeriosis, lepra bubalorum, glanders, epizootic lymphangitis, rabies, Newcastle disease, fowl pox, foot-and-mouth disease, toxoplasmosis, and many parasitic diseases.

2. Institute of Animal Husbandry at Bogor: This facility is a part of the Agricultural Experiment Station under the Ministry of Agriculture. An organizational outline of the institute gives an insight to the types of activities in which the staff has been engaged.

   a. Department of animal husbandry technology with sections for investigation of the acclimatization of farm animals, pasture research, housing of farm animal research, and artificial insemination.

   b. The department of livestock breeding, consists of sections for: investigation of the characteristics, capacity, production, and improvement of cattle and buffalo breeds, horse breeding, goat and sheep breeding, and hog breeding.

   c. The department of poultry breeding has sections for investigation of poultry egg hatching, poultry management research, investigation of the characteristics of egg production, etc., of poultry breeds, and improvement of Indonesian chicken and duck breeds.

   d. The department of animal nutrition has sections for: investigation of the digestibility coefficient of feeds, values of feeds and rations, feeding standards for farm animals, investigation of new feeds for farm animals, and values and benefits of commercial feed preparations, especially their vitamins and microelements.

e. The department of animal industry deals with research on milk and dairy products, research on eggs, wool research, and animal hides research.

f. The department of mixed farming has sections for soil improvement, livestock economics, animal feed production, and study of mixed farming on dry soils.

g. The department of chemical investigation in animal husbandry has the following sections: analysis of cattle feeds, microbiology, investigation of toxic elements of feeds, and soil and plant analysis.

h. The extension department of the institute at Grati, East Java, has sections for livestock and poultry breeding, and farm management.

3. Institute of Animal Virus Diseases at Surabaja, also known as the Foot-and-Mouth Disease Institute: This Institute was developed with assistance from the Food and Agriculture Organization in 1957. It is considered the most modern, best-equipped veterinary medical research facility in all of Indonesia. Foot-and-mouth disease vaccine production and research are the chief programs and goals of this institution.

4. Zoonoses Laboratory, Padjadjaran State University at Bandung: This recently established facility, which receives support from the World Health Organization, is conducting research on toxoplasmosis, listeriosis, and leptospirosis.

Since independence of the country was established, most of Indonesia's research in veterinary medicine has been coordinated by the Indonesian Academy of Sciences, the Ministry of Education, and the Ministry of Agriculture which had also distributed federal funds for research. Currently, however, due to the nation's serious economic situation, budgeted funds for research are virtually nonexistent. Some assistance has been furnished by FAO, WHO, USAID, the Ford Foundation, Rockefeller Foundation, etc., but little is available now. Lack of funds for travel, glassware, chemicals, reagents, journals, etc., are acute problems for the Indonesian researcher. The Australian Government has recently presented some much needed equipment to the Institute of Animal Diseases at Bogor. However, the chief impediment to progressive research in Indonesia is and always has been lack of financial support.

In spite of the limitations of support, some modest yet meaningful research is being conducted. A list of investigations in progress at the College of Veterinary Sciences, Institute of Agricultural Sciences, Bogor, include the following: Evaluation of laboratory diagnostic procedures for anthrax, hydrogen peroxide as a milk preservative, comparative macro- and microanatomic studies on water buffalo and several breeds of cattle, distribution and control of avian coccidiosis in Java, the use of DDVP (O,O-dimethyl O-2,2-dichlorovinylphosphate) on animals with ectoparasites, prevalence of rabies in pound dogs, and livestock census for Indonesia.

IV. The Future of Veterinary Medicine in Indonesia

Like most developing countries, Indonesia's primary problem is hunger. The rapid population growth and unusual geographic distribution of the Indonesian people pose some difficult problems. The nation is lacking in food production and the continuing high birth rate makes it unlikely that it will be self-sufficient for years to come. Absence of foreign exchange, lack of effective programs for birth control and transmigration of people, and inadequate food production, processing, transportation, and marketing create tremendous challenges for the new political regime.

Against this background, veterinary medicine can and must make contributions to more efficient and greater animal production. Improvement in livestock breeding, nutrition, and management and the prevention of animal diseases are essential (Mansjoer, 1965b). Important animal diseases which require further investigation and augmented control programming are the following:

1. Anthrax is estimated to cause annual losses of $6,500,000. A number of human cases have been documented. Better systems of vaccine production and distribution are needed (Boer and Djaenoedin, 1950; Mansjoer, 1961a).

2. Hemorrhagic septicemia of cattle, buffalo, and swine, causing an estimated annual loss of $12,000,000 is widespread (Oetojo, 1958). The vaccine produced in Bogor induces transient immunity and many cases of postvaccinal anaphylaxis.

3. Brucellosis of cattle and swine is estimated to take an annual toll of $10,000,000. Transmission to man is not uncommon in Indonesia. It is especially prevalent in dairy herds in East Java.

4. Blackleg occurs sporadically in Central and East Java.

5. Tuberculosis prevails chiefly in Holstein-Friesian cattle. Bali and Madura breeds of cattle appear to be highly resistant. Tuberculosis has been diagnosed in buffalo and swine (Lobel et al., 1936). A few human cases of animal origin have occurred.

6. Glanders still occurs sporadically in horses. No human cases have been documented.

7. Epizootic lymphangitis has occurred sporadically in horses in several regions of Indonesia.

8. Foot-and-mouth disease extracts an annual toll of $18,000,000. Only type O virus has been isolated (Boer, 1941). Human cases were observed

during the Japanese occupation. The immunity from the Frenkel type vaccine produced at Surabaja is limited to 6 months. Field trials of experimental vaccine containing live suckling mouse-adapted virus accidentally introduced the disease to the island of Bali in 1964.

9. Newcastle disease is estimated to cause annual losses of $20,000,000, which is devastating Indonesia's poultry industry (Mansjoer, 1961b). More effective and stable vaccines are needed (Soegeng, 1966). Human cases of the infection have been documented.

10. Helminthic diseases of livestock, i.e., fascioliasis, cysticercosis, stephanofilariasis, hemonchiasis, ascariasis, and trichinosis, cause an estimated annual loss of $600,000,000. Parasitisms are the most important of all animal diseases in Indonesia (Tandjung, 1955).

11. Protozoan diseases, e.g., surra, piroplasmosis, anaplasmosis, trichimoniasis, are widespread and will require additional efforts toward detection and control.

12. Rabies is widespread throughout the islands and was only recently introduced to the islands of Bali and Buton. West Irian is the only rabies-free area. Dogs are the chief reservoir and many human, livestock, and wildlife cases occur (Ressang, 1959; Ressang et al., 1963).

13. Leptospirosis is widespread in swine. Human cases have been documented (Soeratno, 1964).

14. There are several little-known diseases of animals which merit intensive study:

   a. Purwokerto disease affects buffalo in Central Java, causing emaciation, vesicular dermatitis, diarrhea, mesenteric lymphadenopathy and, occasionally, hemorrhagic gastroenteritis. The infection is transmissible experimentally by blood transfusion and is considered by some to be a mild variant of rinderpest. A similar disease, Penjaki Djembrana, now occurs in buffalo in North Sumatra and in cattle and buffalo in Bali.

   b. Bali disease affects only the Bali breed of cattle and is characterized by dry eczema followed by severe necrosis of skin and superficial mucous membranes.

   c. Lepra bubalorum is a leprosy-like illness of water buffalo and occasionally cattle (Lobel, 1934). The causative agent is an acid-fast bacillus which has not been cultured or transmitted by artificial means.

   d. Other diseases include crippling osteoarthritis affecting buffalo in Tapanuli, North Sumatra, severe keratoconjunctivitis of horses in Menado, Celebes, and of goats in several parts of Indonesia, and a new disease of cattle in Djember, East Java, typified by nervous excitation and sudden death.

Intensification of efforts to improve animal production through breeding procedures, further development of artificial insemination programs, as well as nutrition and marketing research, are as important to Indonesia as investigation and control of animal diseases (Lubis, 1955, 1961; Napitupulus, 1960). The new government of Indonesia will embark on a 5-year plan in 1969 for the economic and social development of the country. Financial assistance is anticipated from many nations including the U. S. A., The Netherlands, France, West Germany, and Japan. Obviously justified is expenditure of a portion of these funds for research in animal production and disease investigation and control. It is hoped that Indonesia's capable veterinary scientists, practitioners, and educators will be granted sufficient support to apply their talents and energies to the struggle to solve the problems of this developing nation.

REFERENCES

Boer, E. (1941). Investigations on foot-and-mouth diseases. *Nederlandsch-Indische bladen voor diergeneeskunde* **53**, 127.

Boer, E., and Djaenoedin, R. (1950). Anthrax of man. *Hemera Zoa* **57**, 147.

Dieben, C. P. A. (1939). Primitive diergeneeskundige Gebruiken in Oost Java in ethnologisch verband. *Nederlandsch-Indische bladen voor diergeneeskunde* **51**, 251.

Kraneveld, F. C. (1957a). Veterinaire varia van Indonesie. No. I. Inleiding. *Hemera Zoa* **64**, 324.

Kraneveld, F. C. (1957b). Veterinaire varia van Indonesia. No. II. Engie gegevens over de eerste invoer van paarden op de Banda-eilanden. *Hemera Zoa* **64**, 341.

Kraneveld, F. C. (1957c). Veterinaire varia van Indonesie. No. III Buffels zonder horens. *Hemera Zoa* **64**, 390.

Kraneveld, F. C. (1958). Veterinaire varia van Indonesie. No. IV. Een flitsbeeld over de geschiedenis der diergeneeskunde van Ned. Oost Indie gedurende de periode 1820–1940. *Hemera Zoa* **65**, 96.

Lobel, L. W. M. (1934). Lepra bubalorum. *Nederlandsch-Indische bladen voor diergeneeskunde* **46**, 290.

Lobel, L. W. M., van der Schaaf, A., and Roza, M. (1936). Differentiation of the types of tubercle bacilli from the cow, buffalo and pig in the Dutch East Indies. *Nederlandsch-Indische bladen voor diergeneeskunde* **48**, 315.

Lubis, D. A. (1955). The problem of livestock feeding in Indonesia. *Hemera Zoa* **62**, 302.

Lubis, D. A. (1961). The possibilities for improving poultry breeding in Indonesia. *Hemera Zoa* **68**, 1.

Mansjoer, M. (1961a). Anthrax in man and animals in Indonesia. *Communicationes Veterinariae (Bojor, Indonesia)* **5**, 61.

Mansjoer, M. (1961b). Newcastle disease in Indonesia. *Communicationes Veterinairiae (Bojor, Indonesia)* **5**, 1.

Mansjoer, M. (1965a). Developmental of animal health in Indonesia (1945–1965). *Research in Indonesia 1945–1965* **III**, 173.

Mansjoer, M. (1965b). The influence of animal health and the control of infectious diseases for development of animal husbandry in Indonesia. *Bogor Symposium on Animal Husbandry, 1965.*

Napitupulus, B. (1960). The possibilities of milk production in Indonesia. *Hemera Zoa* **67**, 95.

Oetojo, R. P. (1958). Contribution to the knowledge of biological habits of *Pasteurella septica* variants in Indonesia. Doctoral Thesis, Institute Pertanian Bogor.

Ressang, A. A. (1959). Rabies—the incurable Indonesian wound. *Communicationes Veterinariae (Bogor, Indonesia)* **4**, 1.

Ressang, A. A. (1962). The concept of veterinary public health in Indonesia. *Communicationes Veterinariae (Bogor, Indonesia)* **6**, 1.

Ressang, A. A., Fischer, H., and Muchlis, A. (1959). The Indonesian veterinarian. *Communicationes Veterinariae (Bogor, Indonesia)* **3**, 55.

Ressang, A. A., So Ik Gwan, and Soehardjo, H. (1963). Bats, rodents and rabies in Indonesia. *Communicationes Veterinariae (Bogor, Indonesia)* **7**, 33.

Schoute, D. (1937). Occidental therapeutics in the Netherlands East Indies during three centuries of Netherlands settlement. *Publications of the Netherlands East Indies Public Health Service.*

Seyffers, S. M., and Van Dulken, H. (1941). Over een wijze waardelepaling van varkens op Nias. *Nederlandsch-Indische bladen voor diergeneeskunde* **53**, 1.

Soegeng, D. (1966). Tissue culture modification of Newcastle disease virus. Doctoral Thesis, Institute Pertanian Bogor.

Soeratno, P. (1964). Studies on leptospirosis: A zoonotic disease with economic and public health significance in Indonesia. Doctoral Thesis, Institute Pertanian Bogor.

Tandjung, A. R. (1955). Parasitic worms found in mammals and birds in Indonesia. *Hemera Zoa* **62**, 229.

Tojib, H. (1962). Results of the conferences between the schools of veterinary medicine and of animal husbandry. Gadja Mada University, Jogjakarta, 7.

A Review of Recent Developments in Veterinary Science in the Federal Republic of Germany *

KURT DIETER STOTTMEIER

National Communicable Disease Center, Atlanta, Georgia

I. Introduction: The Changing Concept of the Veterinary Profession

The rapid development of industrialized nations during the 1950's and 1960's not only has created new professions, but also has changed the responsibilities and goals of traditional professions in European countries. According to Eckerskorn (1965), the veterinarians of today have to adapt to the industrialization of agriculture and to the industrialized production of food. The modern practitioner has to cooperate with the government program for veterinary medicine in the prevention and control of certain diseases, which requires compulsory foot-and-mouth disease vaccination, tuberculin testing, brucellosis blood sampling, and general animal health services. Although compulsory prophylaxis represents an important factor in a practitioner's income, the prophylaxis naturally results in fewer

* Dr. James H. Steele has served as Coordinator of this article.

treatments of animals which was formerly the principal purpose and income source of veterinary medicine. Fifty percent of the 9450 West German veterinarians are private practitioners, but the number of veterinarians employed as state officers and researchers is increasing.

Major achievements in veterinary medicine, like the eradication of bovine tuberculosis in West Germany, were possible because of the development of regulatory and research programs. Only through the cooperation of the government, the community of farmers, and state and private veterinarians can campaigns of disease eradication succeed. These organized programs are vital for the food production of a growing nation.

II. Veterinary Schools in the Federal Republic of Germany

There are 4 veterinary medical schools in West Germany. The College at Hannover is an independent school. The others—Berlin, Giessen, and Munich—are components of the universities and are called faculties for veterinary medicine. These three schools operate as a group of institutes which are responsible for teaching and carrying on research. The Veterinary College of Hannover is organized in departments for teaching, replacing the traditional institutes which continue to be the research centers. Hannover also has adopted the college year during which the students attend classes most of the year instead of the traditional semesters which allowed long vacation periods. All educational institutions are supervised by the State Ministry of Cultural Affairs. However, self-administration is granted to each university or college, and university constitutions rule the life of teachers and students on the campus; no state authority is effective on university grounds without the permission of the rector. The rector is elected by the professors, who are heads of institutes. He is "the first among equals" and represents the highest authority in the university. The Senate, the Council, or other parliamentary bodies are the legislature of the university. Members are elected from among the professors, their assistants, or other teachers' and students' associations. The students of West German universities and colleges send elected representatives to student parliaments which form the "General Student Committees" (ASTA). The ASTA represents the students in university institutions, parliaments, and in the German Student Association.

Table I demonstrates the continuously increasing number of veterinary students from 1958 to 1967. In 1967, there were 2147 students studying veterinary medicine in West Germany; more than 80% of the students have finished their studies successfully, many of them after a minimum requirement of 4½ years of studies (Herter, 1968).

After the first year of study, the student may apply to be examined

TABLE I

Numbers of Students at the Veterinary Medical Schools in Berlin, Munich, Giessen, and Hannover in 1958, 1963, and 1967[a]

Year	German students		Foreign students		Total
	Male	Female	Male	Female	
1958	1269	210	104	7	1590
1963	1294	293	127	12	1726
1967	1538	404	182	23	2147

[a] Data adapted from Herter (1968).

in physics, chemistry, zoology, and botany. After the second, he may be examined in anatomy, histology, embryology, physiology, biochemistry, and physiology of nutrition. On passing these examinations, the student may enter the so-called area of clinical study. The first part of the final veterinary examination may be undertaken after 3 years of study, providing the following lectures and courses were subscribed and attended: general pathology, clinical propaedeutics, general medicine, general surgery, general therapy, general obstetrics, pharmacology and toxicology, animal husbandry and genetics, animal nutrition and general agriculture (including a 2-week course on an experimental farm).

A student may apply for examination after another year of study of contagious diseases, bacteriology, mycology, virology, parasitology, animal hygiene, radiology, and drug prescription in the second part of the veterinary examination. The third and last part of the examination may be taken after working 6 weeks in an animal clinic or an abattoir and 3 months with a private practitioner. Further studies in pathology, medicine, surgery, radiology, and in clinical medicine are also required. These subjects include diseases of the eyes, diseases of young animals and poultry, and study of artificial insemination, meat and milk hygiene, statistics, history of veterinary medicine, contagious disease control, veterinary medical law and insurance, and diseases of experimental animals. After passing all of the veterinary examinations, the student may apply for a veterinary license which is valid nationally and permits the graduate to practice veterinary medicine according to the regulations and the constitution of the German Veterinary Association, of which he becomes a member. Negotiations are under way for reciprocal recognition of academic degrees acquired in the Common Market countries by all members, i.e., Germany, France, Italy, The Netherlands, Belgium, and Luxembourg. The veterinary examination is called a state examination which means that the government supervises the study and the examination procedures. The goal of the veterinary profession is as follows:

1. Treatment and medical care of animals, as well as the prophylaxis of their diseases and illnesses.
2. Supervision of production of food for man from animals.
3. Protection of human health from zoonoses, contamination of and intoxication by food.

The degree, doctor medicinae veterinariae (Dr. med. vet.), is acquired by the presentation of a scientific thesis and an additional doctoral examination. Qualification for the Dr. med. vet. is undertaken voluntarily by the student. The veterinary state examination is the only requirement for a veterinary license; the same examination is necessary for the Dr. med. vet. These regulations of the Federal Law Bundes-Tierärzteordnung (1965) became effective in 1965.

III. Distribution of Veterinarians in Different Fields of Their Profession

Table II indicates that the number of veterinarians employed in offices, abattoirs, and institutes during this century is increasing, while the number of private practitioners is decreasing. However, the number of veterinarians has increased each year since 1900, with the exception of 1925. This fact is even more striking since the data for 1958 to 1967 apply only to western Germany which lost almost all of its agricultural regions after World War II.

The figures in Table II reveal that 4429 veterinarians i.e., 52%, in this country of approximately 58 million inhabitants are in private practice; federal and state employment is 10%; abattoirs, 10%; veterinary schools, 6%. Data concerning the economic situation for practitioners only are available (Schulz, 1968). The majority, i.e., 60%, earn

TABLE II

DEVELOPMENT OF THE VETERINARY MEDICAL PROFESSION IN GERMANY FROM 1900 TO 1967[a]

Type	Number of veterinarians in year:				
	1900	1925	1937	1958[b]	1967[b]
Practitioner	4000	4800	4600	5757	4429
Armed Forces	650	200	400	2	44
Employees[c]	3350	2500	3000	2381	5120

[a] Data adapted from Schulz (1968) and Herter (1968).
[b] Federal Republic of Germany.
[c] In abattoirs, institutions, and offices.

an income of U. S. $7,500–$12,500 and 40% receive more than $12,500 annually. A total of 9454 veterinarians hold licenses in West Germany.

The veterinary profession is supervised by the state governments and is regulated by state laws, similar to those for medical doctors, dentists, and pharmacists (Chamber laws). Self-administration is granted to those professions within limits of the state laws. Each licensed veterinarian has to join at least one of the 12 veterinary chambers which are present in each West German state. The decisions of the chambers are reached by majority vote and constitute the professional law for the members, providing they are in agreement with existing state laws. All veterinarians are obliged to pay membership fees, to have insurance, to fulfill professional duties, to study recent achievements in veterinary medicine, and to support and assist, on their request, the Public Health Services and government agencies.

The major obligations of a veterinarian are mutual respect toward all colleagues, professional discretion, eschewal of professional advertisement, and advanced training in accordance with the chamber regulations. There are other professional associations for which membership is not compulsory. The veterinary chambers of the states and the other free associations founded the "Deutsche Tierärzteschaft" in 1954; it is the top organization of veterinarians in West Germany. This organization publishes the official organ of the chambers, the "Deutsches Tierärzteblatt," a monthly periodical.

This organization has the task of representing the veterinarians of the nation and to cooperate with government and public officials. It combines the efforts of all chambers and associations in promoting the advancement of veterinary medicine in Germany. The organization maintains close contacts with international and foreign institutions, organizations and associations of similar nature, particularly those of Europe. It supports the integration of the veterinary profession within the Common Market countries. The latter activity remains one of the major goals of the veterinarians of the Federal Republic of Germany.

IV. The Veterinarian and Economy, Food Control, and Meat Inspection

Veterinarians, with special expertise, control food hygiene and food production in the Federal Republic of Germany. The protein needs for 58 million people in West Germany are supplied by meat, milk, eggs, and fish. Food of animal origin represents the most important part of human diet in Europe. The per capita consumption of meat was 63 kilograms in 1962–1963 versus 29.3 kilograms in 1873 and 15.3 kilograms in 1816 (Schulte, 1966). The importance of veterinarians as food hygienists has increased in relation to the improvement of protein supply. Since a housewife in West Germany spends more than 50% of her household budget for food of animal origin, she wants to purchase good quality (Schulte, 1966). The veterinarian's responsibility is protecting the consumer from food adulteration, food intoxication of all kinds, and misleading food offers and advertisements. Hygienic supervision has increased in importance as more food is prepared, cut, and packed industrially, thus depriving the housewife of the opportunity to inspect the raw product. Twenty-five veterinary institutes are maintained by the 10 states of West Germany; these are the official laboratories for food control which are able to perform laboratory work in anatomy, histology, physiology, pathology, bacteriology, and serology (Schulte, 1966) (Bundesminister für Gesundheitswesen, 1968).

Violations of the laws by food producers or dealers have been uncovered by these institutes in about 10% of the investigations. One of the institutes reported 349 (14.2%) cases of violations out of 2462 samples of meat and sausages investigated in one year. The common violations were of cheap quality meat for the production of sausages indicated to be of high quality. Most of the veterinary investigators are employed as full time state officers. The investigations are made in cooperation with medical doctors and chemists who hold similar posts in food inspection and control in the state governments.

The city of West Berlin inhabited by 2.2 million people represents an isolated area and is cited as an example. Thirty veterinarians have control of 25,000 food producers or dealers. Facilities are examined, and food samples are purchased for laboratory examination. About 114,000 employees in the food industries are examined physically, bacteriologically, and by x-ray annually in order to prevent the spread of diseases by food distribution. Approximately 200,000 kilograms of food of animal origin were confiscated by veterinarians in West Berlin in 1964 as being unfit for human use (Scheunemann, 1966).

The meat and food inspection of West Germany is regulated by federal laws which have their origin in pre-World War II laws. These federal laws with their amendments and decrees try to cope with the problems of the integration of the European Common Market. Details of the recent amendments (1968) of the meat inspection law are found in the Deutsches Tierärzteblatt (Gesetze und Verordnungen, 1968).

Meat inspection is an official function in Germany and is supervised by the state veterinarian. Lay meat inspectors have to undergo special training and are appointed only if no veterinarian is available for this function. However, such inspectors are employed principally for the inspection of pork for trichinosis, to which every pig carcass is subjected.

TABLE III
ANIMALS SLAUGHTERED AND INSPECTED BY VETERINARIANS OR MEAT INSPECTORS
IN 1966[a]

Animals	Numbers
Oxen	112,802
Bulls	1,519,903
Cows	1,275,758
Heifers	786,904
Cattle (total)	3,695,367
Calves (younger than 3 months)	1,672,606
Pigs	24,679,036
Sheep	430,370
Goats	15,892
Horses	29,601

[a] Data adapted from Statistisches Bundesamt (1966).

Meat inspection and artificial insemination are the only fields of veterinary medical science where nonveterinarians may substitute for veterinarians after special training.

Table III lists the number of animals slaughtered in West Germany in 1966. About 25 million pigs and more than 5.3 million head of cattle were inspected by veterinarians or under veterinary supervision. The commercial and "home" slaughtering of native and imported animals provided 3.53 million tons of meat in 1967; this was 2.2% more than for 1966. Pork was first (66%), followed by beef (31%), and veal, mutton, goat, and horse meat (Statistisches Bundesamt, 1966).

Table IV depicts the number of entire animal carcasses per thousand which were wholesome only under restrictions or were unfit for human use. Some meat is rendered fit for human use by freezing or cooking which destroys bacteria or parasites. Poor quality meats are usually condemned because of excessive water or blood content especially those of emergency slaughtered sick animals (Statistisches Bundesamt, 1966).

TABLE IV
SLAUGHTERED ANIMALS WITHHELD BY VETERINARY MEAT
INSPECTION IN 1966 IN THOUSANDS[a]

Examination	Cattle	Calves	Pigs
Unfit for human use	3.4	5.8	1.1
Fit under restrictions	1.7	0.2	4.8
Poor quality	31.3	13.3	4.0

[a] Data adapted from Statistisches Bundesamt (1966).

Table V lists reasons for meat rejection by the veterinarians in the Federal Republic of Germany in 1966. No specific diagnosis was established in the majority of the rejected carcasses. There were more than 6500 cases of sepsis, almost 4000 cases of icterus, and 3000 cases of dropsy. The data indicate that cysticercosis of cattle is much more frequent than trichinosis of swine. The usefulness of the compulsory inspection of all pork for trichinosis is under consideration in Germany. The occurrence of Salmonella in food and in animals will be discussed later.

The figures given in Table V do not include the numbers of animal organs which were rejected due to only local manifestations of disease.

From slaughtered cattle, exclusive of calves, 362,324 lungs, 556,146 livers, and 259,369 other single organs were rejected for various reasons in 1966. The data on rejections of organs of pigs were 7.8 million lungs, 645,839 livers, and 582,874 other organs. Unfit for human use were 678,775 kg. of beef (meat, bones, and fat), 35,624 kg. of veal (meat, bones, and fat), and 760,681 kg. of pork (meat, bones, and fat). Further details were given by the Statistisches Bundesamt (1966).

TABLE V

NUMBER AND SPECIES OF ANIMAL CARCASSES DECLARED UNFIT FOR HUMAN USE ON
VETERINARY INSPECTION IN 1966[a]

Reason for rejection	Cattle	Calves	Pigs[b]	Sheep	Goats	Horses
Anthracis, clostridial, and pasteurella infections	57	63	68	2	0	0
Sepsis	1586	2033	2944	102	7	49
Salmonellosis or presence of Salmonella	732	922	517	17	1	26
Erysipelothrix rhusiopathiae infection	—	—	1023	—	—	—
Brucellosis	3	3	5	0	0	0
Listerellosis	4	0	4	5	0	0
Cysticercosis	582	40	20	8	2	0
Swine influenza	—	—	245	—	—	—
Hog cholera (swine fever)	—	—	1745	—	—	—
Icterus	552	913	2357	76	4	6
Dropsy	1060	650	1122	235	11	49
Tumors	2011	136	907	14	1	35
Bad quality	1229	465	3463	82	6	33
Putrefaction	2107	1706	3852	190	11	108
Cachexia	1322	1217	3654	421	19	32
Miscellaneous	1463	1623	5347	140	37	101
TOTAL	12,708	9771	27,280	1292	99	439

[a] Data adapted from Statistisches Bundesamt (1966).

[b] Trichinosis was detected only in 7 swine.

Of imported meat examined in 1966, 124,726,176 kg. of beef, 18,879,104 kg. of pork, and 3,165,275 kg. of other meat products were found to be fit, i.e., wholesome for human consumption. In contrast, 243,945 kg. of beef, 110,531 kg. of pork, and 1,975 kg. of other meats were declared unfit for human use.

Special frontier abattoirs were established by law in order to slaughter animals immediately after importation and to inspect imported meat as required by German laws.

West Germany is a major importer of agricultural products from the world market; she buys products from all meat-exporting countries of the world, particularly from Common Market countries like France and The Netherlands. The data were provided by the Statistisches Bundesamt (1966).

V. The Veterinarian in Administration and the Animal Health Services. The Private Practitioners

Service for agriculture is rendered by veterinary officers of the federal and state governments and districts, veterinary state institutes, veterinarians employed by the Animal Health Services of the Agricultural Chambers of the states, veterinarians of the artificial insemination cooperatives, and private practitioners. According to Eckerskorn (1965), 750 veterinarians are responsible for the control and eradication programs for diseases like bovine tuberculosis, brucellosis, and rabies. Due to advances in veterinary medicine, the veterinary administration devotes increasing attention to the control of food production and disease prevention and prophylaxis. The veterinary administration of pre-World War II governments worked mainly as veterinary police against outbreaks of animal diseases, while today's administration aims to cooperate with the farmers, to develop certain agricultural specialties by subsidies, and to integrate German agriculture with the Common Market.

The veterinary state institutes, already mentioned, serve both as laboratories for meat and food investigations and for the diagnosis of diseases transmittable from animal to animal or from animal to man. A major task of the institutes is the annual serologic testing of cattle for brucellosis. The veterinary institutes do not perform basic research, but they are equipped with modern facilities to detect new viral diseases and to trace sources of radioactive contamination of animals and feed (Eckerskorn, 1962).

Approximately 350 veterinarians are employed by the cattle artificial insemination cooperatives and by the Animal Health Services for this work. More than 3 million cows and heifers were artificially inseminated in 1966, i.e., 47.2% of all cows and heifers in West Germany (Scheunemann, 1967).

The veterinarians employed by the Animal Health Services are responsible for the prophylaxis of animal diseases, a field not emphasized by either veterinary state officers or private practitioners (Eckerskorn, 1965). This situation adapts the veterinary profession to the requirements of industrialized food production by exclusive specialization in animal disease prophylaxis. The majority of veterinarians, approximately 4500, work in general private practices or in specialized practices in support of agriculture. As mentioned earlier, state supervision of practitioners exists only in the field of meat inspection, while the veterinary chambers of the states supervise the private practitioners.

The veterinary schools with their institutes and the Federal Research Institutes serve as reference laboratories under certain circumstances.

VI. Occurrence of Animal Diseases and Methods of Their Control

Since only certain animal diseases are notifiable according to the German law (Tierseuchengesetz), the data obtained were about these diseases. The Food and Agriculture Organization–World Health Organization–Office of International Epizootiology Animal Health Yearbook (1966a) has dealt with the occurrence of animal diseases in the world in terms of "low incidences," "widespread," "occurs exceptionally," and others. Incidences of animal diseases in the Federal Republic of Germany were given by the Animal Health Yearbook of 1966.

Data concerning the occurrence of 9 diseases notifiable in West Germany from January through March 1968 are given in Table VI (Statis-

TABLE VI

INCIDENCES OF CONTAGIOUS ANIMAL DISEASES WITHIN A 3-MONTH PERIOD[a]

(January 1, 1968 through March 31, 1968)

Disease	Numbers of infected communities		Numbers of infected farms	
	New infections	Total	New infections	Total
Foot-and-mouth disease	6	3	8	5
Brucellosis	68	73	87	87
Swine fever	49	7	59	7
Newcastle disease	1	0	3	0
Rabies	801	1080	Occurs mainly in wild fauna	
Anthrax	3	2	3	2
Tuberculosis (bovine)	49	56	53	59
Malignant foulbrood	0	58	0	99
Arcariasis	51	557	125	835

[a] Data adapted from Statistisches Bundesamt (1968) and Bundesernährungsministerium (1968).

tisches Bundesamt, 1968). Animals on 87 farms were infected with brucellosis, and on 59 with bovine tuberculosis out of 1 million cattle breeding farms, i.e., less than 0.01%. Rabies has been the most widespread disease, 1080 communities in West Germany having the infection in 1968. The prevalence of swine fever is low in Germany due to the strict slaughter policy in the west and slaughter and vaccination policies in the east. Anthrax and Newcastle disease occur rarely in Germany. According to Fritzsche (1968), the other poultry diseases such as infectious bronchitis, Gumboro disease, and mycoplasmosis, which also affects swine, are increasing in incidence and importance in the West German state of Rhineland-Pfalz. Problems encountered in this state are the occurrence of "new" viral diseases such as mucosal disease and rhinotracheitis of cattle.

1. Rabies

Rabies in wild fauna represents a major threat to human health in both parts of Germany. Eckerskorn (1966a) reported 37 deaths from 1945 to 1966; 32 fatal cases of rabies occurred in East Germany and 5 in West Germany. Dogs, cats, foxes, and cattle were the sources of these infections. The disease crossed the Oder River, representing the Eastern frontier of East Germany, spreading toward the West in 1947. Within 2 to 3 years, the disease had spread through East Germany and advanced to Schleswig-Holstein in the north and Lower Saxony in central Germany. By 1958, the Rhineland and, by 1964, Bavaria and Baden-Württemberg were infected with rabies (Goerttler, 1968).

Table VII indicates the continuing increase of rabies in the Federal Republic of Germany from 1746 cases in 1958 to 3913 in 1965. The state

TABLE VII

INCIDENCES OF RABIES IN THE FEDERAL REPUBLIC OF GERMANY FROM 1958 TO 1964 AND BAVARIA FROM 1951 TO 1966[a]

Year	Domestic animals (%)			Wild fauna (%)			Occurrences
	Dogs	Cats	Cattle	Foxes	Deer	Other (%)	
Bavaria							
1951–66	5.2	6.0	1.5	72.7	11.1	2.7	5629
Federal Republic of Germany							
1958	5.5	5.8	5.8	64.5	12.7	3.7	1746
1960	5.4	6.9	6.8	59.7	17.4	2.6	2991
1962	5.3	7.0	8.9	61.9	12.2	2.8	3186
1964	5.2	11.9	5.7	59.3	13.8	3.6	3096
1965	6.3	12.0	7.4	58.3	11.3	4.0	3913

[a] Data adapted from Beck and Osthoff (1966) and Eckerskorn (1966b).

of Bavaria reported 5629 cases of rabies within the period 1951 to 1966 (Beck and Osthoff, 1966; Eckerskorn, 1966b).

Table VII shows that 12 to 25% of the rabies cases were among domestic animals, while the majority of cases were observed in foxes, i.e., 58 to 72%. The incidences of rabies in deer or other wild animals are almost as high as those among domestic animals. The data compiled in Table VI reveal that the more than 1000 West German communities infected in 1968 offer a major problem to be solved by veterinarians in cooperation with the entire population of the involved communities.

2. FOOT-AND-MOUTH DISEASE

Foot-and-mouth disease is a serious deterrent to the German agriculture and economy. The data in Table VIII, obtained from the Food and Agriculture Organization–World Health Organization–Office of International Epizoology (1965), the Food and Agriculture Organization–World Health Organization–Office of International Epizoology (1966a), Eissner and Böhm (1967), and Eissner and Böhm (1968) show the incidences of foot-and-mouth disease in West Germany from 1965 through 1967. Cattle and swine were affected throughout the year in 1965; also, sheep and goats were affected in 1966 and sheep in 1967. The annual revaccination of all cattle older than 6 weeks was made compulsory after the development of trivalent (OAC) vaccine. In West Germany, nearly 14 million head of cattle were vaccinated during the spring of 1966. The cost of this particular campaign was estimated to exceed 12 million U. S. dollars. The campaign was promoted and subsidized by some state governments. Most of the vaccine, i.e., 13 million doses, was produced locally; some vaccine was imported from Great Britain, France, and Italy. Accord-

TABLE VIII
FOOT-AND-MOUTH DISEASE FROM 1965 THROUGH 1967[a]

Year	Species affected	No. of outbreaks	Time of outbreaks	Specimens identified			Vaccination	
				Typ O	Typ A	Typ C	Species	Typ
1965	Cattle, swine	15,942	All year	62	23	407	Cattle, swine	OAC
1966	Cattle, swine, sheep, goats	4,689	All year	1285	36	273	Cattle, swine	OAC
1967	Cattle, swine, sheep	3,350	All year	470	1	0	?	?

[a] Data adapted from Eissner and Böhm (1967, 1968) and Food and Agriculture Organization—World Health Organization—Office of International Epizoology (1965, 1966c).

ing to Eissner and Böhm (1968), foot-and-mouth disease in cattle has been brought under control by extensive OAC revaccination in recent years. However, the immunity of swine does not develop as well, and Böhne (1966) supports the slaughter policy in combination with a monovalent (C) vaccination as an optimal measure. Other precautions and restrictions were not as effective due to frequent purchase, sale, and transport of swine within Germany.

The law provides for compulsory slaughter of all diseased animals.

3. Salmonella and Salmonellosis

The occurrence of Salmonella organisms in man, animals, food, feed, and water has been recorded in West Germany by the Federal Institute of Health in West Berlin and is reported annually (Pietzsch and Bulling, 1968). The data presented in Tables IX, X, and XI were collected from the 1967 annual report. West Germany has intensified its fight against Salmonella since World War II; the high rate of food imports from all over the world after the war resulted in increased occurrence of many different Salmonella types unknown to pre-World War II Germany. A reference laboratory was established in the West Berlin institute, in order to cope with the Salmonella problems in West Germany's increasing imports, international traffic, and trade. Salmonella strains are isolated, identified, and collected, and tracing of sources of Salmonella infections is undertaken by this laboratory. The Federal Institute cooperates closely with all veterinary and medical state laboratories and with officials who furnish data needed for the annual analysis of the Salmonella situation in West Germany.

Table IX shows the prevalence of *Salmonella typhimurium* and *S. dublin* in 84,000 samples of cattle excrement (5.5%). A high incidence (3.5%) of these Salmonellae was also observed in 42,011 animal organs. More than 30 different types of Salmonella were found in 245,229 samples

TABLE IX

Isolations of Salmonella from Domestic Animals in 1967[a]

No. of specimens examined	No. of positive specimens	Positive samples (%)	No. of types involved
245,229 Meat	2690	1.1	33, predominantly *S. typhimurium*
42,011 Organs	1453	3.46	and *S. dublin*
273,959 Feed	255	0.09	54, predominantly *S. typhimurium*
83,911 Excrements	4592	5.47	and *S. dublin*
159,988 Food and water	574	0.36	22

[a] Data adapted from Pietzsch and Bulling (1968).

TABLE X

INCIDENCES OF ENTERITIS IN CATTLE AND FIRST ISOLATIONS OF SALMONELLA FROM SPECIMENS OF CATTLE EXCREMENT IN 1967[a]

Animals infected	No. of primary isolations	Predominant Salmonella			Excretors eliminated				
		Type	No.	%	No.	S. typh.	S. dubl.	Other
Cattle	2015	S. dublin	1248	61.9	312	5	249	58
Calves	598	S. typhimurium	570	95.3	22	4	18	0

[a] Data adapted from Pietzsch and Bulling (1968).

of meat or meat products. The overall incidence was approximately 1% of the samples tested. The most common of the Salmonella types have been involved regularly every year since 1956. Only 0.5% of 159,988 water and other food samples examined yielded 22 different types of Salmonella. Even though the percentage of Salmonella isolations in feed was less than 0.1% of 273,959 samples, the 54 different types isolated indicate their importance as contaminants of feed, particularly of imported fish meal, as a major source of rare Salmonella types.

Table X lists the incidence of infectious salmonellosis among cattle. More than 2000 primary isolations of Salmonella were made from cattle in 1967; of these, 1248 (62%) were S. dublin. S. dublin had infected 249 of 312 Salmonella-excreting cattle which were eliminated during 1967. In contrast, S. typhimurium was isolated from 570 of 598 calves examined. S. dublin was excreted by 18 of 22 calves that were eliminated.

TABLE XI

INCIDENCES OF SALMONELLOSIS IN MAN IN 1967[a]

No. of instances investigated	Salmonella types	Sources
1	S. derby	Sausage
6	S. bovis-morbificans	Food
8	S. typhimurium	Salami
80	S. brandenburg	Sausage
4	S. bareilly	Dutch chicken
1	S. infantis	U.S. chicken
163	S. thompson	Chicken
1	S. isangi	Sausage
300	S. braenderup	Cantine kitchen
160	S. typhimurium	Roast
724		

Total cases: 8102
Total deaths: 26

[a] Data adapted from Pietzsch and Bulling (1968).

Table XI lists the types and incidences of investigated Salmonella infections as well as the total cases and deaths in man for 1967. The sources of infection were identified in less than 10% of the cases. Sausage, the most common meat product in Germany, was the major source of Salmonella, followed by chicken. Chicken meat and products are now being inspected closely for evidence of Salmonella (Pietzsch and Bulling, 1968).

4. Eradication of Bovine Tuberculosis

The pre-World War II attempt to eradicate bovine tuberculosis by slaughtering bacteriologically positive cattle was abandoned in the early fifties, because of the difficulties in detecting animals excreting *Mycobacterium bovis*. The official introduction of a new eradication program based on the detection, separation, and eradication of all tuberculin-positive reacting animals, was delayed until 1952. Only 10% of the 11.5 million cattle in West Germany failed to react to the tuberculin test in 1952. Of these nearly 90% infected cattle, few had clinical manifestations. A national program, supported by the federal government, the farmers, and the veterinarians to eradicate tuberculosis was initiated in 1952. Participation by the farmers was encouraged by a bonus paid for milk from tuberculin test negative cows. This noncompulsory approach toward eradication was successful and, within a period of 5 years, 60% of the cattle were free of tuberculosis. Thereafter, a law made participation compulsory for farmers who kept tuberculous cattle in a district where 66% of the cattle herds were free of tuberculosis. This measure was adopted from similar eradication campaigns in North America, northern Europe, and Great Britain where bovine tuberculosis had been virtually eradicated before the German campaign started (Wagener, 1967).

The success of the German bovine tuberculosis eradication program is dramatized by the decreasing percentage of tuberculin-reacting cattle herds which was as follows (Rosenberger, 1967):

1952	90%	1958	26%
1955	64%	1959	15%
1956	52%	1960	7%
1957	40%	1961	0.3%

West Germany was practically free of bovine tuberculosis by 1968 (Table VI). Reinfections with *Mycobacterium bovis* rarely occurred. However, tuberculin reactions due to infections with human or atypical mycobacteria are of increasing concern. After eradicating *Mycobacterium bovis* from cattle, West Germany shares the problem with other developed countries of distinguishing specific and nonspecific tuberculin reactions.

The economic loss caused by bovine tuberculosis in West Germany was estimated to be more than 70 million U. S. dollars annually. No data exist as to the economic loss of public health, but, according to Schwarz (1963), bovine tubercle bacilli represented the source of infections in 5% of all pulmonary tuberculosis of man and in 25% of all extra-pulmonary cases. The cost of eradication to the German federal and state governments, the U. S. Marshall Plan, and the farmers was over 500 million U. S. dollars. This amount has already been recovered by increased production and value of animals, not to mention the public health benefits.

5. BOVINE LEUKOSIS AND OTHER VIRUS DISEASES

The tumoral form of leukosis in cattle has been observed in 0.02% of all slaughtered cattle in the Federal Republic of Germany. The hematologically demonstrable stage of the disease was about 20 times more frequent (0.4–0.5%) in cattle over 2 years of age. South Germany's mountain breeds are practically free of the disease (Tolle, 1966). Diagnosis by means of an electronic white blood cell counter is based on persistent lymphocytosis revealed by two blood counts at an interval of 4 to 6 months. When the diagnosis of leukosis has been confirmed, the elimination of affected animals is encouraged and subsidized (Food and Agriculture Organization–World Health Organization–Office of International Epizoology, 1966b). The occurrence of "new" viruses, PPLO, and Miyagawanella in the cattle of West Germany was reported by Bögel (1966). His summary gives the following picture of the "new" disease in West Germany.

"New" pathogenic agents were isolated from cattle with mucosal lesions and examined during the past 8 years. Among them were the viruses of (a) mucosal disease (MD), (b) infectious bovine rhinotracheitis and infectious pustular vulvovaginitis (vesicular coital exanthema) (IBR/IPV), (c) parainfluenza, type 3 (PI-3), and (d) a rhinovirus, several enteroviruses, and Miyagawanella. PPLO and other tetracycline-susceptible agents were isolated by the tissue culture technique, but are not yet identified.

Neither adenovirus nor antibodies were found in the cattle of West Germany. Infections by IBR/IPV viruses were rare in both southern and northern Germany (Federal Republic). The cattle in northern Germany were frequently infected by the MD virus within the first two years of their lives. The herds were infected by this virus at 1 to 2 year intervals in the north, and at 5 to 10 year intervals in the south; the cycle of infection was interrupted frequently for unknown reasons. Outbreaks of MD occurred frequently in northern Germany. Approximately 9% of the animals in certain herds in southern Germany are serologically positive.

Immunoprophylaxis by protection of healthy animals with a live vaccine or hyperimmune serum are common measures in herds prone to this infection.

Virus PI-3 is more widespread than the MD and the IBR/IPV viruses. Calves become infected early and, due to maternal antibodies or a developing immunity or both, seldom show any manifestations of the disease. A different situation prevails in southern Germany where the herds are reinfected every other year. This interrupted cycle of infection renders calves susceptible to the PI-3 infection, and enzootics can occur which involve several herds or those of entire communities. The PI-3 virus has been a common cause of respiratory syndrome enzootics in southern Germany. The rhinovirus, the enteroviruses, and the Miyagawanella occurred commonly and were frequently isolated. Only the latter caused enzootics, the other viruses being of low pathogenicity and recognizable only in cases of mixed infections.

VII. Veterinary Research in the Federal Republic of Germany

1. THE VETERINARY COLLEGE OF HANNOVER

The Veterinary College of Hannover, founded in 1778, has long been considered the outstanding veterinary college of Germany, and one of the leading schools of the world. As mentioned earlier, the veterinary schools of Germany are responsible not only for teaching and research, but also for routine and reference work for public and private institutions, practitioners, farmers, and for agriculture in general. There are 23 institutes and clinics at the Hannover College (Land-und Hauswirtschaftlicher Auswertungs-und Informationsdienst e.V., 1966), which make it impossible to review or even to mention all research projects of this school. However, the Institute for Anatomy is known for its comprehensive research, the results of which appear in the three-volume Handbook of Anatomy. The Institutes for Physiology and Physiological Chemistry investigate the protein metabolism of domestic animals, the fate of certain fatty acids and lipids ingested by animals, and the influence of different qualities of fat and vitamins on the biochemistry of the macroorganism. The Institute for Pathology does diagnostic reference work (4000 to 5000 specimens per year) and also carries on electron microscopic research of the animal cell. A histochemical section of the Institute studies disturbances in the metabolism of tissue. The Institute's staff investigates the rheumatoid-disease-complex in cooperation with the animal clinics of the college. The research of the Virological Institute is focused on the European swine fever (hog cholera) and the mucosal disease viruses. A vaccine against influenza of horses is being developed. The Institute for

Food and Meat Hygiene investigates microbiologic processes involved in the production of foods of animal origin, the occurrence of Salmonella in food, the disinfection of food-manufacturing plants, and the nature of nonspecific food intoxications. The Clinic for Diseases of Cattle has a special interest in leukosis, parasitic diseases (liver fluke, lung and stomach worms), and tetanies of cattle as well as other agriculturally important problems. The students have the opportunity to study the diseases of approximately 3000 cattle, which are treated annually at the clinic. The recently established Institute of Poultry Diseases emphasizes the increasing importance of poultry meat in the human diet. In order to fight coccidiosis more successfully, research is being done to cultivate the parasites *in vitro*. Another new institute, founded in 1955, is the Institute for Artificial Insemination and Andrology which does research in the field of semen conservation. The number of artificially inseminated cows has increased to almost 50% in West Germany. The Institute for Pharmacology, Toxicology and Pharmacy has focused research on the importance of pharmacologic effects of nutrition *in vivo*, the pharmacologic impact of sexual organs, and the toxicology of pesticides and insecticides. The Hannover College was the first veterinary school of West Germany to establish an Institute for Statistics and Biometry. The Institute for Animal Husbandry studies the influences of genetics and environmental factors on the economic efficiency of cattle and swine; it does reference work and research in the field of hereditary defects in domestic animals. Other institutes of the college carry out research in the fields of enzymatic diagnosis of heart and muscle diseases of swine, the influence of plant estrogens on bovine gynecology, the metabolism of electrolytes studied by artificial kidneys in small domestic animals, hygienic production of milk, immunity of animals against cestode parasites, and synthesis of enzymes and peptides.

More information about veterinary research in Hannover and other places in West Germany is given in "Die Deutsche Veterinärmedizinische Wissenschaft" (Land-und Hauswirtschaftlicher Auswertungs-und Informationsdienst, 1966).

2. THE VETERINARY SCHOOL OF THE FREE UNIVERSITY IN BERLIN

The Free University of Berlin was founded in 1948 with American support after the communistic take-over of Humboldt University in East Berlin following World War II. Since 1952, the Veterinary Faculty has carried on the tradition of the "Schola Veterinaria Berolinensis" of 1790; its faculty is aware of the veterinary faculty at the Humboldt University located on the other side of the Berlin Wall which claims to be the only legal successor of the old veterinary school. In East Berlin and Leipzig are the two veterinary schools of East Germany. The research by the faculty in West Berlin will be discussed briefly. The Institute for Pathology receives over 2000 reference specimens annually. Research is centered on the pathology of the mammary gland, tumors and kidney diseases in animals. The Institute for Pharmacology and Toxicology has research projects on the mode of action of different drugs. Basic research by electron microscopy is performed in a special section of the Institute for Veterinary Hygiene. Also being investigated is the DNA structure of bacterial chromosomes, the cytology of pathogenic bacteria, and the role of phosphates, K and Na ions, and carbohydrates in the metabolism of bacteria, particularly their importance to the chromosomes and their mitosis. The Institute for Parasitology is engaged in toxoplasmosis research and immunologic studies of nematodes and tick infestations. The Institute conducts clinical research work in Near East countries. German veterinarians aid in applying new methods in developing countries to enhance the economic efficiency of domestic animals. National recognition has been earned by the Institute for Food Hygiene under the leadership of Professor Lerche, who is a governmental adviser and chief expert in adapting the German laws of food and meat inspection to the necessities of modern industrialized nations. The microbiology and the quality of food are missions of this Institute. The establishment of the new Institute for Meat Hygiene and Abattoirs in 1962 was a measure of the emphasis put on food and meat research by the Berlin faculty. The clinic for small domestic animals treats dogs and cats belonging to West Berlin's 2.2 million inhabitants. The clinic is renowned for the diagnosis of liver and kidney diseases, lipid metabolism malfunctions, heart and circulation problems, and for its electroencephalographic studies. Surgery has made great advances, and a large clinic has developed along with the technical advances of modern instrumentation. Basic research in orthopedics and dentistry by the Institute of Radiology, Orthopedics and Dentistry has supported the surgical development. Modern methods of human medicine have been adapted to the needs and problems of domestic animals to open an entirely new field in veterinary medicine, and many valuable racing horses, private and police horses, as well as numerous dogs have been saved.

3. The Veterinary School of the University in Giessen

The veterinary school (Faculty of Veterinary Medicine) at the University of Giessen has a tradition of almost 200 years of scientific research in cooperation with the different faculties. The first lecture in veterinary science was given in Giessen in 1777. The University of Giessen carries the name of Justus Liebig, who developed the synthetic fertilizers and whose basic research work is well known all over the world. Since his days, interfaculty cooperation among veterinary medicine, medicine, agriculture, and science has constituted a traditional obligation in Giessen. A comprehensive report about the work of the veterinary faculty was given by Rieck (1968) and Ulbrich (1967).

The Institute of Physiology does research in the fields of hematology and nutrition. Erythrocytes are investigated under conditions of severe disease or physical exercise. The genetics of lymphocytes and their proliferation is studied in cooperation with the Medical Research Center, Brookhaven, New York, U. S. A.

The Institute for Biochemistry represents another example of interfaculty cooperation where 3 veterinarians, 3 chemists, a physicist, and a mathematician study the *in vivo* effect and metabolism of vitamin E. They also assay hormonal and antihormonal additives to feeds. Emphasis is on natural sciences and infectious diseases as demonstrated by the fact that the school in Giessen has 3 institutes; namely, those of Hygiene and Infectious Diseases, Bacteriology and Immunology, and Virology. The research of the first institute is focused on the etiology of leukosis and the analysis of chromosomes in human beings and animals. Analysis of human chromosomes is done in close cooperation with the Clinic for Children's Diseases of the Faculty of Medicine. Other microbiologic research is on mycoplasmosis of swine and in virology with "new" infective agents. Laboratory methods are being developed for the isolation and identification of mucosal disease, parainfluenza and rhinotracheitis viruses, and the Miyagawanella agent in cattle, as well as equine influenza viruses, A1 and A2, rhinopneumonia and other herpes viruses, and the rhinoviruses of horses. Another link between veterinary medical and other faculties is through the comprehensive research on the hygiene of solid and liquid waste disposal. This research not only helps to solve sewage problems in modern animal confinement units, but it also represents a contribution toward solving waste disposal problems of expanding urban areas in densely populated West Germany. Composting and incinerator methods for disinfecting human and animal liquid and solid wastes and their use in agriculture as manure or soil conditioners are under study. A member of the Institute is a consultant for the World Health Organization in this field and worked for the U. S. Public Health Service in 1968 (Ulbrich, 1967).

The Institute of Bacteriology and Immunology is doing basic research in the field of pathogenicity of *Staphylococcus aureus* and other bacteria. The Institute of Virology also does basic research on the structure and multiplication of myxo-, arbo-, and papovaviruses and the problems of molecular biology.

The Institute for Pharmacology and Toxicology was founded in 1964, before which veterinary students were taught in the corresponding institute of the medical faculty. The Microbiological Institute and the Pharmacological Institute are in the same building with the corresponding Institute of Medical Pharmacology in order to facilitate interfaculty cooperation. The Institute participates in a special program of the West German Research Council to study the nature of mushroom poisons. A unique institute, the "Tropeninstitut," was founded in 1961; its members, from 5 different faculties, are united for germane research on agricultural, nutritional, and economic problems of developing countries. There are teaching facilities to aid German nationals who are in research abroad and to help foreign postgraduate students in Germany. The interfaculty institution is directly supervised by the rector and the senate of the Justus-Liebig-University. Social economics, geography, nutrition, agriculture, and veterinary medicine represent the faculties at the Tropeninstitut. The research of the tropical veterinary medicine, which is a part of the Faculty of Veterinary Medicine, is focused on water buffalo, tropical cattle, and camels (Fischer, 1966). Furthermore, the economic exploitation of the game reserves of Africa, the cattle, sheep, and goat husbandry of Thailand, Malaysia, and parts of Africa are under investigation. The life cycle of rickettsia and *Aegyptianella pullorum* in ticks and mammals, respectively, is another project in tropical veterinary medicine. Projects are planned or are in operation in Turkey, Columbia, and Kenya.

As this brief report reveals, the University of Giessen and the veterinary school are traditionally orientated toward close cooperation among the scientific, medical, agricultural, and veterinary medical disciplines with special emphasis on problems of modern civilization and human nutrition at home and abroad.

4. THE VETERINARY SCHOOL OF THE UNIVERSITY IN MUNICH

The only veterinary school in southern Germany is located in Munich, the capital of Bavaria. Founded in 1790, the veterinary school has developed rapidly and represents now, in spite of the severe damage inflicted by World War II, one of the best equipped veterinary schools in Europe (Land-und Hauswirtschaftlicher Auswertungs-und Informationsdienst e.V., 1966). It is a model of what foreign assistance can give to rehabilitate a school. The school was reconstructed and equipped under the Marshall Plan.

Students are taught zoology and parasitology at the Bavarian Biological Research Institute which covers not only veterinary parasitology and antiparasitic drugs, but also the biologic aspects of sewage, water and fishes, and general zoology. The Institute of Histology and Embryology investigates, in cooperation with medical research centers, the morphology of immunobiologically active cell systems after transplantation of organs. Other research is done on the structure of skin and hair of domestic and wild animals for differential purposes. The Institute of Physiology studies the metabolism of vitamins and drugs and the nutrition of animals using isotopes and germ-free domestic animals. The Institute for Animal Husbandry and Hereditary Research has facilities of a research farm in order to determine the mutual influence of genetics and environment on growth, health, aging, reproduction, and productivity of domestic animals. This work is closely coordinated with that of the Institute of Genetics. Basic research in the analysis of chromosomes and in oncology and teratology is also done by the Institute of Pathology. Since 1965, a special Institute of Oncology has participated in international research projects, particularly those of the World Health Organization. Special attention is paid to tumors of the nervous system and their development. The basic research of the Microbiology Institute is concerned with the importance of the interferons in the pathogenesis of infectious diseases and the penetration of cells by virus and viral reproduction. Bacterial and fungal infections and diseases are being studied separately in research projects focused on etiology, epidemiology, and immunology of fungal and bacterial infections with special emphasis on prophylaxis. The Animal Hygiene Institute was separated from that of Microbiology in 1964. It is responsible for the study of optimal animal productivity under optimal environmental conditions. Temperature and climatic conditions, feed additives, and intoxications of animals by toxic synthetic materials and substrates in the rural environment represent a wide range of research projects of this institute. The Institute for Food Inspection has devoted its research efforts toward the harmonization of the European food law within the Common Market countries. Parallel to microbiologic tests, indicators for the quality of packed food as well as methods to control errors in the production of cheese are under study. The differentiation of proteins of meat products, the radiologic effects on food, and the radioactive contamination and decontamination of food are projects of this institute. This is interfaculty cooperative research, but it is predominantly performed by the Institute of Pharmacology, Toxicology and Pharmacy. Here, research on the protection of human beings and animals from radiation by drugs has had priority. Experimental neuropharmacology and electroencephalography are new fields to be expanded.

The animal clinics in Munich are for the areas of veterinary medicine, surgery, and gynecology. The diseases of domestic poultry and wild birds are covered by an institute conducting research on blood groups of poultry. The Institute for Palaeo-anatomy, Domestication and History of Veterinary Medicine is unique in West Germany and the world. This institute studies the process of the domestication with all its biologic and cultural repercussions. Furthermore, historic manuscripts on veterinary medicine are collected and evaluated.

The veterinary school at Munich represents a part of one of the biggest universities of West Germany. According to the tradition of general education, the different faculties offer a wide range of scientific lectures in order to encourage students to choose lectures and to attend courses of interest to them. Students of similar or related faculties as well as students of philosophy or arts who are interested in certain aspects of medicine, veterinary medicine, or science are eligible to attend. An example is the Institute of Comparative Tropical Medicine where students of different faculties attend lectures on the animal pox viruses as well as trypanosomiasis, babesiosis, and piroplasmosis in man, and domestic and wild animals.

5. OTHER RESEARCH CENTERS

The federal research centers play an important role in the veterinary medicine of West Germany. The veterinary section of the Max-von-Pettenkofer Institute (Bundesgesundheitsamt) is the central veterinary institute of the country. The section offers veterinary scientific advice and expert opinions to all government agencies and is largely engaged in the preparation of veterinary and agricultural laws and decrees of the federal government. Veterinary reference laboratories are established to study the epidemiology, pathogenesis, and diagnosis and control of viral diseases, i.e., rabies, bovine leukosis, and hygiene of food so as to prevent the transmission of tuberculosis, salmonellosis, toxoplasmosis, and leptospirosis. Other laboratories work in zoology, bacteriology (Salmonella and Brucella Center of West Germany), serology, pathology, veterinary chemistry and disinfection. The veterinary central laboratory represents a part of the Bundesgesundheitsamt (Federal Public Health Agency) which is located, with other sections such as medicine and public health, pharmacology, physiology, and drug and food chemistry, in West Berlin.

There are 17 more federal research centers in the biologic and agricultural field in West Germany (Höcherl, 1967). The work of the Federal Institute for Milk Research in Kiel, the Federal Research Institute for the Husbandry of Small Animals in Celle, the Federal Research Institute for Meat Research in Kulmbach, and the Federal Research Institute for the Virus Diseases of Animals in Tübingen will be alluded to since these institutes work predominantly in the veterinary field. The Institute for Milk Research is organized to investigate milk production and the hygiene, microbiology, chemistry, and physics of milk as well as the economy and the marketing and engineering of milk and milk products. Research is supported by a center of statistics and documentation and an experimental farm. The entire field of herbage and feed, the production of milk, and the marketing of the products is covered by research projects of this institute which is specially known as the Streptococcus Center of Germany, as a laboratory leading in the electronic evaluation of the cell and bacterial content of milk, and as a radiologic research and investigation center in the agricultural field (Bundesanstalt für Milchforschung Kiel, 1967).

The Research Center for the Husbandry of Small Animals formulates scientific bases for the breeding, care, and feeding of small animals. The center is concerned with the qualitative improvement of poultry and fur farming products. A special section investigates microbiologic, parasitic, and genetic problems of poultry with special attention to avian leukosis. The Institute for Meat Research controls the hygienic production of meat and meat products in West Germany. It is especially concerned with the protection of the consumer and in improving the position of domestic meat and meat products in international competition. The Institute covers the entire field of meat production and marketing and is organized in sub-institutes for meat production, technology, bacteriology and histology, chemistry, physics, and biochemistry. The Institute represents the office of the Codex Committee for meat and meat products of the Joint Food and Agriculture Organization–World Health Organization Codex Alimentarius Commission which is concerned with the standardization of slaughtered animals and carcasses to facilitate and stimulate international trade. Furthermore, the nature and control of food additives and residues in meat products are of increasing concern to meat importing countries (Bundesanstalt für Fleischforschung in Kulmbach, 1966).

The Federal Research Institute for the Virus Diseases of Animals was founded after World War II. The pre-World War II center for virus diseases was located on the Island of Riems in the Baltic Sea, which is now being used by the East German Government for similar purposes. The Institute was founded to protect German agriculture from viral diseases. Methods for the isolation, identification, diagnosis, and control of viral diseases, particularly foot-and-mouth, are developed, evaluated, and improved. Commercial viral vaccines are evaluated. Current research besides that on foot-and-mouth disease is focused on rabies, influenza of horses, rinderpest (in cooperation with French institutions), myxomatosis, carp pox virus, infectious rhinotracheitis of cattle, Marek's disease and avian leukosis, bovine leukosis, leukemia of mice, swine fever (hog cholera), and tumor research. The institute cooperates with similar institutes in England (Weybridge), Denmark (Lindholm), Austria (Vienna), Chad (Farsha), Senegal (Dakar), and with the OIE in Paris and the WHO in Geneva (Bundesforschungsanstalt für Viruskrankheiten der Tiere in Tübingen/N., 1966).

The Paul-Ehrlich-Institute for experimental therapy represents the central laboratory for the standardization of sera, vaccines, tuberculins, and antibiotics; the latter is a World Health Organization project (Land- und Hauswirtschaftlicher Auswertungs-und Informationsdienst e.V., 1966). The veterinary section of the Bernhard-Nocht-Institute for tropical diseases in Hamburg contributes to international research on piroplasmosis, brucellosis, rabies, malaria, psittacosis, and arboviruses (Land-und Hauswirtschaftlicher Auswertungs-und Informationsdienst e.V., 1966).

Veterinary institutes are located at the Friedrich-Wilhelm-University of Bonn (anatomy and physiology of domestic animals), the Johann-Wolfgang-von-Goethe-University in Frankfurt (zoonoses research), the Georg-August-University in Göttingen, and at the agricultural college of Hohenheim. These institutes teach certain veterinary aspects and often represent the veterinary reference laboratory for a particular area of the state; they may, however, specialize in certain areas such as the zoonoses (Land-und Hauswirtschaftlicher Auswertungs-und Informationsdienst e.V., 1966).

Veterinary research in West Germany is represented professionally by the German Society for Veterinary Medicine, a society of researchers promoting and encouraging research and organizing meetings. Meetings have been held in Bad Nauheim every other year since 1955; different topics are discussed. The tumor and cancer problem in domestic animals with special attention to avian and bovine leukosis was reviewed in 25 papers in 1967 (Deutsche Veterinärmedizinische Gesellschaft, 1968). The different diseases of young domestic animals were the topic of 24 papers given in 1965. The disturbances of the fertility and metabolism of domestic animals, the control of contagious diseases, the diagnoses of animal and poultry diseases were discussed in other scientific lectures and papers since 1955 (Deutsche Veterinärmedizinische Gesellschaft, 1966).

VIII. Conclusions

This article tries to picture the changing concepts of the veterinary profession in West Germany. With advances in industrialized food production, the veterinary profession has gradually shifted its emphasis from the treatment of horses, cattle, swine, and other domestic animals to the eradication and prophylaxis of diseases, and to food hygiene and food production. The agricultural development within the Common Market countries, particularly the disappearance of many small farms in West Germany, necessitated the eradication of bovine tuberculosis and brucellosis and more effective immunoprophylactic control of foot-and-mouth disease, since the concentration of more animals on larger farms increases the risks of infectious and parasitic diseases. This development started with the eradication campaigns against tuberculosis and brucellosis in the 1950's. Today's efforts are directed toward prophylactic measures to protect the achievements of control and eradication campaigns and to stabilize the favorable situation. Besides rabies in wild animals, foot-and-mouth disease is the nation-wide problem. Hopefully, control of the latter will be solved by the immunoprophylactic program including annual OAC vaccination. The establishment of Animal Health Services for cattle, sheep, swine, and poultry and the employment of veterinarians exclusively in the field of prophylaxis exemplifies the development which have been described. Routine vaccinations, testing for tuberculosis and brucellosis, and other measures to prevent reinfections of the livestock will be the prime tasks of veterinarians in the field. Artificial insemination will remain an important activity. Veterinary medicine has proved its abilities to cope with the problems of this industrialized nation, the present favorable situation having been achieved after a most destructive war, occupation, and loss of the predominantly agricultural territory in the East.

ACKNOWLEDGMENTS

Dr. James H. Steele, Chief, Veterinary Public Health Services, has initiated and encouraged the present work. His valuable advice, criticism, and support made this article possible. The author is also indebted to the Bundesminister für Gesundheitswesen and the Bundesminister für Ernährung, Landwirtschaft und Forsten, particularly to Min.-Rat Dr. W. Eckerskorn, who furnished valuable information and reprints. The author acknowledges gratefully the help and assistance of Die Deutsche Tierärzteschaft and its president, Dr. Schulz. Professor Dr. Kurt Wagener of Hannover supported the work by valuable suggestions and advice. Statistical data of importance were forwarded by the Statistisches Bundesamt, Wiesbaden, West-Germany. Special interest in this article was shown by the Veterinärmedizinische Fakultät der Justus Liebig-Universität; particularly, Professors Rieck and Ulbrich furnished information, reprints, and reports about the Giessen faculty. Other information about the veterinary schools came from the Veterinärmedizinische Fakultät der Freien Universität Berlin, Tierärztliche Hochschule Hannover, and the Veterinärmedizinische Fakultät der Universität München. Veterinary research was summarized by the Deutsche Veterinärmedizinische Gesellschaft e.V., who generously furnished the congress reports. Information about animal diseases were sent by Professor Fritzsche of the Landes- Veterinäruntersuchungsamt für Rheinland-Pfalz and Dr. Beck of the Bayrische Landesanstalt für Tierseuchenbekämpfung. The author thanks Mrs. Helga Stottmeier for her comprehensive reference work used in this article.

REFERENCES

Beck, G., and Osthoff, F. (1966). Ein Beitrag zur Tollwutsituation. *Tierärztliche Umschau* **21**, 441–447.

Bögel, K. (1966). Epizootologie et prophylaxie sur le territoire de la République Fédéral d'Allemagne des maladies a virus des bovides affectant les muqueuses. *Bulletin Office international des Epizooties* **66**, 355–388.

Böhne, F. (1966). Die Maul-und Klauenseuche in Niedersachsen. *Deutsche tierärztliche Wochenschrift* **73**, 121–124.

Bundesanstalt für Fleischforschung in Kulmbach. (1966). Jahresbericht 1966.

Bundesanstalt für Milchforschung in Kiel. (1967). Jahresbericht 1967.

Bundesernährungsministerium. (1968). Tierseuchenbericht. *Berliner und Münchener tierärztliche Wochenschrift* **81**, 185.

Bundesforschungsanstalt für Viruskrankheiten der Tiere in Tübingen/N. (1966). Jahresbericht 1966.

Bundesminister für Gesundheitswesen. (1968). Verzeichnis der für die amtliche Lebensmittelüberwachung tätigen tierärztlichen Untersuchungsämter. *Gemeinsames Ministerialblatt* **19**, 122–123.

Bundes-Tierärzteordnung. (1965). Sammlung des Bundesrechts, Bundesgesetzblatt III 7830-1. *Bundesgesetzblatt* Part I, 416–418.

Deutsche Veterinärmedizinische Gesellschaft. (1966). *Bericht des 6. Kongresses, Bad Nauheim, April 1965. Zentralblatt für Veterinärmedizin* **13**, 89–222.

Deutsche Veterinärmedizinische Gesellschaft. (1968). *Bericht des 7. Kongresses, Bad Nauheim, April 1967. Zentralblatt für Veterinärmedizin* **15**, 1–200.

Eckerskorn, W. (1962). Zukünftige Aufgaben der Staatlichen Veterinäruntersuchungsämter. *Deutsches Tierärzteblatt* **11**, 39–43.

Eckerskorn, W. (1965). Zur Frage einer sachgerechten Zuordnung der Veterinärmedizin im heutigen Wirtschafts-und Sozialgefüge. *Tierärztliche Umschau* **20**, 103–107.

Eckerskorn, W. (1966a). Die Wildtollwut als Problem der staatlichen Tierseuchenbekämpfung. *Deutsche tierärztliche Wochenschrift* **73**, 150–155.

Eckerskorn, W. (1966b). Information concernant le développement et la situation de la rage en République Fédéral d'Allemagne depuis 1950 et les mésures prises dans la lutte antirabique. *Bulletin Office international des Epizooties* **65**, 3–11.

Eissner, G., and Böhm, H. O. (1967). MKS-Typendiagnosen in der Zeit von. 1.1.66 bis zum 31.12. 66 in der Bundesforschungsanstalt für Viruskrankheiten der Tiere in Tübingen/N. *Deutsches Tierärzteblatt* **15**, 118–119.

Eissner, G., and Böhm, H. O. (1968). MKS-Typendiagnosen in der Zeit vom 1.1.67 bis zum 31.12.67 in der Bundesforschungsanstalt für Viruskrankheiten der Tiere in Tübingen/N. *Deutsches Tierärzteblatt* **16**, 96–100.

Fischer, H. (1966). "Institut für Tropische Veterinärmedizin. Ein Tätigkeitsbericht 1961/1966." Das Tropeninstitut der Justus Liebig-Universitat, Giessen, Germany.

Food and Agriculture Organization—World Health Organization—Office of International Epizoology. (1965). "Animal Health Yearbook 1965," p. 274. Rome, Italy.

Food and Agriculture Organization—World Health Organization—Office of International Epizoology. (1966a). "Animal Health Yearbook 1966," pp. 125–191. Rome, Italy.

Food and Agriculture Organization—World Health Organization—Office of International Epizoology. (1966b). "Animal Health Yearbook 1966," p. 257. Rome, Italy.

Food and Agriculture Organization—World Health Organization—Office of International Epizoology. (1966c). "Animal Health Yearbook 1966," p. 272. Rome, Italy.

Fritzsche, K. (1968). Personal communication.

Gesetze und Verordnungen. (1968). Gesetz zur Änderung des Durchführungsgesetzes EWG-Richtlinie Frisches Fleisch und des Fleischbeschaugesetzes. *Deutsches Tierärzteblatt* **16**, 199–202.

Goerttler, V. (1968). Tollwut der Füchse durch Impfung der Hunde bekämpfen? *Das Tier* **8**, 28–29.

Herter, R. (1968). Statistische Untersuchungen über die westdeutsche Tierärzteschaft. *Deutsches Tierärzteblatt* **16**, 139–142.

Höcherl, H. (1967). Neuordnung der Forschung im Bereich des Bundesernährungsministeriums. *Deutsches Tierärzteblatt* **15**, 448–450.

Land-und Hauswirtschaftlicher Auswertungs-und Informationsdienst e.V. (1966). "Die Deutsche Veterinärmedizinische Wissenschaft," pp. 9–93. Hans Meister K. G., Kassel, Germany.

Pietzsch, O., and Bulling, E. (1968). Verbreitung der Salmonella-Infektionen bei Tieren, tierischen Lebens-und Futtermitteln in der Bundesrepublik Deutschland einschl. Berlin (West). *Bundesgesundheitsblatt* **11**, 233–239.

Rieck, G. W. (1968). Personal communication.

Rosenberger, L. (1967). Personal communication.

Scheunemann, H. (1966). Nahrungsmittelüberwachung in der Praxis. *Das Parlament* No. 35, 29–31.

Scheunemann, H. (1967). Die Rinderbesamung in der Bundesrepublik 1966. *Deutsches Tierärzteblatt* **15**, 266.

Schulte, F. (1966). Tierärzte als Sachverständige. *Das Parlament* No. 35, 27–28.

Schulz, H. (1968). Grundlagen des Veterinärwesens. *Communication of the Deutsche Tierärzteschaft* (unpublished).

Schwarz, W. (1963). "Rede auf der Kundgebung anlässlich der Bekanntgabe der Tuberkulose—Freiheit der deutschen Rinderbestände am 27.1.1963." Grüne Woche, Berlin, Germany.

Statistisches Bundesamt. (1966). "Land-und Forstwirtschaft, Fischerei." Fachserie B, Reihe 3, Viehwirtschaft. IV. Schlachttier-und Fleischbeschau, pp. 1–36. W. Kohlhammer GMBH, Stuttgart und Mainz, Germany.

Statistisches Bundesamt. (1968). "Statistisches Jahrbuch über Ernährung, Landwirtschaft und Forsten der Bundesrepublik Deutschland," p. 120. W. Kohlhammer GMBH, Stuttgart und Mainz, Germany.

Tolle, A. (1966). Übertragung, Diagnose und Prophylaxe der Bovinen Leukose in der Bundesrepublik Deutschland. *Bulletin Office international des Epizooties* **66**, 757–774.

Ulbrich, F. (1967). *Tätigkeitsbericht* des Institutes für Hygiene und Infektionskrankheiten der Tiere der Justus Liebig-Universität Giessen für die Zeit vom 1.4.64 bis zum 31.3.67 (unpublished).

Wagener, K. (1967). Personal communication.

Author Index

Numbers in italics refer to the pages on which the complete references are listed.

A

Abadie, S., 52, *55*
Abaza, H. M., 177, *187*
Ablashi, D. V., 119, 126, *139, 148*
Able, M. E., 336, *350*
Absolon, K. B., 174, *205*
Abt, D., 337, 338, 339, 340, *350, 351*
Ackerman, L. V., 325, 330, *350*
Adams, J. C., 241, *252*
Adams, R. D., 170, 171, *206*
Adams, W. E., 174, *207*
Adler, H. E., 126, *139*
Afzal, H., 267, *299*
Akcasu, A., 158, *187*
Akers, T. G., 109, 113, 120, 128, *140*
Alarcon-Segovia, D., 166, *187*
Alberts, J. O., 89, *102,* 125, 139, *143*
Aldersberg, D., 156, *189*
Alexandre, G. P., 176, *194*
Alexander, G. I., 1, *24*
Alford, W. C., 91, *102*
Alger, N. E., 52, *58*
Alicata, J. E., 53, *56*
Allam, M. W., 184, *187,* 327, *350*
Allcroft, W. M., 93, *94*
Almeida, J. D., 107, 109, 111, 112, 124, 125, 134, *140, 147*
Almgard, L. E., 175, *187*
Alper, C. A., 157, *187*
Altland, P.D., 168, *194*
Altman, B., 175, *187*
Altman, I., 159, *189, 191*
Altszuler, N., 211, 213, 215, 217, 218, *259*
Alvord, E. C., 171, *187*
Amelung, D., 76, *94*
Amend, J. R., Jr., 161, 177, *195*
Amos, B., 183, *187*
Anand, R. S., 239, 249, *254*
Andersen, A. D., 167, *193*
Anderson, E., 222, 223, 225, 227, 237, *256*
Anderson, J. M., 178, *187*
Anderson, L. J., 168, 169, *187*
Andre-Schwartz, J., 185, *203*

Andrews, M. F., 92, *94*
Andrews, S. B., 19, 22, *25*
Angell, M. E., 169, *187*
Annison, E. F., 213, 220, 222, 223, 225, 228, 231, 232, 234, 235, 238, 241, 243, 244, 249, *252, 253, 257, 260*
Anson, R. J., 1, *24*
Apella, E., 79, *94*
Appel, M. J. G., 170, *188*
Appelhanz, J., 73, *103*
Appleton, G. S., 121, 138, *143, 147*
Apostol, J. V., 174, *202*
Apostolou, K., 178, *196*
Arey, L. B., 158, *188*
Arkins, J. A., 160, *188, 189*
Armstrong, D. G., 210, 233, *253, 258*
Armstrong, R., 276, *298*
Arrocha, R., 174, *188*
Asmar, J., 126, *146*
Asmundson, V. S., 84, *94, 96*
Atkinson, M. R., 231, *255*
Attaran, S. E., 174, *188*
Augustinsson, K-B., 78, *94*
Austen, K. F., 157, *188*

B

Bach, F. H., 180, 181, *188*
Bachrach, H. L., 264, 268, *299, 302*
Baer, R. L., 162, *188*
Baile, C. A., 231, *253*
Bailey, W. S., 345, *350*
Bain, B., 182, *188*
Baird, G. D., 247, 248, *253*
Baker, E., 159, 160, *188*
Baker, J. A., 35, *55,* 153, *188*
Baker, J. R., 2, 4, 5, 7, 9, *23,* 31, *59,* 84, *99*
Baker, K. P., 316, *350*
Baker, N., 211, 213, 215, 216, 217, 252, *253, 259*
Baldelli, B., 282, *305*
Baldini, M., 165, *188*
Baldwin, D. E., 282, *300*
Baldwin, D. S., 166, *198*
Baldwin, E., 50, *55*

393

Zimmerman, C. E., 178, *207*
Zimmerman, G. L., 55, *59*
Zimmerman, H. J., 65, 66, 82, *97, 103*
Zinkle, J. G., 76, *103*

Znamensky, M. S., 174, *207*
Zook, B. C., 168, *195,* 334, *354*
Zühlke, V., 161, 177, *195*
Zukoski, C. F., 174, 175, 176, *202, 207*

Subject Index

A

Acid phosphatases, use in diagnosis, 79

Aldolase (ALD), levels of in various species, 66

Alkaline phosphatase
serum activity of in dogs, 91
use in diagnosis, 79

Allergy, in dogs, 159–160

Amino acids, gluconeogenesis from in ruminants, 239–241

Amyloidosis, in dogs, 157

Arginase, serum activity of
in dogs, 91
in horses, 92

Arthropods, as vectors of foot and mouth disease virus, 279–281

Autoimmune hemolytic anemia, in dogs, 165

Autosensitivity disorders, in dogs, 164–172

Avian infectious bronchitis, (AIB), 105–148. (See also Infectious bronchitis virus.)
classification of, 108–110
definition of, 106–107
diagnosis of, 132–137
economic and public health significance of, 107
history of, 107–108
incidence and distribution of, 108–129
prevention and control of, 137–139
synonyms for, 107
treatment of, 137

B

Berlin, veterinary research done at Free University of, 382–383

Birds, as vectors of foot and mouth disease virus, 278–279

Blood
enzyme removal from, 75–77
enzymopathies of cellular elements in 86

Bone neoplasms, in cats and dogs, 327–331

C

Bronchitis, avian infectious type, *see* Avian infectious bronchitis

C-reactive protein, in dog serum, 156

Cat
hypervitaminosis A in, 1–27
serum enzymes in liver pathology of, 88–90
tumors in, 309–354
as vector of foot and mouth disease virus, 276

Cattle
glucose entry rates in, 222–228
in pregnant and lactating animals, 228–231
serum enzymes in liver pathology of, 93

Central nervous system, serum enzymes in pathology of, 87

Chickens, avian infectious bronchitis in, 105–148

Chicken embryo extract (CEE), for nematode cultivation, 36–40

Chimpanzees, serum enzymes in liver pathology of, 93

Chondrosarcomas, in cats and dogs, 328, 330–331

Colitis, in dogs, 172

Complement activity, in dog serum, 155–156

Coonhound paralysis, in dogs, 171

Cori cycle, in ruminants, 242–244

Creatine phosphokinase (CPK)
assay of, 69
serum activity of
in dogs, 91
in horses, 92
use in diagnosis, 82–84

D

Dehydrogenases, isoenzymes of, 79

Demyelinating leukoencephalopathy, in dogs, 170–171

Dermatitis, in dogs, 162–163